FEMALE HEALTH AND GYNECOLOGY

WOMEN'S STUDIES PROGRAM
UNIVERSITY OF DAYTON
ST. JOSEPH   414

Executive Editor: Richard A. Weimer

Production Editor: Michael J. Rogers

Art Director: Don Sellers, AMI

Illustrator: Joe Vitek

Pathology photographs: Andrew G. Smith, PhD
                        Department of Clinical Pathology
                        University of Maryland Hospital

Photography: George Dodson

Typesetting by: Carver Photocomposition, Arlington, Virginia

Typeface: Palatino (text) and Friz Quadrata Bold (heads)

Printed by: Fairfield Graphics, Fairfield, Pennsylvania

FEMALE HEALTH AND GYNECOLOGY

across the lifespan

SANDRA L. TYLER, RN, MS
School of Nursing
University of Maryland
Baltimore, Maryland

GAIL M. WOODALL, RN, BS
Family Planning Nurse Practitioner
University of Maryland
College Park, Maryland

Robert J. Brady Co. • Bowie, Maryland 20715 • (301) 262-6300
A PRENTICE-HALL PUBLISHING AND COMMUNICATIONS COMPANY

Female Health and Gynecology: Across the Lifespan

Library of Congress Cataloging in Publication Data

Tyler, Sandra L., 1943-
    Female health.

    Includes index.
    1. Gynecologic nursing.   I. Woodall, Gail M.,
1936-   II. Title.   [DNLM: 1. Gynecology—
Nursing texts.   2. Human development—Nursing
texts.   WY 156.7 F329]
RG105.T94   618.1   81-17041
ISBN 0-89303-031-7   AACR2

Prentice-Hall International, Inc., London
Prentice-Hall of Australia, Pty., Ltd., Sydney
Prentice-Hall of India Private Limited, New Delhi
Prentice-Hall of Japan, Inc., Tokyo
Prentice-Hall of Southeast Asia Pte. Ltd., Singapore
Whitehall Books, Limited, Petone, New Zealand

Printed in the United States of America

82 83 84 85 86 87 88 89 90 91 92 10 9 8 7 6 5 4 3 2 1

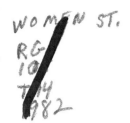
WOMEN'S HEALTH PROGRAM
UNIVERSITY OF DAYTON
ST. _____ 24

TABLE OF CONTENTS

PREFACE

When women find themselves talking with other women, the conversation will often turn to gynecology and its related issues. If a female nurse is present, she often finds that she is looked to for answers and advice. It is assumed that she is knowledgeable in all aspects of health care. Although people often consider female nurses to be a "double authority" on women's health by virtue of both gender and profession, male nurses may also be confronted with these issues.

A nurse practicing in any area of health care will at times work with women. They frequently bring their gynecological needs and questions to her. These questions also arise in non-professional settings. They come up at club meetings, over the backyard fence, at the PTA, and the grocery store. All of these women want answers and the nurse seems a comfortable and trustworthy source.

Unfortunately, the nurse may not possess much gynecologic expertise. Nursing education of the reproductive system typically focuses on obstetrics and serious disease processes. Some nursing curricula are beginning to reflect an awareness of the need for more information about gynecology, reproduction, sexuality, and women's health. However, most nurses are poorly prepared to answer questions related to such common concerns as vaginitis, contraception, menstruation, and menopause.

When caught in this situation, what does the nurse do? One of a combination of approaches may be used to find the needed information. The nurse may look for answers in a magazine article or reference book. A physician or a nurse-specialist may be approached for information. Many choose to just "wing it."

These approaches, excluding "winging it", have some merit although they all fall short of both nurse and client need. Reference or textbooks are often restricted to anatomy and physiology. They may be directed at the nurse working in the women's health specialty area, may not be designed for ready reference, and content is often difficult to relate to a clinical situation. They are usually large, clumsy, and expensive. Magazine articles are scarce, have limited scope, and may not relate adequately to a specific question or situation. The physician is generally disease-oriented and often leaves out the interpersonal aspect which is important to the client. The nurse-specialist for female health is a rarity. Even when one can be found, she is often very busy with a heavy patient load and many professional requests. "Winging it" is, of course, neither professional nor prudent, and may prove to be dangerous.

An inadequate knowledge base makes it easy to minimize, ignore, or overlook concerns of femininity, sexuality, and/or minor gynecologic problems. These concerns are often treated as if they were isolated issues, yet they pervade all aspects of a woman's life. Women will keep looking for comprehensible and integrated answers and information. It is a professional responsibility as well as a personal satisfaction to provide this information.

The purpose of this book is to provide a resource about female health and development for the professional nurse. It is primarily intended for the nurse who feels a lack of gynecologic knowledge. It builds onto the body of knowledge which was provided by the basic nursing program. It helps the nurse answer questions regarding basic physiology while incorporating concepts of femininity, sexuality, and self-esteem. It provides an approach for the nurse who may be uncomfortable with sexuality and reproductive issues. It summarizes and consolidates a great deal of information in order that it may remain a practical, useful resource book.

To meet these objectives, the material is presented in a developmental sequence. Because we feel that health and prevention of illness are of primary importance, we have placed them first. We believe that health care must be delivered to a whole person. "Wholeness" consists of the psychosocial as well as the physical. It includes the entire lifespan, past, future, and present. Because we believe this, our book has a developmental approach and integrates biopsychosocial aspects throughout.

This book is about women because our nursing practices have focused on women, and because in these practices we have found a need for a resource book with a comprehensive approach. Thus, we discuss health care, nursing, and the female client at all ages. However, we feel that a comprehensive, "holistic" approach to male health care is equally important. Health care is inadequate unless it is delivered with respect and consideration for the complete individual. We have found this approach useful in our nursing practices and hope that by sharing it, others will benefit.

Contributing Authors

KATHRYN J HENDERSON, RN, MS
  Assistant Professor
  School of Nursing
  University of Maryland

L COLETTE JONES, RN, PhD, NP
  Assistant Professor
  Acting Chairperson, Primary Care Department
  School of Nursing
  University of Maryland

ROSE M MAYS, RN, MS, CPNA
  Associate Professor
  School of Nursing
  Indiana University

SUSAN SHREVE McCARTER, RN, BS
  Director of Community Education and
  Director of Menopause Program
  Women's Medical Center
  Washington, D.C.

ETHEL HALE NAUGLE, RN
  Freelance Health Information Consultant
  Formerly Administrator for Sigma Reproductive Health Clinic,
    Rockville, Maryland
  Freelance Author

NANCY M O'HARA, MA
  Community Health Educator
  Division of Health Education and Promotion
  Prince George's County Health Department
  Cheverly, Maryland

PEGGY H ROEDER, BS
  Public Health Librarian
  Prince George's County Health Department
  Cheverly, Maryland

CARMINE M VALENTE, MA (PhD candidate)
Director of Health Education and Promotion
Prince George's County Health Department
Cheverly, Maryland

JANET STEARNS WYATT, RN, MS, NP
Assistant Professor
Primary Care Department
School of Nursing
University of Maryland

ACKNOWLEDGMENTS

Special thanks to:

BOB WOODALL and FORREST TYLER

For their continuous love and support throughout this project. (Also for their help in cooking, cleaning, child care, sewing, shopping and washing *ad infinitum.*)

SHANE, KAREN, and CHRIS WELLS

For sharing so much of their mother's time with Sandy; for sacrificing some family activities and being willing to do many things on their own. (And for a small fee, helping type and number manuscript pages.)

BETH TYLER

For cover design inspiration. In addition, her encouragement and interest helped a lot.

ROBERT WEINFELD, MD and KENNETH TRAVERS, MD

For innumerable hours taken from their OB-GYN practices and otherwise busy lives to read, critique, explain, and to debate with us ideas in the manuscript. We asked for their input because of their extensive knowledge of gynecology, high standards of practice, and special awareness of and sensitivity to women's health needs.

SHIRLEY WETHERALD, RN

For reviewing the manuscript from a nursing perspective, asking pertinent questions, and helping us maintain our focus.

UNIVERSITY OF MARYLAND LESBIAN AND BISEXUAL WOMEN'S GROUP and the WHITMAN-WALKER CLINIC OF WASHINGTON, D.C.

For taking the time to give us insight into the special health concerns of gay women.

RICHARD WEIMER

For listening, supporting, and encouraging our ideas without interrupting our writing. (And for showing remarkable self control when we missed a deadline or two.)

MIKE ROGERS

For the overall appearance of our book and for his undeviating calm throughout the entire editorial process.

DON SELLERS, BERNARD VERVIN, JOE VITEK, and GEORGE DODSON

For illustrating our ideas so creatively, and for maintaining their good humor throughout our numerous requests for changes.

There is no way to repay these people for the help that they have given. We know now why authors say in their acknowledgements "This book could not have been written without the help of . . ." Finally we want to thank each other. The contribution from each has been equal. In addition, when one of us was discouraged the other encouraged. We've learned from each other and in so doing have strengthened our friendship.

Section I

PRELIMINARY ESSENTIALS

Patient Bill Of Rights

1. The patient has the right to considerate and respectful care.
2. The patient has the right to obtain from his physician complete current information concerning his diagnosis, treatment, and prognosis in terms the patient can be reasonably expected to understand. When it is not medically advisable to give such information to the patient, the information should be made available to an appropriate person in his behalf. He has the right to know, by name, the physician responsible for coordinating his care.
3. The patient has the right to receive from his physician information necessary to give informed consent prior to the start of any procedure and/or treatment. Except in emergencies, such information for informed consent should include but not necessarily be limited to the specific procedure and/or treatment, the medically significant risks involved, and the probable duration of incapacitation. Where medically significant alternatives for care or treatment exist, or when the patient requests information concerning medical alternatives, the patient has the right to such information. The patient also has the right to know the name of the person responsible for the procedures and/or treatment.
4. The patient has the right to refuse treatment to the extent permitted by law and to be informed of the medical consequences of his action.
5. The patient has the right to every consideration of his privacy concerning his own medical care program. Case discussion, consultation, examination, and treatment are confidential and should be conducted discreetly. Those not directly involved in his care must have the permission of the patient to be present.
6. The patient has the right to expect that all communications and records pertaining to his care should be treated as confidential.
7. The patient has the right to expect that within its capacity a hospital must make reasonable response to the request of a patient for services. The hospital must provide evaluation, service, and/or referral as indicated by the urgency of the case. When medically permissible, a patient may be transferred to another facility only after he has received complete information and explanation concerning the needs for and alternatives to such a transfer. The institution to which the patient is to be transferred must first have accepted the patient for transfer.
8. The patient has the right to obtain information as to any relationship of his hospital to other health care and educational institutions insofar as his care is concerned. The patient has the right to obtain information as to the existence of any professional relationships among individuals, by name, who are treating him.
9. The patient has the right to be advised if the hospital proposes to engage in or perform human experimentation affecting his care or treatment. The patient has the right to refuse to participate in such research projects.
10. The patient has the right to expect reasonable continuity of care. He has the right to know in advance what appointment times and physicians are available and where. The patient has the right to expect that the hospital will provide a mechanism whereby he is informed by his physician or a delegate of the physician of the patient's continuing health care requirements following discharge.
11. The patient has the right to examine and receive an explanation of his bill regardless of source of payment.
12. The patient has the right to know what hospital rules and regulations apply to his conduct as a patient.

1

Nurses and Clients

In 1972 the American Hospital Association published a Patient's Bill of Rights. This document was developed to inform people of what they have a right to expect when entering a health care institution. The overall goal was to improve the quality of care. The wording infers that most of these mandates are aimed at the physician, client, and institution.

Because of the strategic position of the nursing role in the delivery of health care, the nurse is often the one who assumes the responsibility of protecting and guaranteeing these rights. This is done in any setting by a variety of methods including direct intervention and advocacy, education, interpretation of information, and coordination, monitoring, and evaluation of care. The knowledge base and skills needed to accomplish these and other activities of nursing are highly sophisticated in today's Western cultures.

Nursing and the delivery of nursing care is not just the accomplishment of a series of tasks, although tasks may be included as a part of nursing. Rather nursing is an ongoing process which is continuously being reshaped by its components—the nurse, client, and environment. The nurse assumes a leadership role in the shaping of this ongoing process of health care.

The leadership role of nursing requires the coordination of an enormous amount of information. Thus order and clarity of thought are essential tools for a nurse approaching any health care situation. The scientific method of problem solving provides this orderly approach. Nursing's application of this method is called *the nursing process* [5].

The four steps of the nursing process include assessment, planning, implementation and evaluation [4]. Although the process will be primarily involved in a given step at a given time, it is important to recognize the interplay among the steps. For example, while in the planning stage it is probable that assessment and implementation may also be somewhat involved. However it is important for the nurse to maintain the focus of that stage, that is, in this example to continue the planning [1].

Each step of the nursing process requires specialized skills and tools. Although a skill may have special application in one particular step, it will often be used throughout the whole process. A way to make this idea clearer is with a schematic representation. In Table 1-1, we have categorized some of the skills used in the nursing process, demonstrating their probable area of emphasis. Each nurse will be able to identify additional concepts relevant to accomplishment of the nursing process.

ASSESSMENT

Assessment or data gathering provides for the collection of all pertinent information. This will ensure an accurate definition of the problem by both the nurse and the client. The data base includes the client's description of the problem, relevant personal information, the nurse's basic knowledge, and her observations. Data gathering is accomplished by communication skills, interviewing techniques, careful listening, and physical assessment. Finally, the gathered data is analyzed in order to arrive at an accurate definition of the prob-

Table 1-1. *Schematic representation of some nursing skills used during application of the nursing process. Order of emphasis may vary with the situation.*

Skills and tools	Assessment	Planning	Implementation	Evaluation
Observation	X		O	O
Listening	X	O	O	O
Communication	X	X	X	X
Interview	X			
Physical assessment	X		O	O
Organization	O	X	O	O
Leadership	O	O	X	O
Coordination	X	X	O	O
Negotiation		X	O	
Technical	X	O	X	
Education/Teaching	O	X	O	
Insight/Accountability	O	O	O	X
Referral		X	O	
Consultation			X	
Review				X

X = Skill emphasized in this step
O = Skill also important in this step

lem. This type of critical thinking can be accomplished only with adequate theoretical knowledge [4].

PLANNING

The next step involves formulating a plan to deal with the problem. The nurse and client review various alternatives for solving the problem and then choose an approach that best meets the client's needs. The plan will include activities which involve both the client and nurse. Short and long term goals are usually established, as well as criteria for meeting these goals [4]. For example, an obese woman who must lose 20 pounds may elect to set a short-term goal of a weight loss of 2 pounds per week.

IMPLEMENTATION

Implementation, the third step, occurs when the client and nurse put the agreed-upon plan into action. Data is reassessed during this phase and modifications may be made in the original plan. Although many different nursing interventions may be used, emphasis is placed on clients assuming as much responsibility for their own care as possible. Nursing interventions in this step may range from sophisticated technical skills to merely answering questions [4].

EVALUATION

The final step of the nursing process is evaluation. This critically important step again involves both nurse and client. A review of what was accomplished will focus and reemphasize what each learned during the process. In addition, it provides a way of identifying what remains to be done, thus starting the next cycle of the nursing process [4].

Evaluation of the nurse's role and accomplishments throughout the process is equal in importance to evaluation of the client's accomplishments. As professionals, nurses are accountable for their actions and therefore must look critically at what they do. In this way evaluation serves to promote professional growth and improve health care delivery.

THE PARTICIPANTS

A theme central to the nursing process which must be concretely defined is the mutual involvement of both nurse and client. Nurses cannot presume to know what is best for the client. Rather they serve as resources for clients who are in a better position to make their own decisions and assume responsibility for their own care.

A third, often overlooked, participant is the environment. Any individual's environment includes physical surroundings and social and cultural networks. In this abstract sense the environment includes both supportive and destructive elements which may either help or interfere with resolution of the problem. (Figure 1-1.)

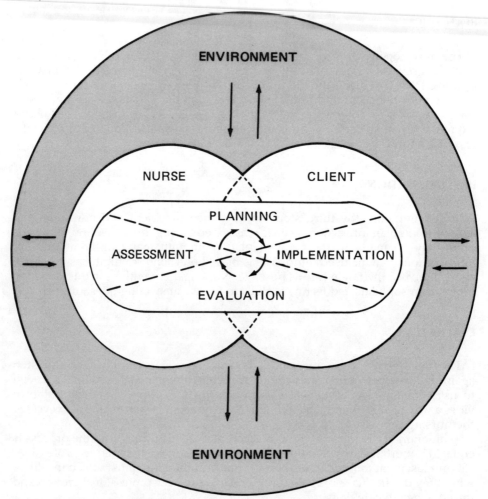

Figure 1-1.   Schematic representation of the participants in the nursing process.

THE NURSING PROCESS AND THIS BOOK

Nursing becomes such a part of one's identity that people often ask health-related questions in sometimes unlikely places. For example, nurses who work in cardiology have found that they must also deal with sexuality. All nurses are asked questions that do not relate to their specialty area at some time or other.

Quality health care, a product of the nursing process, assumes an adequate knowledge base. Lack of knowledge limits the scope and application of the nursing process. In order to answer questions or deal with problems in an unfamiliar area, knowledge must be increased or the client must be referred. If the choice is made to obtain the appropriate information, the nursing process can then be utilized.

This book is meant to serve as a resource for all phases of the nursing process dealing with gynecologic matters. It is hoped that it will assist with assessment, precipitate planning, initiate implementation, and encourage evaluation.

A study of anatomy and physiology offers basic information used in all phases of the nursing process. During assessment, this information is used to distinguish normal from abnormal states. A health care plan cannot be made without a good understanding of anatomy and physiology. Teaching the client how her body functions is only one of many ways that this information is used in implementation. Evaluation involves reassessment and measurement of change; therefore, basic knowledge is necessary for this step also.

Since this book is about women and their health, and since basic information precedes and is essential to the nursing process, both prenatal development and normal anatomy and physiology have been placed in the first section. In this way it can be used as a basis for the information which follows, or it can be read separately by those who wish only to review that material.

Pregnancy and childbirth is an important aspect of normal development for many women. However, for the most part we have not included this information for a number of reasons. Obstetrical information is extensive and so adequate treatment of this subject would not be consistent with the goals and format of this book. Although many women do not experience pregnancy, all women at some time must deal with various gynecologic concerns. Yet it is often difficult to find information on gynecologic issues while obstetric information is readily available. Therefore, the major focus of this book is gynecology.

Normal physical and psychosocial development throughout the life span is knowledge which is needed in all steps of the nursing process. It is especially relevant to assessment for the establishment of "normals." Planning must often include preparation for anticipated changes. This information also provides guidelines for implementation and evaluation.

We have divided the developmental information into the major stages of a woman's life cycle. This necessitates the overlapping of information at times although each stage provides a different perspective. For example, physiological information is used as a basis for explaining changes that occur throughout life; it also provides a basis for understanding various types of contraception.

The chapters concerned with health issues provide information needed for all steps of the nursing process. The emphasis placed on any one step will be defined by the situation. An example might be a woman asking for information about vaginal discharge. A quick assessment might reveal either that a much more detailed assessment must be done or that she merely wants some information. Planning and implementation may include referral, gynecologic examination and/or supplying the needed information. Evaluation will be as detailed as the situation requires.

Throughout life, various aspects of female health become issues which must be dealt with or understood. They may or may not present problems. Because the approach to a child with a gynecologic concern is often different from the approach used with an adult and because the issues themselves may differ, we have separated them. Because the gynecologic issues for an adolescent, a young adult, and an older adult woman are often similar we have included them in one section. We have attempted to include the most common health situations that women encounter, although our list is not inclusive. It is hoped that the nurse will be able to draw on these examples and apply the knowledge to similar situations.

Nurses are often asked technical questions about gynecologic surgery or examination procedures. Concerns may range from what to expect during pelvic examination to issues surrounding a mastectomy. Many nurses may be unfamiliar with these procedures yet will want to offer support and education. The last section gives information related to some commonly encountered examples. This, plus the material in the rest of the book, by necessity cannot be inclusive. In addition, research constantly makes new information available. Those who wish additional information or those who wish to check for updated information in the future will find referrals and sources in the last chapter.

A basic assumption that health care providers often make is that their clients are heterosexual. This assumption, like any unconfirmed assumption, may lead to many problems. For example, protocol may "insist" that a pregnancy test be done prior to other examinations when the complaint is a missed period. The result for both lesbian women and health care providers is embarrassment and delay in treatment of any underlying pathology. The same result may occur when the health care provider insists on contraception for the sexually active lesbian.

Embarrassment and delayed treatment are two of many reasons health care providers must be sensitive to the needs of women who have chosen alternate life styles. Both as a means of consciousness-raising and as clarification where assumptions may exist, we have indicated similarities or differences of health care needs of the lesbian or bisexual woman from those of the heterosexual woman.

The words "girl" and "lady" suggest asexuality and dependency [3]. Words can be very powerful and we choose not to attribute these qualities to prepubertal or postmenopausal women. It is our belief that a woman is a sexual being whether she is one minute or 99 years old and that sexuality is an integral part of her being. Therefore we have elected, instead, to use the terms "female" and "woman" interchangeably and at all ages. In addition, childhood and aging have been given as much emphasis as have the reproductive years.

In the past few years there has been increasing interest in natural remedies. These remedies include such things as dietary measures, specialized exercises, yoga and meditation, therapeutic touch, self-hypnosis, visual imagery, and herbal medicine. We recognize the value of a balanced life style including good nutrition, rest and exercise as being basic to good health. Even so, health problems occur for most everyone at some point in life. If a person rejects traditional medical treatment or finds that it does not help, they may ask for information about natural remedies. We have included a few of these. If more information is desired, resources can be found in chapter 25.

REFERENCES

1. Bower FL: The Process of Planning Nursing Care. St. Louis, C. V. Mosby Co., 1972
2. Brossart J: The gay patient: what you should be doing. RN, April, 1979
3. Lerner HE: Girls, ladies, or women? The unconscious dynamics of language choice. Comprehensive Psychiatry, 17:2, March-April 1976
4. Marriner A: The Nursing Process, 2nd ed. St. Louis, C. V. Mosby Co., 1979
5. Yura H and Walsh MB: The Nursing Process, 2nd ed. New York, Appleton-Century-Crofts, 1973

2

Prenatal Development

K ATHRYN J. H ENDERSON, S ANDRA L. T YLER, and G AIL M. W OODALL

A review of basic reproductive embryology serves several purposes. It provides a way to understand the normal reproductive and sexual development of a woman. It also gives a basis for understanding deviations from normal. Gender similarities and differences of women and men are clarified by a knowledge of common embryonic beginnings.

Normal sexual development begins with the chromosome pattern which determines whether the gonads will become ovaries or testes. Subsequent genital development depends upon hormones which are derived from the fetus and the mother.

NORMAL DEVELOPMENT

The sex chromosome pattern of the embryo is normally either an XX for a female or an XY for a male. To obtain this end result, the ova carry single X chromosomes. Because the sperm may donate either an X or a Y to the pairing, the male parent determines the sex of the offspring.

Sex differentiation begins about the fifth or sixth week after conception. (Figure 2-1.) Three sets of structures are involved in this differentiation process: the *gonads*, the *internal sex organs*, and the *external sex organs*. Development of each is separate and does not guarantee or predict the development of the others. Sexual differentiation also involves the *central nervous system*. Although research is inconclusive at this time, it bears mentioning because of its implications.

Gonads

At the fifth or sixth gestational week, primordial germ cells arise extragonadally. They migrate to the genital ridges and are then enclosed by the primitive gonad. At this point, it is impossible to differentiate a male from a female gonad, and so they are referred to as indifferent gonads [4].

In the presence of two X chromosomes, these indifferent gonads become ovaries. If a Y chromosome is present, they become testes. In the genetic female, the

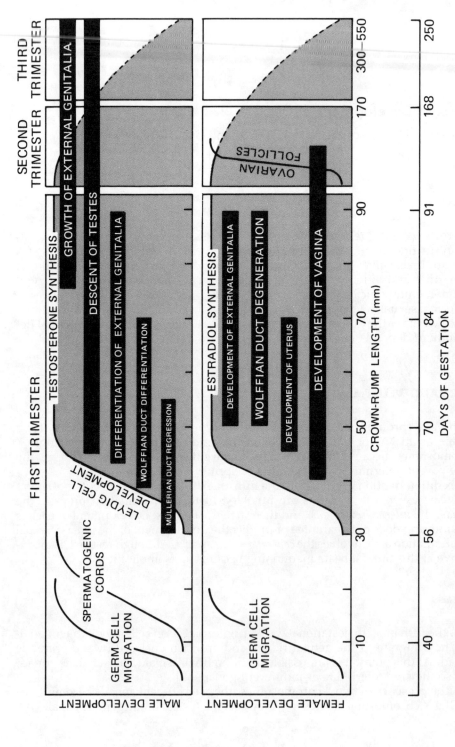

Figure 2-1. *Relation between differentiation of the gonads and the anatomical differentiation of the human male and female embryos. Used with permission from Science magazine, Vol. 211 No. 4488, March 20, 1981.*

germ cells will migrate to the cortex portion of the ovary while the medulla becomes a vascular stroma.

Internal Genitalia

By the seventh week of gestation, two sets of rudimentary structures are present in all embryos. (Figure 2-2.) These are the Müllerian and Wolffian ducts and they are the precursors of the internal sex organs. Secretions from the fetal gonads will determine which of these ducts develop and which fade.

Secretions from the testes will cause the Wolffian ducts to evolve into the vas deferens, the seminal vesicles and the ejaculatory ducts, while the Müllerian ducts atrophy. Without testicular secretions, the Müllerian ducts will develop into Fallopian tubes, uterus, and upper vagina while the Wolffian ducts fade. This is probably also influenced by circulating maternal and placental hormones [4].

There are two secretions from the testes which are essential for normal male development. One is an androgen-like substance which stimulates proliferation of the Wolffian ducts. However, the body must be able to respond to androgen before these ducts will develop. The second secretion is responsible for *prevention* of Müllerian duct development. It is called the Mullerian Inhibiting Factor (MIF) [9].

Both of these secretions are local in effect. That is, secretions from each of the testes will stimulate or inhibit development of Wolffian structures on that side only. In the absence of testicular secretions, Müllerian duct development will proceed.

External Genitalia

The precursors to the external genitalia appear at about the third week. They remain bipotential until about the eighth week, when hormonal influences begin to differentiate them. At this time, there is a genital tubercle above a urogenital slit. Urethral folds and labioscrotal swellings are found on either side. (Figure 2-3.)

Influenced by androgen, the genital tubercle will become the corpora cavernosa and glans of the penis. The urethral folds fuse and form the urethra, which then becomes enclosed in the penis. The labioscrotal folds fuse in the midline and become the scrotum.

In the absence of androgen, the genital tubercle becomes the corpora cavernosa and glans of the clitoris. The urethral folds remain separate, forming the labia minora while the labioscrotal swellings become the labia majora. The urogenital slit differentiates into the lower vagina and urethra. Thus, the lower vagina is formed as a part of the external genitals [9].

The seventh gestational week is a critical period in the development of the external genitalia. If the female embryo is exposed to androgen at this time, the external genitals will be masculinized even though normal internal genitals may develop. Insensitivity to, or inadequate amounts of, androgen in the male will result in incomplete development of the external genitals.

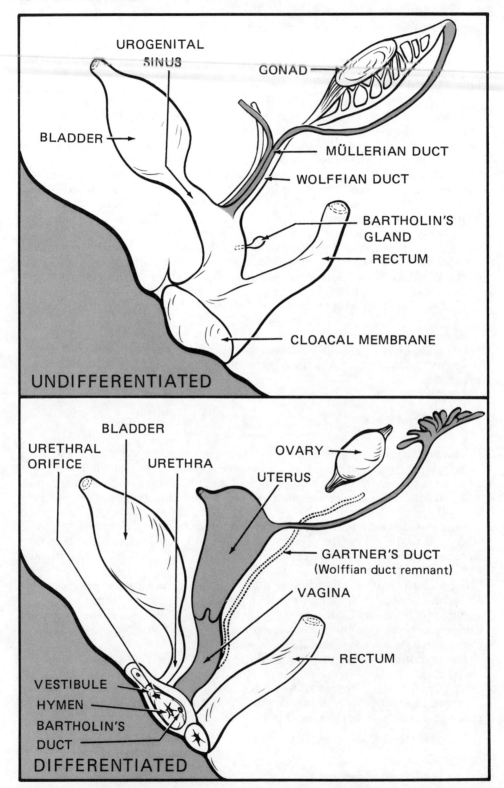

Figure 2-2.   Prenatal development of the female genital tract.

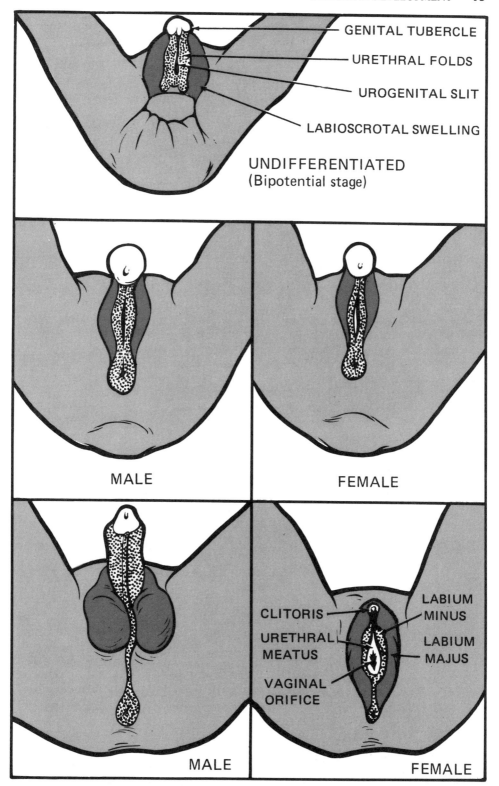

Figure 2-3.   Prenatal development of the male and female external genitalia from the undifferentiated state.

The common tissue origin of the external genitals would suggest that similar or comparable physical sensations are experienced by both sexes. However, many people speak of the penis and scrotum as being the earmark of a male, while forgetting some or all of the comparable structures in the female. A study of the childrearing practices of several hundred Cleveland area parents found that they often said, "a boy has a penis, a girl does not." Sometimes the vagina was mentioned. The word clitoris was not mentioned by a single parent [7].

To define a female as not having a penis is to imply that women are lacking in some way. To define her by only mentioning the vagina may imply that her main function is to be able to receive the penis for purposes of procreation. To mention the other structures is to begin the process of teaching children that their genitals are a source of pleasure and pride. It has been suggested that a highly functional word, vulva, be used more commonly to summarize the female external genitalia. Using this word with children would then require further explanation, in itself a highly valuable activity.

Central Nervous System Differentiation

Ongoing research is exploring the effects of fetal hormones on the brain. Some of this research theorizes that the brain is a bipotential structure as are some of the genital precursors. An element of this theory is that the presence or absence of androgen determines the form of gender behavior. That is, androgens produce aggressive behavior; lack of androgens result in passive behavior. This would ensure complementary copulating behaviors, procreation, and survival of the species. Other researchers are exploring differences in male and female verbal and spatial abilities, response to sensory stimuli, and ability to handle stress [3, 6, 8].

At this time the available research is generally inconclusive. Many factors enter into sexual behavior and it becomes extremely difficult to separate physical from cultural and psychological influences. Care should always be used when interpreting results from any type of research. It is easy to draw presumptive conclusions and then use them to further one's cause, be it feminism versus male superiority or bisexuality versus homosexuality [8].

DEVELOPMENTAL ABNORMALITIES

Sexual Ambiguity

Historically, an ambiguity about the sex of a child at birth has been referred to as hermaphroditism. This term comes from the names of the Greek god and goddess of love, Hermes and Aphrodite, and implies mixed gonads. This rare condition came to be known as *true hermaphroditism*.

All other sexual ambiguities were referred to as *pseudo-hermaphroditism*. Trying to classify male and female pseudo-hermaphrodites led to a great deal of confusion. In addition, the "pseudo" part of this label implies "false" whereas the resultant problems are just as realistic in either case.

It is well-known that labeling has a negative impact on people. This, plus the confusion that exists when using these terms, has led many health professionals to replace them with the phrase, "sexually ambiguous genitalia." This term has less negative impact, yet is adequately descriptive.

The origin of sexual ambiguities may be chromosomal or hormonal or both. At fertilization, a chromosome may be lost or one or more may be gained. There may be too much or too little androgen present for normal development. Finally, the male fetus may not be able to respond to androgen. We will discuss the most common problems resulting from these conditions as they relate to females.

Turner's Syndrome

The chromosome pattern of XO (a single X) results in the well-known characteristics of Turner's syndrome. These include absence of ovaries (gonadal dysgenesis), sexual infantilism, and, obviously, infertility. Since there is no Y chromosome, the individual is female. Physical characteristics include short stature and a webbed neck. Other congenital anomalies may include coarctation of the aorta, renal abnormalities and mental retardation. Occasionally the diagnosis is not made until puberty, when failure to menstruate initiates a medical investigation.

Mosaicism

Mosaicism is a condition in which a variety of abnormal chromosome combinations can be found within the cells of an individual. Various combinations occur and are written as X/XY, XX/XY, X/XX, X/XX/XXX. Characteristic conditions, such as mental retardation or a range of physical defects, exist for each of these. Occasionally individuals with Turner's syndrome show mosaicism. Another condition associated with mosaicism is Kleinfelter's syndrome. More information about mosaicism or its related syndromes can be found in Langman's *Medical Embryology* or Speroff, Glass and Kase's *Clinical Gynecologic Endocrinology and Infertility.* (See chapter 25 for information regarding genetic counseling.)

Adrenogenital Syndrome (Masculinized Female)

Individuals with adrenogenital syndrome are genetically female with an XX chromosome pattern. They have normal ovaries, uterus, tubes, and upper vagina. However, they were exposed to androgen at the critical time (seven weeks) with resultant masculinization of the external genitals. The source of this androgen can be fetal or maternal. The mother may have an adrenal tumor or may have taken progestins at the critical time (seventh gestational week). The child may have adrenal hyperplasia or an adrenal tumor.

If diagnosed at birth or shortly thereafter, treatment is aimed at changing the external genitals to a female phenotype. These females then grow up to be fertile, normally functioning women. If diagnosed any time after eighteen months, male socialization is so complete that they should continue to be reared as males. Medical and surgical treatment will be necessary to complement this, but they will be normally functioning, although sterile, males [9].

Testicular Feminization (Androgen Insensitivity)

Testicular feminization is a condition in which the individual has a normal XY chromosome pattern. Although the testes produce sufficient androgen, the fetal body is unable to respond to that androgen. Therefore, the Wolffian ducts do not develop nor are the external genitals masculinized. The testes do produce MIF, thereby also inhibiting development of female internal genital organs.

These individuals will be sterile whether raised male or female. It is difficult to surgically create a functional penis and impossible to supply it with erotic sensitivity. Surgical intervention to create female genitalia is much more successful. Therefore, individuals with this syndrome are generally raised as females.

Incompletely Masculinized Males

Incompletely masculinized males have an XY chromosome pattern. Although they have testes, the external genitals are incompletely masculinized and fall anywhere on a spectrum from being slightly to completely feminized. This syndrome can be brought about by three different conditions:

Absent or defective MIF.
Insufficient androgen.
Inability of the body to respond to androgen.

The factors may appear singly or in combination. The individual's particular syndrome will vary accordingly; for example, an individual may be born with both male and female internal genitals.

DISCUSSION

Social and psychological influences play as great or greater a part as the physical influences on a person's gender identity. As mentioned earlier, attempting to change a child's sex after the age of eighteen months is not recommended because of the difficult adjustment for both the child and parents [5]. The intertwining of the physical with the psychosocial elements of an individual become more complex and difficult to separate throughout the life span. The important issue is not just whether the Müllerian or Wolffian ducts developed, but what meaning the individual assigns to all life experiences.

This chapter has summarized basic physical reproductive embryology. We realize that our review of both normal and abnormal development is limited; if further information is desired, we suggest Langman's *Medical Embryology* [4] or Speroff's *Clinical Gynecologic Endocrinology and Infertility* [9].

REFERENCES

1. Diamond M: Human Sexual Development: Biological foundations for social development. *In* Beath FA (ed): Human Sexuality in Four Perspectives. Baltimore, Johns Hopkins University Press, 1976
2. Federman DD: Abnormal Sexual Development: A Genetic and Endocrine Approach to Differential Diagnosis. Philadelphia, W.B. Saunders Co., 1968
3. Goleman D: Special abilities of the sexes: Do they begin in the brain? Psychology Today, 12, November 1978, p. 120
4. Langman J: Medical Embryology, 3rd ed. Baltimore, Williams and Wilkins, 1975
5. Money J and Erhardt A: Man and Woman, Boy and Girl. Baltimore, Johns Hopkins University Press, 1972
6. Parlee MB: The sexes under scrutiny: From old biases to new theories. Psychology Today, 12, November 1978, p. 66
7. Project on Human Sexual Development: Family life and sexual learning: A study of the role of parents in the sexual learning of children. Cambridge, MA, 1978
8. Science, Vol. 211 No. 4488, March 20, 1981 (Special issue entitled Sexual Dimorphism)
9. Speroff L, Glass RH, Kase NG: Clinical Gynecologic Endocrinology and Infertility, 2nd ed. Baltimore, Williams and Wilkins, 1978

3

Reproductive Anatomy and Physiology

Anatomy

THE BREAST

The female breast is cone-shaped with an axillary tail. (Figure 3-1.) It protrudes from the second or third rib to the sixth or seventh rib on the anterior chest wall, and extends from the edge of the sternum across to the anterior axillary line. In addition, a thin layer of breast tissue continues to the clavicle, chest midline, and across the axilla to the latissimus dorsi.

The shape of the breast varies according to genetics, age, obesity, and exercise of the underlying chest-wall muscles. Age and obesity contribute to a more pendulous shape, exercise and muscle development to a "cone" shape. Evidence does not support the idea that breastfeeding will result in pendulous breasts [8]. Normally, one breast is smaller than the other, but the pair will be symmetrical in shape.

The nipple and areola lie about center of the flattened chest and are pigmented. The amount of pigmentation is related to estrogen levels and decreases as the woman ages. It increases as puberty approaches, with pregnancy, or with the use of exogenous estrogen regardless of the age of the woman [1].

Having developed from the ectoderm, the breast is a specialized cutaneous gland whose various tissue structures are so closely interwoven and interinvolved that they are impossible to dissect. These structures include a gland and ductal network, fat, connective tissue, fascia, blood vessels, nerves, and lymph. The glandular tissue is organized into lobes, lobules, acini, and ducts.

Gland and Ductal Structures

Leading from the nipple and back into the breast are approximately twenty excretory ducts. (Figure 3-2.) Each of the ducts widens and becomes a lactiferous sinus just behind and extending into the nipple. During lactation this is where milk is stored prior to its excretion through tiny pin-sized openings in the nipple. As the duct is traced back into the breast it begins to branch again and again, finally forming tiny collecting ducts.

Acini. The collecting ducts terminate in blind-sac structures called acini. These are highly specialized tissues that produce milk during lactation. Acini are composed of two types of cells. Epithelial cells line the interior cavity and are responsi-

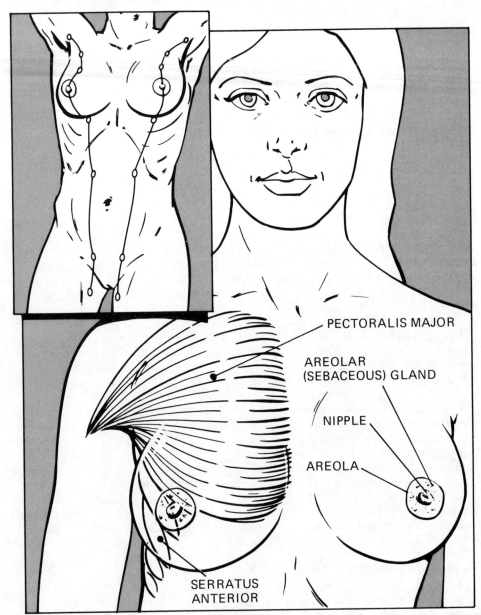

PECTORALIS MAJOR

AREOLAR
(SEBACEOUS) GLAND

NIPPLE

AREOLA

SERRATUS
ANTERIOR

Figure 3-1.   Placement of breast on anterior chest wall. Inset shows mammary line and possible location of accessory breast tissue.

ble for producing milk during lactation. A layer of myoepithelium (muscle) cells surrounds the epithelial cells. Contraction of these cells forces the milk out of the acini and into the ducts.

Lobule. The numerous acini associated with one branch of an excretory duct are called a lobule. They resemble a bunch of grapes attached to a stem. There are

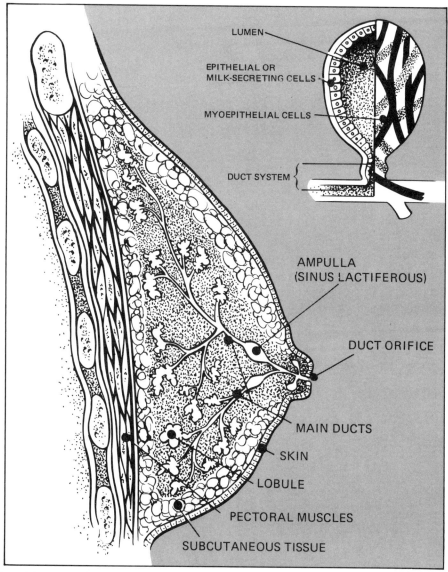

Figure 3-2. Details of gland and ductal structures of the breast. Inset shows cross section of acini and duct system.

from ten to one-hundred lobules per lobe.

Lobe. A lobe consists of all the glandular tissue (lobules) that drains into one excretory duct. There are approximately twenty lobes per breast. Both lobes and lobules are structural units.

In addition, glandular, collagenous, connective, and other tissues (such as nerves and blood vessels) are found both intra and interlobularly. Also, varying amounts of fat and connective tissue surround the breast as a whole.

Support Structures

The chest wall is formed by the various tissues that cover the anterior rib cage. (Figure 3-3.) It contains two separate fascia coverings, superficial and deep. The deep fascia covers the chest muscles. Anterior to this, the breast tissue lies between two layers of superficial fascia. Jagged projections from the deep layer of superficial fascia extend through the breast tissue to the exterior layer of superficial fascia. These projections, named Cooper's ligaments, provide movable sup-

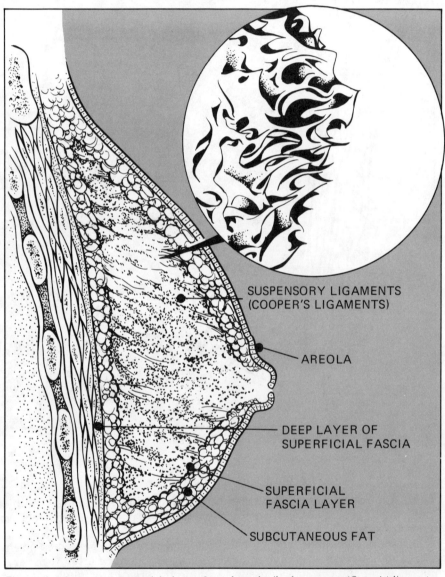

Figure 3-3.   Support structures of the breast. Inset shows details of suspensory (Cooper's) ligaments.

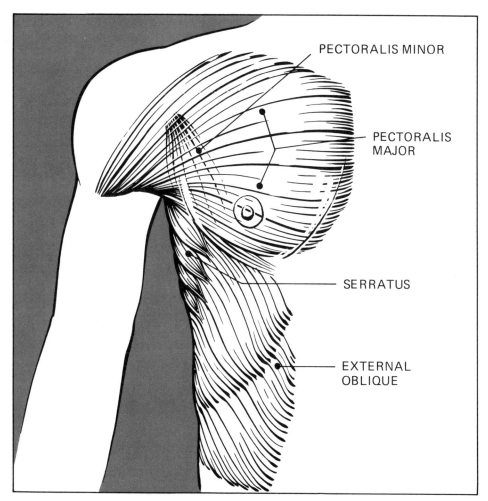

Figure 3-4.   *Major muscles of the chest wall.*

port to the breast tissue. A tumor growing on or near one of these ligaments will cause it to shorten and produce a dimpling effect on the skin of the breast.

A space separates the posterior layer of superficial fascia from the deep fascia which covers the chest muscles. This space provides for more movability of the mammary glands. Suspensory ligaments cross this space to connect the superficial and deep fascias. Sometimes breast tissue will follow these ligaments and may be found scattered among the muscle fibers. This is why some surgeons argue for more extensive removal of tissue during mastectomy for carcinoma.

The major chest muscles covered by breast tissue include the pectoralis major, serratus, external oblique, and pectoralis minor. (Figure 3-4.)

Coordinating Structures

Blood. Oxygenated blood arrives at the breast via two major routes. Branches of the *internal mammary artery* emerge near the sternum at the first, second, third, and fourth interspaces. These branches travel through the pectoralis major muscle to the outer edge of the breast. The *axillary artery* is the second major vessel to send blood via its branches to the breast. (Figure 3-5.)

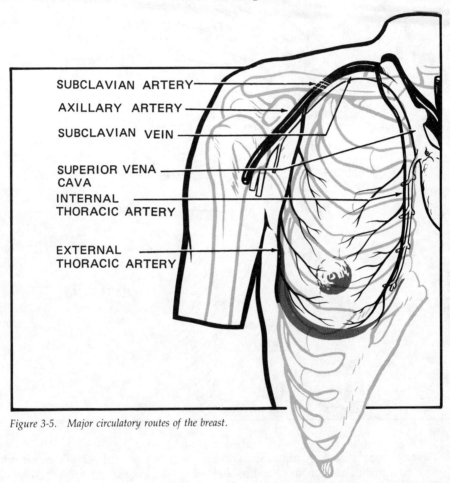

SUBCLAVIAN ARTERY

AXILLARY ARTERY

SUBCLAVIAN VEIN

SUPERIOR VENA CAVA

INTERNAL THORACIC ARTERY

EXTERNAL THORACIC ARTERY

Figure 3-5. Major circulatory routes of the breast.

There are also two major venous routes for removing deoxygenated blood from breast tissues named the caval system and vertebral veins.

The *caval system* is made up of both superficial cutaneous veins and deep veins. The superficial veins will either follow a transverse pattern across the breast toward the sternum or a longitudinal pattern toward the sternal notch. Finally, they drain into the superficial veins of the neck and then directly into the jugular vein.

The deep veins include the perforating branches of the internal mammary, the axillary vein, and the intercostal vein. These veins communicate directly with the pulmonary capillary network, the venous system of the pectoral muscle and the vertebral veins, respectively.

The *vertebral veins* parallel the caval system. However, in addition to draining the chest wall, this venous system also receives blood from the vertebrae and their adjacent muscles, the spinal cord, the pelvic bones and upper femurs, the upper humeri, shoulder and shoulder-girdle bones, and the skull. In turn, it empties directly into the superior vena cava.

Haagensen notes that because this system is without valves and because pressure within it is low, a retrograde flow of blood easily occurs. Even slight changes in intraabdominal pressure will cause a back-and-forth movement of blood within the vertebral veins. The relevance of this is that it provides a venous pathway for metastasis of breast cancer to those related areas, that is, lungs, pelvis, vertebrae, or skull [7].

Lymph. As with the pelvis (and rest of the body), the lymphatic pathways generally follow the veins. Many nodes are involved in draining the lymph from the breast and chest wall. The major ones include the external mammary nodes, scapular nodes, central nodes, axillary nodes, Rotter's nodes (also called internal and external pectoral nodes), subclavian nodes, and the internal mammary nodes. Collecting tubules connect these nodes throughout the chest. (Figure 3-6.)

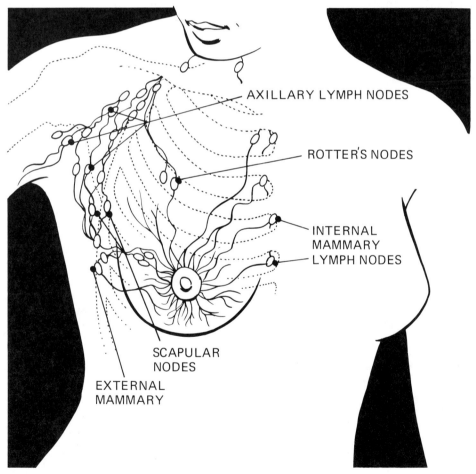

Figure 3-6.   Lymphatic system of the breast.

Although the lymph flow travels in all directions, the main direction is toward the axilla. From here, lymph trunks travel medially, connecting with ducts from the other parts of the chest wall, to finally empty into the jugular and subclavian veins. This establishes a very short route for cancer cells to enter the general circulation.

Nerve supply. The functions of the mammary glands are under control of the neuroendocrine system. The breasts receive innervation from both the central and autonomic nervous systems. The nipple and areola are supplied with sensory nerve endings that respond to touch and pressure. The rich supply of mixed nerve fibers along with a venous plexus results in the nipple and areola being erectile tissue. Thus the entire breast, including the nipple and areola, respond as a unit to sexual stimulation. A detailed description of this response pattern can be found in chapter 22.

More deeply, the upper breast is innervated by sensory fibers branching from the cervical plexus. The lower breast area receives sensory nerve branches from the thoracic nerves. Note that these same thoracic branches also innervate the skin of the upper arm. A severance of the sensory nerve supply to the breast during mastectomy or trauma will result in anesthesia of the upper arm.

THE PELVIS

External Genitalia

Vulva is a collective term referring to the many external landmarks, structures, and organs of sex and reproduction. These structures include the mons veneris, labia majora and minora, clitoris, vestibule, urethral meatus, periurethral glands (Skene's glands), vaginal introitus, hymen, vulvovaginal glands (Bartholin's glands), and perineum. Many of these structures are cutaneous tissue and subject to the same manifestations of health and disease as is the skin of other areas of the body. In addition, some structures contain glandular epithelium and are subject to disease states typical of that tissue. (For example, both squamous and adeno-carcinoma affect vulvar tissue). This similarity of tissue structure reflects the common embryonic origin of these organs. The sexual response of many of these organs is also a reflection of their related tissue structure and blood and nerve supply. (Figure 3-7.)

Mons veneris. The rounded pad of fatty tissue which covers the pubic symphysis is named after the Greek love goddess, Venus. It contains many sebaceous and sweat glands and, after puberty is covered by an inverted triangle of coarse, curly, often dark hair. The amount of fat and hair seems to be controlled by a combination of nutrition, steroids, and genetics as demonstrated by changes appearing after puberty and menopause or with starvation or obesity. This area is a landmark rather than a distinctive structure.

Labia. In addition to being a protective covering for the genitals, the labia have been found to be an important factor in normal urination. Following vulvectomy, uncontrolled "spraying" is a common complaint [8]. The labia also have a sexual function and show marked swelling in response to emotional or physical stimula-

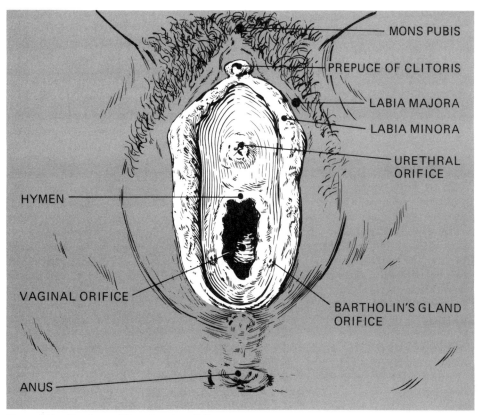

Figure 3-7. Structures of the external genitalia.

tion. The labia consist of two sets of "lips," the labia majora and labia minora.

LABIA MAJORA. The two longitudinal folds of skin that define the vulvar area are the labia majora. Anteriorly, they merge at the midline and form the mons. Their posterior union is called the posterior commissure. In the adult, the skin is covered with hair, contains many sebaceous glands, and may be pigmented. Tissue structure is stratified squamous epithelium with some keratinization, some involuntary muscle fibers, elastic connective tissue and areolar tissue. The round ligament extending from the uterus, inserts into and fuses with the labia majora, becoming part of its connective tissue.

LABIA MINORA. Two thin longitudinal folds of tissue extend bilaterally beneath the labia majora and are called the labia minora. It is perfectly normal for them to project beyond the labia majora either as a result of genetic determination or extensive tissue stretching during vaginal deliveries. At the anterior junction, their overlap forms the *prepuce* (upper fold) and *frenulum* (lower fold) of the clitoris. Posteriorly, they merge at the forchette. The outer surfaces are usually pigmented while the inner surfaces are pink and moist. There are no hair follicles, only a small number of sweat glands, and many sebaceous glands. The surface tissue is stratified squamous epithelium with minimal keratinization. Since this tissue is skin and not mucous membrane, it does NOT secrete mucus.

Clitoris. The clitoris is a 3–4 cm long, cylindrical organ located anterior to the urethra and directly between the overlapping, anterior junction of the labia minora. Its two roots, or *crura,* are attached in the periosteum of the posterior wall of the pubic symphysis. As these crura extend down and forward, they unite and form the body of the clitoris. The terminal portion of the clitoris is the glans, the only part of the structure which is visible.

The erectile tissue of the body of the clitoris is arranged into two corpora cavernosa or "cavernous bodies." These bodies contain many venous channels surrounded by involuntary muscle and numerous sensory nerve endings.

Vestibule. The elliptical space between the labia minora extending from the glans of the clitoris to the posterior hymenal ring is called the vestibule. This area is covered by stratified squamous epithelium and is not an organ, but a landmark.

Urethral meatus. The opening to the urethra sits on a slight elevation and resembles an inverted v (Λ). Its vascular mucosa often everts making it appear even more raised and redder than the surrounding tissue. The tissue which forms the meatus is striated muscle lined by stratified squamous epithelium. The position of the urethral meatus varies. It is commonly found two-thirds of the way between the clitoris and vaginal introitus, but may be located in the anterior wall of the vagina just inside the introitus.

Periurethral glands and ducts (Skene's ducts). Two small openings are found just below the urethra. (Figure 3-8.) These openings lead to a network of ducts which run a tortuous course below and lateral to the urethra, finally terminating in Skene's glands. These glands are correlates of the male's prostate gland, and do not seem to have any function in the female. They are easily infected by gonococcus, and once infected, their structure and location make treatment difficult. At times, cure may be possible only be excision or destruction of the glands. The tissue which lines these ducts is stratified squamous epithelium.

Vaginal introitus. Neither tissue, organ, nor structure, the vaginal introitus is an anatomic landmark and only a name for the external opening into the vagina.

Hymen. An irregular, membranous fold of epithelium and fibrous tissue surrounds and "covers" the vaginal introitus in varying degrees. (Figure 3-9.) This tissue or hymen is described as imperforate, incomplete, absent, or cribriform. Pelvic examination, surgery, childbirth, coitus, insertion of tampons, or exercise may tear the hymen leaving only small bits of tissue. Rarely, an imperforate hymen is so thick that surgical intervention is needed to allow for examination, release of menstrual blood, and/or intercourse.

Vestibular bulbs. The two masses of erectile tissue located on either side of the vaginal introitus are called the vestibular bulbs. They correspond to the corpus spongiosum of the male. Their posterior surface lies against the Bartholin's glands.

Vulvovaginal glands (Bartholin's glands). The small (1–2cm long) glands located just inside the mid to lower vaginal introitus are named Bartholin's glands and are homologous to the male's Cowper's glands. They are lined by a single layer of columnar epithelium. The ducts leading to the glands are lined by transitional epithelium with an invagination of stratified squamous epithelium at the vaginal opening. It was formerly thought that these glands provided lubrication during intercourse but this has since been disproved.

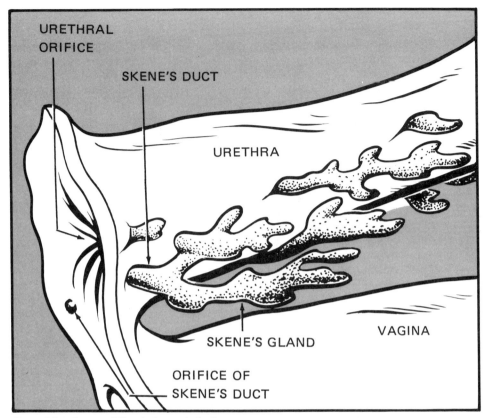

Figure 3-8. System of Skene's duct and glands.

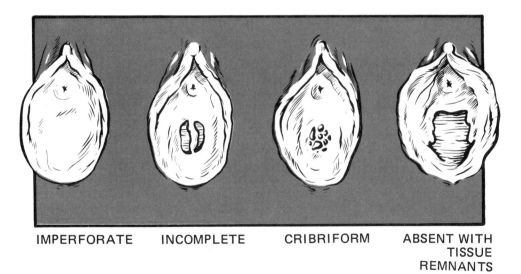

IMPERFORATE   INCOMPLETE   CRIBRIFORM   ABSENT WITH TISSUE REMNANTS

Figure 3-9. Forms of hymenal tissue.

Perineum. The perineum includes the perineal body, the fossa navicularis, and the forchette. The *perineal body* includes the skin and underlying tissue between the vaginal introitus and the anal orifice. It is supported by the transverse perineal muscle and the bulbocavernosa muscle. The *fossa navicularis* is the shallow, boat-shaped depression found posterior to the vaginal introitus. The *forchette* is the low ridge formed by the posterior junction of the labia majora and minora. Both the forchette and fossa navicularis are landmarks.

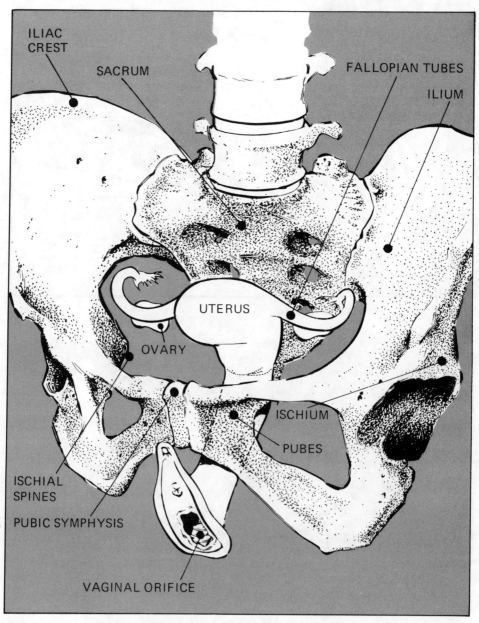

Figure 3-10.   Bony pelvis and genital structures.

All of these areas are highly vascular. An episiotomy done too early during childbirth may result in the loss of a great amount of blood, as can tearing and trauma from childbirth or rape. In addition, faulty repair of an episiotomy or laceration of the perineum during childbirth may result in dyspareunia or pelvic relaxation later in life.

Internal Genitalia

The internal organs of sex and reproduction include the *vagina, uterus, Fallopian tubes*, and *ovaries*. (Figure 3-10.)

Vagina. The vagina is a 9–10cm long, fibromuscular tube, extending back and upward at a 45-degree angle when the woman is in a standing position. It serves as the external genital canal and reaches from the perineum to the internal genital canal which begins at the cervix. The anterior vaginal wall is separated from the urethra and bladder by a thin layer of tissue. This tissue is called the vesico-vaginal septum. The posterior vaginal wall lies against the perineal body and rectum. This tissue is named the rectovaginal fascia. Both the rectovaginal fascia and the vesicovaginal septum are extensions of the same structures. (Figure 3-11).

At its upper end, the vagina attaches to the cervix so that one-third to one-half of the cervix extends into the vaginal canal. This connection forms four pouch-like spaces which are called the anterior, posterior, and two lateral fornices, depending upon their respective position. The posterior fornix is the deepest since the posterior lip of the cervix reaches further into the vaginal canal. Access to the posterior cul-de-sac, and subsequently the abdominal cavity, can be gained through the posterior fornix.

The vaginal "tube" is actually only a potential space with the walls normally being collapsed together. An exception is found in some multiparous woman, where stretching and sometimes tearing of the vaginal support structures during repeated deliveries make the vaginal canal an actual space. Longitudinal ridges found along the anterior and posterior walls are called the vaginal columns. These columns are formed by the fusion of the Müllerian ducts. Numerous prominent elevations or rugae extend laterally from these ridges in young adolescents and adults but tend to disappear with multiparity and aging.

The vaginal walls are composed of four layers of tissue: mucous membrane, connective tissue (sometimes called lamina propria), muscle, and adventitia. Some authors include the lamina propria as a part of the mucous membrane.

MUCOUS MEMBRANE (epithelium). The surface lining of the vagina is approximately six to ten layers of stratified squamous epithelium. This vaginal epithelium lines the entire canal and extends to cover the anterior and posterior lips of the cervix. While the cells contain some keratin, they are not truly cornified even though this term is sometimes incorrectly used.

The vaginal epithelium is highly responsive to estrogen. If adequate estrogen is available, the cells will contain glycogen and thus stain a deep brown if painted with iodine (Schiller's solution). This reaction is so marked that it serves as a test or indicator of normal vaginal cell function. (See chapter 24.)

Cell numbers, size, and structure vary with periodic changes in circulating estrogen. In fact, specific patterns of cell changes are seen with the menstrual

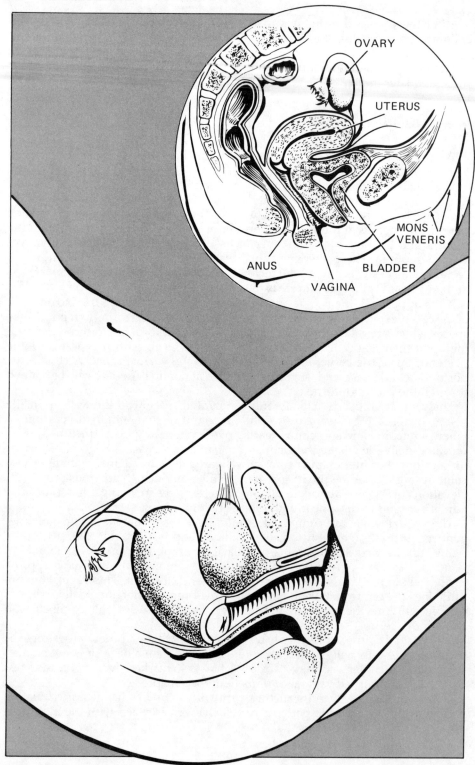

OVARY

UTERUS

MONS VENERIS

ANUS

VAGINA

BLADDER

Figure 3-11.   Uterus and adjoining organs as seen from the side. Inset shows more traditional sagittal section.

cycle, puberty, pregnancy, and menopause. It has not been proved that vaginal epithelial cells are shed cyclically.

The name "mucous membrane" to describe the vaginal epithelium is technically incorrect since this tissue does not contain any mucus secreting glands and, therefore, does not secrete mucus. Common usage persists, however, even though lubrication is provided by secretions from the cervix. In addition, during sexual stimulation, fluid emerges through the walls from the engorged blood vessels of the underlying erectile tissue. This is not, however, true mucus secretion.

Sometimes misplaced endocervical glands, remnants of the Wolffian ducts, or inclusion cysts may be found in the vaginal mucous membrane. When seen microscopically these tissue structures closely resemble malignant cells. Thus during examination of biopsied vaginal tissue the pathologist keeps the normal occurrence of these structures in mind.

CONNECTIVE TISSUE (LAMINA PROPRIA). The lamina propria lies between the muscle and epithelium with projections from the epithelium extending into it. Tough fibers crossing through connect the smooth muscle with a network of numerous thin-walled veins, thereby forming erectile tissue. This connective tissue layer is very dense close to the epithelium and becomes thinner as it nears the muscle.

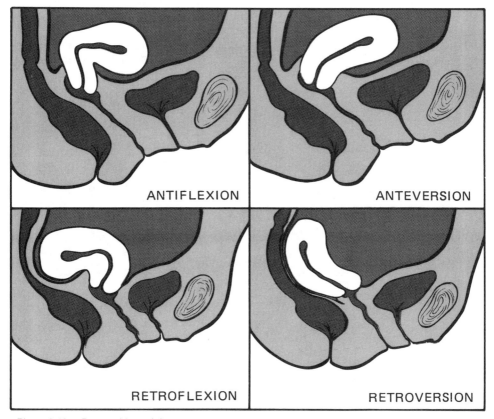

ANTIFLEXION

ANTEVERSION

RETROFLEXION

RETROVERSION

Figure 3-12. Four positions of the uterus.

MUSCLE. There are actually two interwoven layers of smooth muscle within the vaginal wall. The inner layer is circular, extending around the canal. The outer layer is longitudinal continuing from the myometrium of the uterus. Fibroelastic tissue extending from the lamina propria is interspersed throughout adding support to the vaginal wall.

ADVENTITIA. A layer of dense connective tissue with numerous blood vessels covers the muscle and adds further support to the walls. This layer, plus its blood and nerve supply forms erectile tissue. The adventitia blends with the overlying fascia at its outermost edge.

The arrangement of this strong network of muscle, fiber and erectile tissue makes the vagina capable of tremendous dilation and expansion. These qualities are needed for the vagina to fulfill its functions, which include receiving the penis during coitus, providing a protective entrance for seminal fluid to the external os, and serving as a birth canal. In addition, it serves as an excretory duct for menstrual discharge and provides for the examination of the internal genitalia.

Uterus. The uterus is located between the bladder and rectum at about the level of the pubic symphysis. It generally lies at a right angle to the vagina or with a slightly forward tilt. However, since the uterus is suspended rather than rigidly fixed in place its position varies among individuals, as well as within each woman. Various uterine positions are described as anteflexion, anteversion, retroversion and retroflexion. (Figure 3-12.)

The uterus is pear-shaped and hollow with two major segments. The corpus or body is larger (during the reproductive years) and pear-shaped. The cervix is the neck or cylindrical bottom segment. Separating these two sections is a narrowing

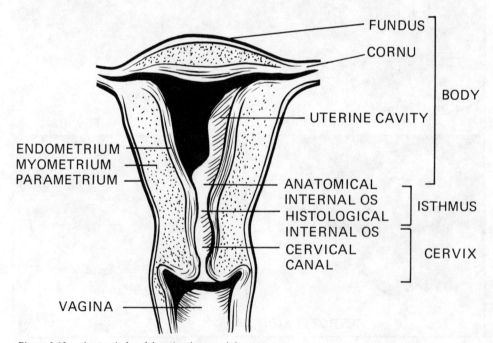

Figure 3-13.   Anatomical and functional parts of the uterus.

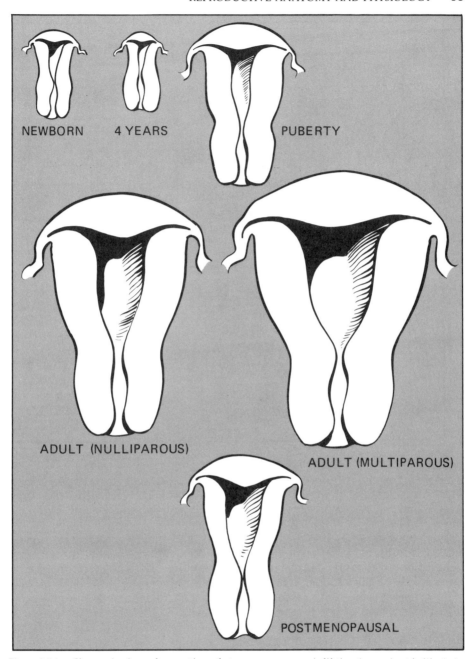

NEWBORN   4 YEARS   PUBERTY

ADULT (NULLIPAROUS)   ADULT (MULTIPAROUS)

POSTMENOPAUSAL

Figure 3-14.   Changes in size and proportions of uterus over a woman's lifetime (approximately life size).

called the isthmus. The rounded top portion of the corpus between the Fallopian tubes is referred to as the fundus. (Figure 3-13.)

During the woman's life span the uterus changes its proportions in response to

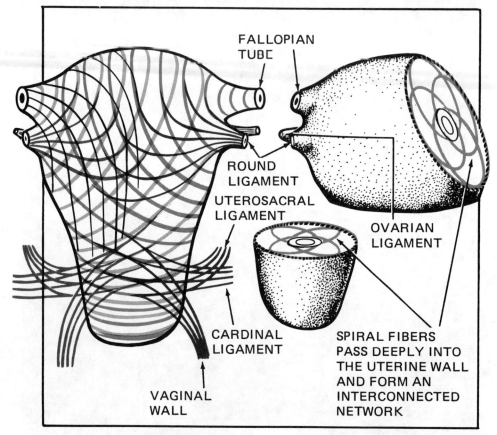

FALLOPIAN TUBE

ROUND LIGAMENT

UTEROSACRAL LIGAMENT

OVARIAN LIGAMENT

CARDINAL LIGAMENT

SPIRAL FIBERS PASS DEEPLY INTO THE UTERINE WALL AND FORM AN INTERCONNECTED NETWORK

VAGINAL WALL

Figure 3-15. Complex network of uterine musculature.

available estrogen. Prepuberty and postmenopause, the corpus is approximately one-third as large as the cervix. During the reproductive years, this ratio is reversed, and the body becomes approximately two-thirds the size of the cervix. (Figure 3-14.)

Many books discuss the cervix and corpus as if they were separate organs. Indeed, the differences in tissue structures and functions make this division seem logical. However, overall normal uterine functioning is dependent upon the complementarity and interdependency of the cervix and corpus.

The *corpus* is composed of three separate layers which form the uterine walls. Each serves a distinct function in reproduction.

PARAMETRIUM (PERITONEUM). The abdominal peritoneum extends down and forms the external covering of the uterus. It becomes so densely attached that it cannot be separated or dissected from the uterine muscle fibers. It folds over the fundus and body, completely enclosing them, and then posteriorly extends down onto the upper cervix. Anteriorly, just above the isthmus, the peritoneal covering is deflected onto the bladder. Laterally, the peritoneal folds extend outward, leave the uterine wall, and become the broad ligaments. This is illustrated in Figure 3-19.

MYOMETRIUM (MUSCLE). The myometrium is composed of three indistinct, inter-woven layers of smooth muscle fiber which are held together by connective and elastic tissues. (Figure 3-15.) In addition, within each of these layers the muscle fibers are further interlaced. The result is a very complex, longitudinal and circular muscle network.

The external layer is composed of longitudinal fibers which have continued onto the uterus from the round and broad ligaments. The middle layer is the thickest. It is made up of circular fibers which continue bilaterally onto the fundus from the Fallopian tubes extending downward until they completely encircle the uterus. The thin, inner layer of myometrium is composed of both oblique and longitudinal muscle strands.

Many blood vessels are arranged within and between the muscle bundles, especially within the circular fibers. This provides a very efficient hemostatic mechanism since contraction of these circular fibers around the vessels will "clamp" them shut. This mechanism is demonstrated during menstruation and following delivery of the placenta after childbirth.

Uterine muscle contractions most often originate in the fundus near the tubouterine junction, sweeping downward toward the cervix. This has lead to speculation about the possibility that "pacemakers" are located at this junction. If such pacemakers exist, they could explain the origin and coordination of uterine muscle contractions. That is, uterine contractions such as labor contractions and even menstrual cramps would originate at these sites and move downward over the uterine wall in a similar, coordinated way [14].

However, distinct pacemaker cells such as those in the SA node of the heart have not been demonstrated. In addition, research has shown that different areas of the uterine muscle seem to serve as pacemakers at different times. Thus, uterine contractions seem to be related to individual myometrial cell excitability with contractions starting and spreading outward from a number of different locations [6]. Progesterone, estrogen, and prostaglandins also influence uterine muscle contractions. These different factors may be a part of a complex system used to coordinate movements of tube, uterus, ligaments, and ovary for optimum positioning at ovulation [8].

ENDOMETRIUM. The endometrium is the specialized epithelial lining of the uterus. It is composed of two layers, the basilar layer and the surface epithelium. The basilar or deepest layer lies next to the myometrium and does not participate in menstrual sloughing. Remnants of the surface glands embedded within are needed for regrowth of the glands following menstruation, as illustrated in Figure 3-22.

The surface epithelium is the outer two-thirds of the endometrium. It is composed of a network of arterial and venous capillaries, secretory glands, and a loose tissue matrix. During the reproductive years, this superficial layer of endometrium will grow and slough off in response to the cyclical changes of the reproductive system hormones.

The *isthmus* is the external narrowing seen between the corpus and cervix. It is defined internally by the internal cervical os. The transition from endometrial to endocervical tissue occurs at the isthmus. A structural feature which becomes important during childbirth is that the myometrium is thinner here, allowing dilation and effacement to occur at the inner os. Therefore, during labor the isthmus is referred to as the lower uterine segment, as is illustrated in Figure 3-13.

The *cervix* is about 2.5cm long and divided into two segments by the vaginal attachments. The upper (supravaginal) cervix lies against the bladder anteriorly and against the rectum posteriorly. Peritoneum covers the supravaginal cervix. The lower (vaginal) portion is covered by the stratified squamous epithelium of the vagina. The external os, located centrally, divides the cervix into anterior and posterior lips.

Circular muscle fibers continuing from the uterine body form the cervical walls. The muscle coat thins as it moves downward so that only a weak, outer muscle layer is present at the lowest portion of the cervix. Connective tissue correspondingly increases [11].

The tissue which lines the cervical canal is called the endocervix. It is a specialized mucous membrane containing tall, mucus-secreting columnar cells, ciliated columnar cells, glands, and a fibrous stroma. It turns out, however, that the endocervical glands are really not glands at all. As described in Novak's *Textbook of Gynecology*, Fluhmann's studies show that the honeycomb appearance of the endocervix is not due to glands but to a complex arrangement of clefts and tunnels which serve to increase the surface area of mucosa and allow for greater secretion of mucus from the columnar cells. Common usage persists, however, and reference is regularly made to endocervical glands [12].

The columnar cells of the endocervix meet the stratified squamous epithelium of the exocervix at the external os. This tissue junction is, thereby, named the squamocolumnar junction. This transition zone may be located at, above, or below the anatomical external os. It is easily identified during speculum examination of the vagina since the endocervix appears more red and glistening than does the epithelial tissue of the exocervix. Outward growth or proliferation of the endocervix is often mistaken for a pathological condition called erosion.

The cervix functions as a canal for birth and for menstrual discharge. In addition, the mucus that is secreted facilitates sperm entry during the fertile phase of the cycle, and then acts as a seal or plug if the fertilized ovum implants. The cervix plays a role in fertility since the properties of the mucus, including pH and viscosity, may serve as initial barriers or facilitators to sperm entry. Finally, cervical mucus can serve as a test for ovarian function since its characteristics are dependent upon estrogen.

Fallopian tubes. The two fibromuscular Fallopian tubes extend bilaterally from the uterus. They exit from the cornu just above the round and ovarian ligaments, extend laterally and then posteriorly in a tortuous 12cm length to finally terminate just in front of the medial surface of the ovary. Both thickness of the tubal wall and lumen size vary throughout the tube. The uterine opening into the tube is about the size of a hairbrush bristle [8].

For descriptive purposes, the tube can be divided into four sections. (Figure 3-16.) The *interstitial* portion extends through the myometrium of the uterus and opens into the uterine cavity. The *isthmus* is the narrowest portion of the tube. It is the short section of the tube just prior to its insertion into the uterine wall. The *ampulla* is the longest portion of the tube, containing thin, dilatable muscular walls. The *infundibulum*, or terminal portion, gives the tubes their trumpet shape. Numerous delicate folds of tissue, or fimbriae, around the small orifice give it a fringed appearance. The longest fimbria is attached to the ovary, keeping the tube in close proximity to the ovarian surface.

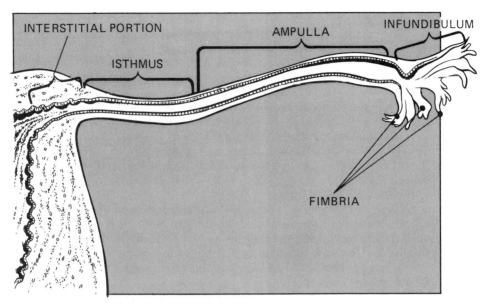

Figure 3-16. Anatomical structure of the Fallopian tube.

The walls of the Fallopian tubes are composed of three layers of tissue:

1. The external covering is an extension of the abdominal peritoneum (broad ligament). It covers and encloses the tubes completely except for the interstitial portion and the fimbrial attachment to the ovary. The area between this layer and the muscle is filled with blood vessels, nerves, and some connective tissue.

2. The intermediate layer is actually two interwoven layers of muscle fibers. The outer, longitudinal fibers are thin and cover a thicker, inner layer of circular muscle fibers. These fibers extend onto, across, and down the uterine walls.

3. The internal layer of the tube consists of longitudinal folds of endometrium-like tissue which enclose the lumen. These tissue folds, or rugae, become more pronounced as they near the fimbria. The cells of this lining are columnar epithelium containing both ciliated and nonciliated secretory cells. Tall, intercolated (or peg) cells interspersed throughout give the epithelium a bumpy appearance.

Tubal function and physiology are closely related. That is, as research investigations proceed, it is becoming clear that the Fallopian tubes function as much more than passive recipients and canals for the ova and sperm. It appears that the tubes play a role in successful fertilization of the ovum, in the early development of the morulla, and in nourishing the embryo during early implantation in the endometrium [8].

Ovaries. The pair of ovaries are found in the true pelvis, one on either side of the uterine fundus. They sit vertically against the peritoneum of the lateral pelvic walls. The appendix is immediately superior to the right ovary. The position of the ovary is not rigid but moves simultaneously with movements of the tubes, the uterus, and various support structures.

The inner, tapered border of the ovary is called the hilus. Blood vessels and nerves interwound with the ovarian ligament enter and leave the ovary here.

Even though the ovaries are described as almond-shaped, both their shape and size varies greatly. In addition, the pair of ovaries may be asymmetrical with the right ovary generally being the larger one.

Surface variations in the adult ovary are caused by newly-ruptured follicles seen as single or multiple reddish swellings as well as by older ruptured follicles appearing as yellow or white swellings. The yellow swellings are called the corpus luteum while the white structures are called the corpora albicans. All of these structures vary in size and, since all are cystic in nature, it is generally accepted that 2.5cm is the lesser parameter of an ovarian "cyst" that would require medical follow-up [8]. Details of this follow-up may be found in chapter 15 (Upper Reproductive Tract Disorders). Excessive bleeding into the follicle at ovulation produces a hemorrhagic corpus luteum cyst. If its thin walls burst there will be resultant bleeding into the abdominal cavity.

Histologically the ovary is composed of two layers of tissue, the cortex and medulla. The cortex composes the outer one-third to one-half of the ovary. It is a tense, elastic tissue containing the follicles and ova which are the functional reproductive tissues. The medulla or inner portion of the ovary is very vascular with loose stroma and no follicles. The ovary is the target organ for pituitary and placental hormones.

The follicle structure is composed of two thecal-cell layers, the theca interna and theca externa. Granulosa cells line the theca interna. The thecal calls are responsible for estradiol production. Under the influence of pituitary hormones, the granulosa cells secrete progesterone [8].

Urinary and Intestinal Structures

The urinary system. The kidneys are located in the posterior abdominal cavity about where the last rib attaches to the vertebrae. The ureters extend down from the kidney to the pelvic floor, then move forward passing about 2cm lateral to the cervix and vaginal fornix. Just as they begin to ascend, they reach the bladder base. (Figure 3-17.)

The urinary bladder is a hollow, muscular sac placed directly behind the pubic symphysis. Its base is in direct contact with the superior vaginal wall. An anteflexed uterine body and fundus will be in direct contact with the superior bladder wall. The tissue lining the inside of the bladder is transitional epithelium. Beneath this epithelium lies a coat of smooth muscle called the detrusor muscle. The outer, superior covering is peritoneum.

The ureters and urethra insert into the base of the bladder in a triangular configuration with the urethra being at the vertex. This area is referred to as the trigone. The detrusor muscle forms a series of loops around the urethral opening creating the internal sphincter.

Opposing parasympathetic fibers innervate the detrusor muscle and internal sphincter. Stimulation of these fibers results in contraction of the detrusor and relaxation of the internal sphincter. Stimulation of sympathetic fibers from the hypogastric nerve which also innervate this area, will reverse this process. Thus, when the bladder walls contract, the internal sphincter relaxes, allowing urine to pass into the urethra. The internal sphincter is normally in a contracted state.

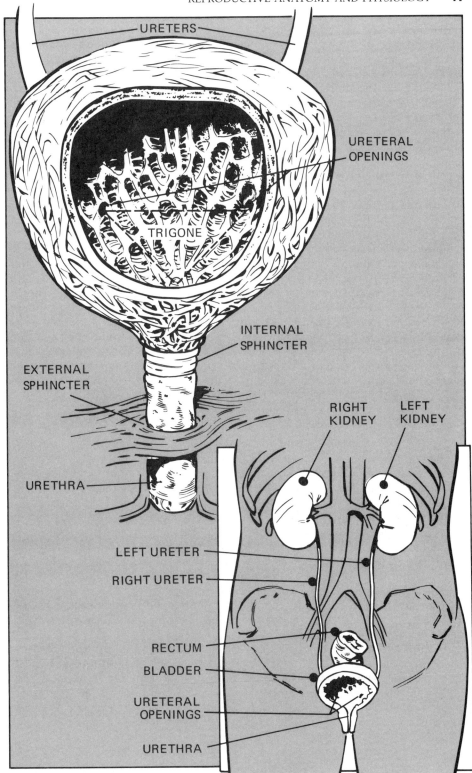

Figure 3-17. Anatomical details of the urinary bladder. Inset shows complete urinary tract.

Just below the internal urethral sphincter, striated muscles surround the urethra and form the external sphincter. Fibers from the pudendal nerve give voluntary control to this sphincter. Since sensory fibers also innervate this area, voiding is a reflex act which is placed under voluntary control. Stretch receptors in the bladder wall are stimulated when 200–300ml of urine has collected. The sensation of a full bladder is received by the central nervous system and interpreted as the desire to void.

The urethra is a short tube, approximately 3–5cm long. It connects the bladder and external meatus, opening onto the perineum. The posterior urethral wall lies against the superior vaginal wall. The urethral walls normally lie flattened together except when the individual is voiding.

The area of the urethra closest to the bladder is lined by transitional epithelium. About one-third of the way down, this tissue becomes stratified squamous epithelium which extends to the meatus. The urethral walls and meatus play a very limited role in control of micturition.

Colon, rectum, and anus. The appendix and cecum are normally found on the right side, just superior to the ovary. From here, the colon generally extends horizontally across the pelvis to the left side. However, since it is very movable, it can be located against the superior or posterior aspects of the uterus or anywhere in between these two locations.

The rectum extends from about the area of the third sacral vertebrae to just beyond the tip of the coccyx. It moves medially across and under the vagina and cervix, finally becoming the anus. The anal sphincter guards the opening of the rectum onto the perineum. This system of continuous, hollow, muscular tubes is responsible for moving fecal wastes from the body.

Spaces

There are two major spaces within the female pelvis. They are created by the deflection of peritoneum from the anterior and posterior uterine surfaces to the adjoining organs. (Figure 3-18.)

Cul-de-sac of Douglas. This "pouch" or space is referred to as the posterior cul-de-sac, rectouterine pouch, or cul-de-sac of Douglas. It is formed as the peritoneum extends downward covering the posterior uterine body, cervix, and vaginal fornix. It then lifts off and reaches across, up, and over the rectum. The space formed between the reflected peritoneal coverings of the cervix and rectum is called the pouch of Douglas. Its major importance is that it allows fairly easy access to the abdominal cavity for examination of pelvic organs by culdoscopy or for drainage of any collected pus or blood from the abdominal cavity. This technique is helpful in diagnosing conditions such as ruptured ectopic pregnancy or pelvic inflammatory disease.

Anterior cul-de-sac. The space between the anterior surface of the uterus and the urinary bladder is called the anterior cul-de-sac or vesicouterine pouch. It is formed as the peritoneum leaves the anterior surface of the uterus about the level of the isthmus, reaches across and extends up and over the bladder. The anterior cul-de-sac is the resultant space formed between the peritoneum which separates the two organs.

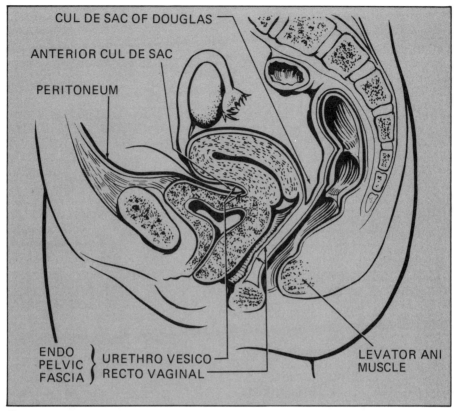

Figure 3-18.   Relationship of peritoneum, endopelvic fascia, organs, and pelvic spaces.

Support Structures

Pelvic bones. The pelvic basin is formed by a fusion of several bones. (See Figure 3-10.) Three bones, the ilium, ischium, and pubes fuse to form each side of the pelvic wall. These two sides are connected in front by a cartilage "joint," the pubic symphysis. In back, another cartilage joint connects the two ilium bones with the sacrum and coccyx.

Several important landmarks are formed by these pelvic bones. The iliac crests, commonly referred to as the hip bones, mark the upper boundary of the pelvis. The ischial spines (what we sit on) mark the lower pelvic boundaries. The ischial spines and tip of the coccyx form the pelvic outlet of the birth canal.

The upper border of the true pelvis is marked by a ridge extending about midway around the inner aspect of this pelvic bowl about the level of the superior pubic symphysis. Beneath this, the pelvis is much narrower, as if it were "the bottom of the bowl." Here, below the level of the pubic symphysis in the true pelvis, the pelvic organs are located.

In addition to providing a bony protection, the pelvic bones provide a place of

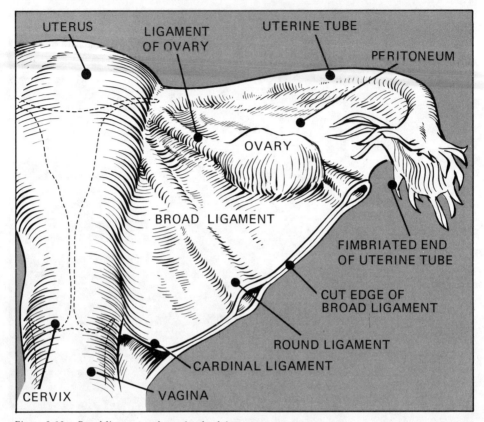

Figure 3-19.   Broad ligament and associated pelvic support structures.

attachment for the various muscles and ligaments of the pelvis. Thus, they also serve as a support structure for the pelvic organs. Finally, and very obviously, a major function of the pelvic bones is to connect the legs and torso of the body.

Muscles, fascia, ligaments. There are many ways to organize the various muscles, ligaments, and tendons of the pelvis. Because there is a great deal of overlapping of these structures, no one system remains "neat" or precise. We have chosen to organize them into three major categories: major pelvic ligaments and peritoneum, pelvic floor, and perineal muscles.

Major Ligaments and Peritoneum

CARDINAL LIGAMENTS OR MACKENRODT'S LIGAMENTS. The cardinal ligaments are actually the base layer of the broad ligaments as they leave the uterine fundus about the level of the isthmus. (Figure 3-19.) Posteriorly, they merge with the uterosacral ligaments, and anteriorly, with the endopelvic fascia. They provide the major support for the cervix and upper vagina thus preventing uterine prolapse. In addition, they enclose the uterine vessels, nerve fibers, and lymphatics.

Laterally, the ligaments fan out and insert onto other fascia and muscles of the pelvic floor, continuing to provide support to the major vessels as they do so.

ROUND LIGAMENTS. The round ligaments are actually muscular bands which are continuous with the uterine muscle. They leave the anterior uterine fundus just below the Fallopian tube, extend laterally between layers of the broad ligament, move through the inguinal canal, and, finally, spread out and terminate in the connective tissue of the labia majora. It was formerly believed that the round ligament held the uterus forward, but this is currently in question. The most important support role of this ligament appears to be during pregnancy when it becomes greatly hypertrophied.

BROAD LIGAMENTS. These wing-like ligaments are actually a double layer of peritoneum which extend from the lateral uterine surface to the pelvic walls. At their upper border, they fold over the Fallopian tubes and ovarian vessels and then continue on to the pelvic wall as the *infundibulopelvic ligament.* Inferior to the tubes, they enclose the round ligament and form the *mesosalpinx.* At the inferior edges, as previously described, they are thickened with connective tissue and become the *cardinal ligaments.* Thus, the broad ligament serves to support most of the pelvic structures.

OVARIAN LIGAMENT. (The infundibulopelvic ligament or suspensory ligament of the ovary). The connective tissue and muscle of the ovarian ligament are continuous with those of the uterus. This ligament originates on the lateral uterine wall between the tube and round ligament and extends as a rounded cord to the ovary. It is enclosed by the broad ligament. Some studies indicate that in addition to anchoring the ovary, it may also play a role in positioning the tube over the ovary to ensure reception of the egg at ovulation [8].

PERITONEUM. It is clear that the abdominal peritoneum serves as more than a partition between the abdominal and pelvic cavities. It is the outermost covering of the bladder, rectum, tubes, and much of the uterus. It forms the anterior and posterior cul-de-sac. It provides support in the form of the broad ligament and its many variations (i.e., mesovarium, infundibulopelvic ligaments, and cardinal ligaments).

Pelvic Floor

There are two divisions of the pelvic floor. The first or upper division can be called the pelvic diaphragm. It includes the endopelvic fascia, uterosacral ligaments, and levator ani and coccygeus muscles. The second or lower division is the urogenital diaphragm [4]. (Figure 3-20.)

PELVIC DIAPHRAGM. The pelvic diaphragm is actually a collective term. As noted above, it is made up of several muscles, ligaments, and fascia. Their interwoven arrangement provides further, reciprocal support. It is interesting to note that these layers are not "fixed" together. This allows them to move across one another, thus facilitating dilation and reclosure of the vaginal canal during childbirth and involution [4].

The pelvic diaphragm actually forms a partition between the pelvic cavity and the perineum. This partition is perforated by the urethra, vagina, and rectum. Each of these tubes cross through the pelvic floor at an angle which enhances the

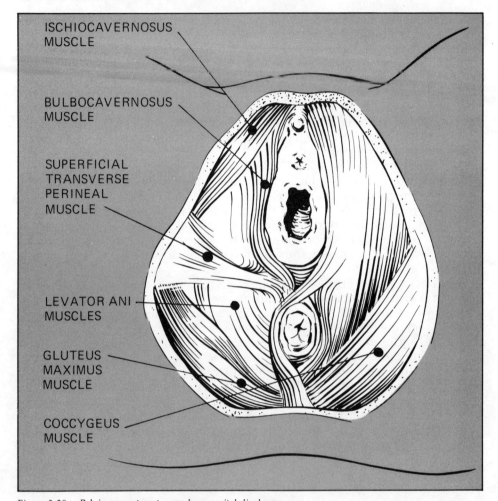

ISCHIOCAVERNOSUS
MUSCLE

BULBOCAVERNOSUS
MUSCLE

SUPERFICIAL
TRANSVERSE
PERINEAL
MUSCLE

LEVATOR ANI
MUSCLES

GLUTEUS
MAXIMUS
MUSCLE

COCCYGEUS
MUSCLE

Figure 3-20. Pelvic support system and urogenital diaphragm.

sphincter-like action of their surrounding muscle.

The first major structure of the pelvic diaphragm is the *endopelvic fascia*. It can be described as three tubes rising from the fascia of the pelvic floor to enclose the bladder and urethra, uterus and vagina, and the rectum. In addition, where these same structures penetrate the pelvic floor, tight "collars" of endopelvic fascia strengthen these potentially weakened areas. This fascia is considered the main support for the bladder and rectum and is the structure utilized for cystocele and rectocele repair.

The *uterosacral ligaments* originate on the posterior uterine wall about the level of the internal os. They form a posterior arch as they extend around the rectum to finally insert on the sacrum. Near the uterus they serve as an insertion for the cardinal ligaments. Their major function is to provide a posterior anchor for the cervix, in effect holding the uterus at a right angle to the vagina. These ligaments are composed of connective tissue, involuntary muscle, blood vessels, lymphatics, and nerve fibers.

The levator ani and coccygeus muscles form a muscular hammock as a base for the pelvic cavity. These muscles extend down from the lateral pelvic walls and then turn inward to either fuse medially or insert into the terminal urethra, vagina, and anus. Just behind the pubic symphysis they fail to meet thus leaving a gap in the pelvic floor.

UROGENITAL DIAPHRAGM. This structure is a strong, muscular partition which extends across the anterior portion of the pelvic outlet, thus closing the gap left by the pelvic diaphragm. It is composed of a pair of deep transverse perineal muscles, blood vessels and nerves, and the urethral sphincter. These structures are enclosed by inferior and superior layers of fascia which fuse with the fascia of the pelvic diaphragm.

Perineal Muscles

The five major muscles of the female perineum correspond to the muscles which form the male perineum. The *ischiocavernosus* muscle inserts into the crura of the clitoris. The *bulbocavernosus muscles* surround the vaginal meatus and cover the vestibular bulbs. They insert anteriorly into the corpora carvernosa of the clitoris. The *perineal muscles and urethral sphincter* are part of the perineal make-up as well as being part of the urogenital diaphragm. The *external anal sphincter* is a part of the perineum as well as of the pelvic diaphragm.

In a collective sense the soft supporting structures of the perineum serve a variety of functions. They cushion, support, and anchor the pelvic viscera and external genitalia. They provide additional protection for these same structures. This protective-supportive role is especially important during pregnancy and childbirth when pelvic organs are additionally stressed. Finally, they provide sphincter muscle activity for the urethral, vaginal, and rectal orifices.

Coordinating Structures

Blood Supply

About the level of the fourth lumbar vertebrate, the aorta bifurcates. The two branches become the right and left common iliac arteries. As they descend bilaterally, they each branch again and form the external and internal iliac (or hypogastric) arteries. The external iliac artery continues downward, finally entering the thigh as the femoral artery.

The internal iliac artery becomes one of the four major vessels to supply blood to the pelvis. The other three of these vessels include the ovarian artery, the superior hemorrhoidal artery, and the middle sacral artery.

The ovarian artery arises directly from the aorta just below the renal arteries. In addition to the ovary and tube, it supplies blood to the broad ligament, ureter,

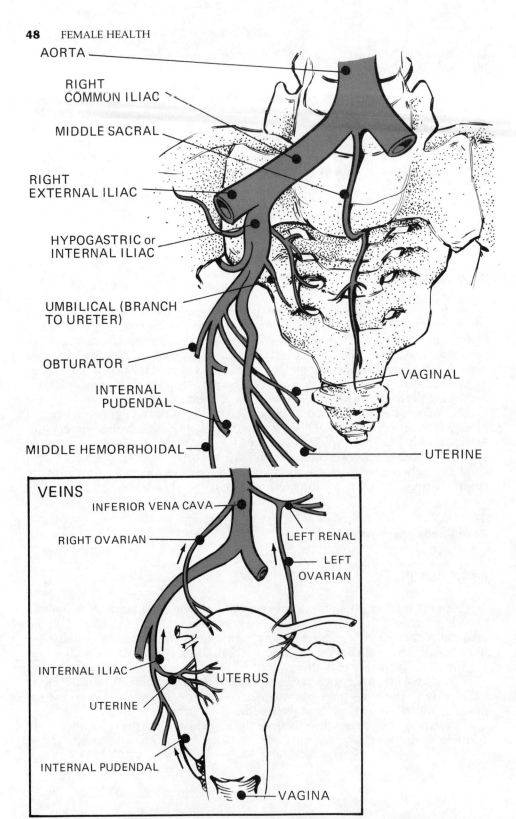

AORTA

RIGHT COMMON ILIAC

MIDDLE SACRAL

RIGHT EXTERNAL ILIAC

HYPOGASTRIC or INTERNAL ILIAC

UMBILICAL (BRANCH TO URETER)

OBTURATOR

INTERNAL PUDENDAL

MIDDLE HEMORRHOIDAL

VAGINAL

UTERINE

VEINS

INFERIOR VENA CAVA

RIGHT OVARIAN

LEFT RENAL

LEFT OVARIAN

INTERNAL ILIAC

UTERUS

UTERINE

INTERNAL PUDENDAL

VAGINA

Figure 3-21. Divisions of the hypogastric artery which supplies blood to the pelvic structures. Inset shows venous drainage.

and round ligament. The superior hemorrhoidal artery anastomoses with the middle and inferior hemorrhoidal arteries to supply the anus, anal canal and perineum with blood. Finally, the middle sacral artery brings blood to the posterior pelvic wall. It is interesting to note that this vessel is actually the continuation of the aorta which has become a small, thin vessel due to the strong development of the common iliac arteries.

The internal iliac artery sends branches to various parts of the pelvis. It has four major branches:

1. The obturator artery supplies blood to the inner and outer aspects of the anterior pelvic wall, including both bony and soft structures.

2. The umbilical artery supplies the ureter and bladder with blood.

3. The vaginal artery forms many branches which anastomose freely with the many branches from the uterine artery. The result is a plexus of vessels surrounding the vaginal walls. This ensures an excellent blood supply and establishes a basis for erectile tissue functioning.

4. The uterine artery reaches the uterus at the level of the internal os. Here it divides and sends out ascending and descending branches. The descending branch supplies the lateral vaginal walls, anastomosing freely with the vaginal artery.

The ascending branch of the uterine artery follows a tortuous pathway up the lateral sides of the uterus to the cornu where it divides, sending one branch to the round ligament and the other to anastomose with the ovarian artery. However, prior to this final branching, the uterine artery sends off many horizontal branches en route over the uterine sides. (Figure 3-22.) These horizontal branches called acuate arteries, encircle the myometrial surface. In turn, branches from the acuate arteries called radial arteries, extend into the myometrium so that every segment of the uterine wall has a rich blood supply.

Once a radial artery reaches the endometrium it forks. The smaller of these forks remains in the basal layer of endometrium ensuring a continued blood supply despite surface endometrial sloughing. It is appropriately called the basilar or straight artery. The second fork is longer, growing to the surface of the endometrium. Any estrogen stimulation causes a rapid growth of these arteries resulting in their having a twisted appearance. Hence, they are called coiled arteries. The coiled arteries show cyclic changes in response to the changing stimulus of reproductive hormone patterns.

The perineal structures receive their primary blood supply from a somewhat different source—the internal and external pudendal arteries. The internal pudendal artery extends from the internal iliac while the external pudendal is a branch from the femoral arteries.

The venous drainage for the pelvic structures generally have similar names and follow routes similar to those of the arteries.

Lymph

The higher pressure within the circulatory system forces serum into the interstitial spaces. This interstitial fluid or lymph surrounds the cells and is responsible for exchanging electrolytes, accumulating waste products, and helping to main-

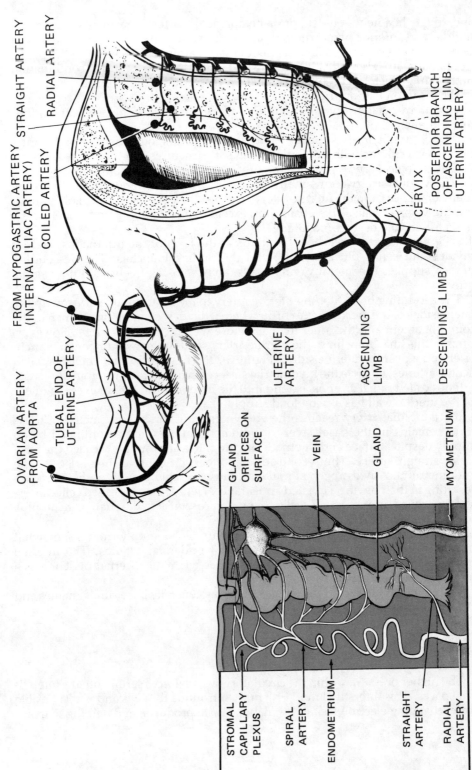

STRAIGHT ARTERY

RADIAL ARTERY

FROM HYPOGASTRIC ARTERY (INTERNAL ILIAC ARTERY)

COILED ARTERY

POSTERIOR BRANCH OF ASCENDING LIMB, UTERINE ARTERY

CERVIX

OVARIAN ARTERY FROM AORTA

TUBAL END OF UTERINE ARTERY

UTERINE ARTERY

ASCENDING LIMB

DESCENDING LIMB

GLAND ORIFICES ON SURFACE

VEIN

GLAND

MYOMETRIUM

STROMAL CAPILLARY PLEXUS

SPIRAL ARTERY

ENDOMETRIUM

STRAIGHT ARTERY

RADIAL ARTERY

Figure 3-22. Detail of blood supply to the uterine wall and ovary. Inset shows endometrial structures and blood supply.

tain the cell environment. The accumulation of this interstitial fluid produces a second pressure gradient which forces the lymph into lymph ductules. Here it joins with lymph from numerous other ductules and is drained to the nearest lymph node.

The lymph nodes serve as filters for removing unwanted particles from the lymph. In addition, they break down waste products such as bacteria or end products of infection. Another function is the development of antibodies, phagocytes, and antitoxins, thus serving as an integral part of the body's defense system. An inherent weakness of this system is that the lymph also transports malignant cells from one part of the body to another leaving them at various lymph nodes and thus facilitating metastases.

The lymph is channeled through a series of vessels passing from node to node until it is returned to the general circulation as serum. These lymph vessels follow the blood vessels rather closely with the nodes scattered in strategic places. The four most important of the pelvic nodes and the areas which they drain are as follows:

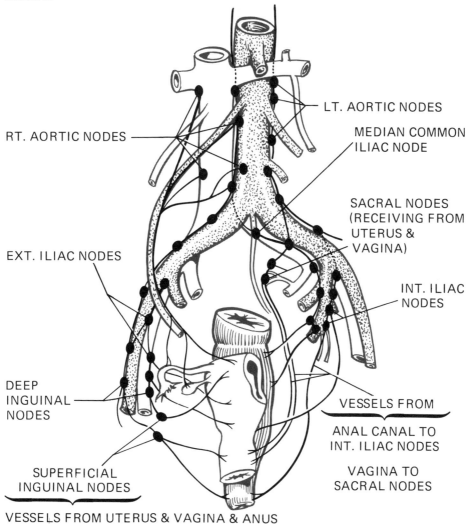

Figure 3-23. *Lymphatic drainage of the pelvic structures.*

The *superficial inguinal nodes* are found in the groin. Lymph from the vulva is filtered here and then drained to the external iliac nodes.

The *external iliac nodes* are located along the external iliac artery. Lymph is received from the inguinal nodes, the glans of the clitoris, urethra, bladder, cervix, and upper vagina. They drain filtered lymph to the lateral aortic nodes.

The *internal iliac nodes* are located along the internal iliac artery and receive lymph from vessels which follow all of the branches of this artery. This lymph is brought to the internal iliac nodes from all of the pelvic viscera. In turn, lymph drains from here to the common iliac nodes.

The *common iliac nodes* are found along the common iliac arteries near the bifurcation of the aorta. Lymph is received from the internal and external iliac nodes and is drained to the aortic nodes.

Nerves

A neuron is composed of the nerve cell (gray matter) with its varying numbers of processes or axons and dendrites (white matter). Axons carry impulses away from nerve cells and are generally longer. The shorter dendrites carry impulses to the nerve cells.

There are two types of nerves. Sensory nerves carry impulses from the periphery of the body to the spinal cord and brain. Motor nerves carry impulses from the brain to the body to bring about muscular contractions or release of secretions from glands. The term mixed nerve refers to a bundle of nerve fibers outside the spinal cord which contains both motor and sensory nerves.

The organization of the nervous system could be represented as follows:

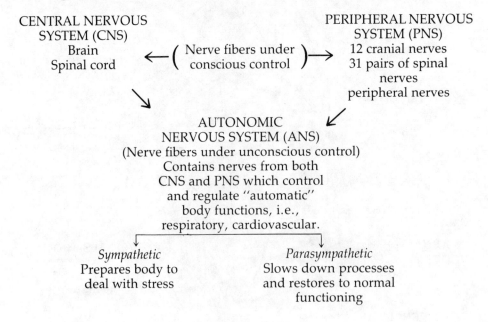

CENTRAL NERVOUS SYSTEM (CNS)
Brain
Spinal cord

← (Nerve fibers under conscious control) →

PERIPHERAL NERVOUS SYSTEM (PNS)
12 cranial nerves
31 pairs of spinal nerves
peripheral nerves

AUTONOMIC NERVOUS SYSTEM (ANS)
(Nerve fibers under unconscious control)
Contains nerves from both CNS and PNS which control and regulate "automatic" body functions, i.e., respiratory, cardiovascular.

Sympathetic
Prepares body to deal with stress

Parasympathetic
Slows down processes and restores to normal functioning

Within the CNS, well-defined groups of neurons in the gray matter are called nuclei. In the peripheral nervous system, the comparable term for groups of neurons is ganglia. A bundle of nerve fibers in the white matter of the CNS is a tract, while in the PNS it is a nerve.

A long sympathetic nerve trunk on each side of the vertebral bodies extends from the base of the skull to the coccyx. Ganglia, scattered along this trunk at regular intervals, send out nerve branches to the organs in respective areas. Fibers extending from the vertebrae in the cranial and the sacral areas provide parasympathetic innervation.

As these various nerve fibers leave the ganglia or spinal cord, they begin to branch and intermingle, forming a mass of nerves called a plexus. Here the nerves are regrouped and rearranged before proceeding to their destinations. Thus, an organ or tissue may be innervated by peripheral nerves under both conscious and unconscious control.

A commonly encountered example helps make this clear. The peripheral motor and sensory nerves of the external urethral sphincters are under the conscious control of the CNS. However, the internal sphincters are under ANS control and can "overrule." If the bladder becomes too full, some urine may be released no matter how strong the willpower of the person.

The pelvis contains some CNS nerve fibers. However, most innervation is from the ANS. Sympathetic fibers extend from the pelvic trunk to the superior hypogastric plexus. This is located near the bifurcation of the aorta. From this, the hypogastric nerve crosses into the pelvis, branches, and forms the pelvic plexus (of the inferior hypogastric plexus). From here, sympathetic innervation is sent to the inner aspect of the Fallopian tube, uterus, vagina, bladder and rectum with some fibers also going to the ovary. Parasympathetic innervation of the pelvic viscera is from the second, third, and fourth sacral nerves.

The ovaries and outer aspect of the tubes receive sympathetic innervation from the aortic and renal plexus (celiac plexus) which is located about the level of L-1. (Figure 3-24.) It sends branches down to the ovarian plexus just above the ovary and near the ovarian artery. It also provides innervation to the broad ligament.

The motor and sensory nerves of the perineal structures arise from S 2-4 and then join to form the pudendal nerve. At the pelvic floor the pudendal nerve sends branches to various sites.

The inferior rectal nerve supplies the external sphincter and skin. The perineal nerve sends superficial branches to the urogenital diaphragm and labia majora. Deep branches are sent to the deep perineal muscles, internal urethral sphincter, and urethra. The dorsal nerve of the clitoris innervates the glans of the clitoris.

The smooth muscle of the viscera with its autonomic nerve supply is more responsive to sensations of stretch and relaxation. The striated muscle and motor/sensory innervation of the external genitalia is subject to conscious control and is also responsive to sensations of pressure and temperature. The common innervation of many pelvic structures provides a basis for understanding the sensations associated with the sexual response cycle, menstrual periods, childbirth and various pathological conditions.

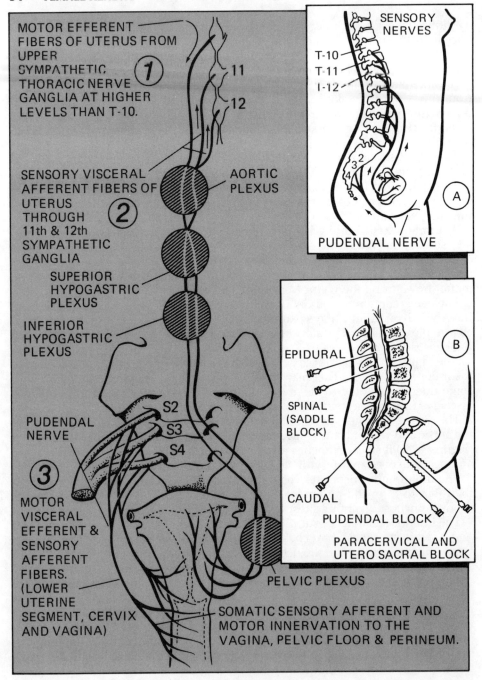

MOTOR EFFERENT FIBERS OF UTERUS FROM UPPER SYMPATHETIC THORACIC NERVE GANGLIA AT HIGHER LEVELS THAN T-10. ①

11
12

SENSORY VISCERAL AFFERENT FIBERS OF UTERUS THROUGH 11th & 12th SYMPATHETIC GANGLIA ②

AORTIC PLEXUS

SUPERIOR HYPOGASTRIC PLEXUS

INFERIOR HYPOGASTRIC PLEXUS

PUDENDAL NERVE

S2
S3
S4

③

MOTOR VISCERAL EFFERENT & SENSORY AFFERENT FIBERS. (LOWER UTERINE SEGMENT, CERVIX AND VAGINA)

PELVIC PLEXUS

SOMATIC SENSORY AFFERENT AND MOTOR INNERVATION TO THE VAGINA, PELVIC FLOOR & PERINEUM.

SENSORY NERVES
T-10
T-11
T-12
3 2
4
PUDENDAL NERVE
Ⓐ

Ⓑ
EPIDURAL
SPINAL (SADDLE BLOCK)
CAUDAL
PUDENDAL BLOCK
PARACERVICAL AND UTERO SACRAL BLOCK

Figure 3-24.   Nerve supply to pelvic organs and the perineum. Inset A shows sensory nerves. Inset B shows areas for administration of regional anesthesia.

Female Sexual and Reproductive Physiology

The first section of this chapter provides an anatomical description of the female breast and internal and external genitals. In essence, this is a picture of a woman's sexual and reproductive organs. The descriptions of the average sizes, shapes, and placement of these organs and the various tissues around them gives a three-dimensional aspect to this anatomical picture, although it remains lifeless. The components which make it all work—organs, muscles, nerves, blood and nutrients—are dependent upon physiological function to give their existence meaning. The purpose of this section, then, is to give life to that three-dimensional picture.

An inherent, semantic reality is that a book cannot really "give life" to an understanding of reproductive function. Although functions can be described as clearly and realistically as possible, a reader's interpretations are what establish the reality. An idea becomes alive for an individual only if it has personal meaning.

Physiology of the breast and pelvic organs described only in terms of reproduction, may subtract life (or interest) from this material for many women. To discuss female functioning only in terms of reproductive physiology ignores the woman who chooses not to have children or perhaps is past menopause. This denies the developmental progress of one and the life-style of the other. For these reasons we have included the physiology of sexual as well as reproductive function.

We have presented physiologic information in a progressive format. This will enable a review and building onto an existing knowledge base, depending upon how much information is needed or desired. Much of the current knowledge of sexual and reproductive physiology is either still speculative, being researched, or not known. Even though this leaves some inevitable knowledge gaps, we hope that the content and presentation will make the anatomical picture come to life.

HORMONE CONTROL OF THE SEXUAL AND REPRODUCTIVE SYSTEM

Many of the functions of sex and reproduction are either directly or indirectly dependent upon hormones. A hormone is a substance which travels from a special tissue through the blood stream to a distant cell-type where it exerts a characteristic effect [8]. The hormones which are actively involved in this physiologic process are secreted by the endocrine system.

The two major endocrine glands involved are the pituitary and the ovary. The hypothalamus produces neurotransmitters which influence functioning of these glands. Because of their functional interrelationships, they are referred to as a unit called the hypothalamic-pituitary-ovarian axis. A fourth major reproductive endocrine gland, the placenta, is present only during pregnancy. Although the thyroid and adrenal cortex have mixed degrees of involvement, reference will be made to them when appropriate rather than including a separate discussion of their involvement.

The hormones are of two types. Either they are steroids which are fat soluble compounds, or they are formed from a protein molecule. The ovaries and placenta secrete steroids, while the hypothalamus and pituitary secrete protein-based hormones. Substances from the hypothalamus are called releasing factors while those from the pituitary are called gonadotropins. The names are derived from their major function.

Once in proximity with the target cells, the hormones act to initiate, change, or discontinue a specific cell function. This function is most often that of controlling the production and release of a second hormone. One of the effects of this second hormone may be to inhibit or increase production of the first hormone. When by its action a hormone ultimately results in increasing production of itself, a positive feedback relationship exists. Negative feedback occurs when production of the first hormone is inhibited.

The chemical composition and the small molecular size of steroids allows them to diffuse across the membrane of their target cells. Once inside the cell, the steroid binds to a special receptor which transports it to the nucleus. Here the steroid initiates a DNA transcription, which in turn activates a specified cell function.

The protein molecule of the gonadotropins and releasing factors are too large to diffuse across the cell membrane. Thus, specific receptor sites are located on the cell wall. The protein molecule of these hormones attaches to the receptor sites. This activates production of an enzyme within the cell which leads to the formation of cyclic AMP. In turn, the cyclic AMP initiates a designated cellular activity.

In the female, the sex steroids include estrogens, progesterone, and androgens or male type hormones including some testosterone. Estrogens are produced at many sites in the body, including the ovary, placenta, adrenal cortex, the brain, and fatty tissue. (Table 3-1)

Testosterone is produced by the ovary and adrenal cortex. Progesterone is produced only by the corpus luteum of the ovary and placenta. All of these hormones are involved in somatic sexual differentiation and the functions of reproduction.

Gonadotropins important to sex and reproduction include follicle stimulating hormone (FSH), leutinizing hormone (LH), and prolactin. The gonadotropins are secreted by the anterior lobe of the pituitary gland along with four other hormones including growth hormone, ACTH, thyroid stimulating hormone (TSH), and melanin-stimulating hormone. The gonadotropins control ovulation and the production and release of the sex steroids by the ovary.

Lastly, luteinizing hormone–releasing hormone (LH-RH) and oxytocin are secreted by the hypothalamus. LH-RH secretions serve to control the release of gonadotropins, FSH and LH which, in turn, act on the follicle to manufacture and release sex steroids. Oxytocin is stored in and released from the posterior pituitary. It brings about smooth muscle contraction especially of breast and uterine tissue.

Thus, the hypothalamus carries out its responsibility to coordinate and respond to messages from the cerebral cortex and the peripheral nervous system. The releasing factors act to maintain the delicate balance and interrelationship of these many hormones. They are brought into play with neuromuscular and psychologic factors for the overall orchestration of female sexual and reproductive functioning. (Figure 3-25.)

The Breast

In Sexual Function. In the United States, breasts are an integral part of an adult woman's sexuality. When the female child is playing "grown-up," she often

TABLE 3-1. Summary of Hormones Involved With Sex and Reproduction.

Tissue of origin	Hormone	Major action and mechanism of control
Hypothalamus	Leutinizing hormone—releasing hormone (LH-RH)	Controls pituitary release of LH. Amount available is controlled by both a positive and negative feedback system with estrogen.
	Prolactin inhibiting factor (PIF)	Prevents pituitary release of prolactin.
	Oxytocin	Stimulates smooth muscle contraction, especially of uterus and breast. Stored in the posterior lobe of the pituitary.
Pituitary: Anterior lobe	Follicle stimulating hormone (FSH)	Stimulates growth of ovarian follicle. Amount available is dependent upon presence of LH-RH and a negative feedback system with estrogen.
	Leutinizing hormone (LH)	Stimulates ovulation and corpus luteum formation. Amount available is dependent upon LH-RH and progesterone.
	Prolactin	Stimulates specialized epithelial cells of the breast to produce milk. Availability is dependent upon absence of PIF and regular breast suckling.

TABLE 3-1. Summary of Hormones Involved With Sex and Reproduction (continued).

Tissue of origin	Hormone	Major action and mechanism of control
Ovary	Estrogen	Stimulates many body changes which are characteristic of the female sex. Called the "female hormone." Target organs are endometrium and breast. Also produced by adrenal cortex, brain, and fatty tissue. Level available depends on FSH and other factors.
	Progesterone	Stimulates gland development of breast and slows smooth muscle activity, especially of uterus. Takes part in many estrogen-related events. Secreted by corpus luteum after ovulation and so is dependent on the presence of LH. Action on hypothalamus results in increase of basal body temperature.
	Testosterone	Stimulates and maintains many growth changes at puberty, especially those characteristics associated with the male sex. In addition, is available for conversion to estrogen if needed.
Local tissue (uterus and ovary)	Prostaglandins (PGE, PGF$_{2\alpha}$)	Stimulates or relaxes smooth muscle contraction and is instrumental in ovulation and menstruation.
Placenta	Human chorionic gonadotropin (HCG)	Important role in maintaining pregnancy.

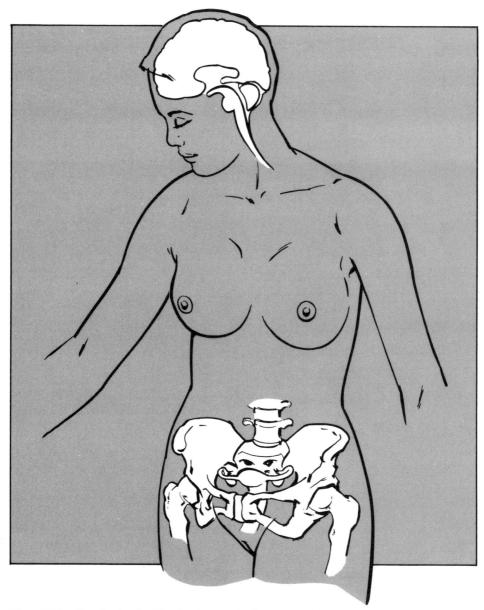

Figure 3-25.   Reproductive physiology involves complex interactions of the brain, breast, and pelvic structures.

stuffs the front of her blouse with socks or washcloths to "look like Mommy."
When she grows up, she finds that, indeed, her breasts do become a part of her
female identity and her sexual responsiveness.

The multitude of sensory nerve endings in the skin of the breast, areola, and
nipple are responsive to touch, pressure, and cold. Exposure to any of these stimuli will elicit a series of neuromuscular and neuroendocrine events. First, an im-

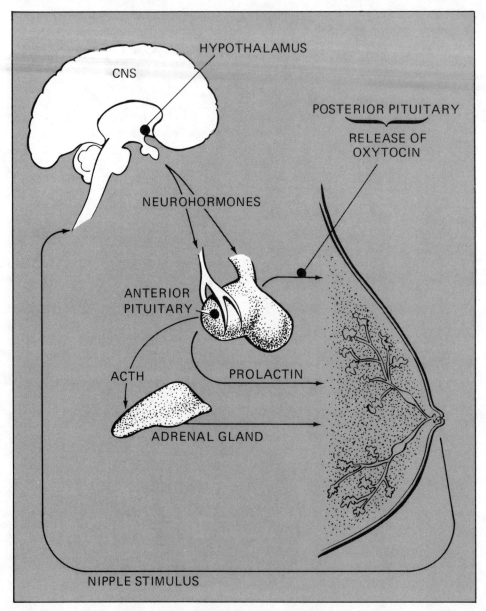

Figure 3-26. Schematic representation of neuroendocrine control of lactation.

pulse will be sent via the sensory nerve (thoracic intercostal nerve branches) to the spinal cord and upward to the hypothalamus. At the hypothalamus, the impulse is coordinated with other messages from the body, and two basic responses are initiated. (See Figure 3-26.)

TISSUE RESPONSE. The hypothalamus directs sympathetic nervous system input to the smooth and skeletal muscle fibers of the breast. There is immediate response from the erectile tissue with resultant erection of the nipple and areola. As stimulation continues, there is some swelling and enlargement of the breast, a deepening of skin color, and increased sensitivity. Much of this response is due to vasocongestion.

CONSCIOUS RESPONSE. The hypothalamus also relays a message to the cortex. This results in conscious awareness and interpretation of the sensations of both breast stimulation and the tissue responsiveness to the stimulation. Because of previous pleasurable experiences, most women will associate and interpret these sensations as pleasurable and desirable. For some women, the sensations are erotic enough that with continued stimulation they experience orgasm. Other women may react with indifference or negatively to breast stimulation. The present situation, past experiences, attitudes, and earlier learning are all included in the woman's overall interpretation and response when breast stimulation occurs.

In addition to cold or tactile stimulation of the breasts, an erotic thought or suggestion may also bring about nipple and areolar erection. However, it is not likely that engorgement, erection, and breast swelling would continue without further and more direct stimuli.

In Reproduction Function. The reproductive role of the breasts is lactation. Lactation, or milk production by the breasts, is dependent upon several hormonal factors and occurs in two consecutive growth stages, puberty and pregnancy.

At puberty the rising levels of estradiol and progesterone stimulate growth and branching of the mammary duct system. In addition, these hormones bring about changes in breast contour by increasing fat deposits, stroma, and connective tissue development. Although each hormone has a specific role, both must be present for pubertal breast development to occur. (Table 3-1.) Although there will be some budding at the terminal ends of the ducts, acini differentiation does not occur at this stage and the breasts are still not capable of lactation [7].

During pregnancy, the second stage of breast development makes lactation possible. Again, combined high levels of estrogen and progesterone bring about further growth and development of breast tissue especially in the first half of pregnancy. The gland tissue grows into the loose stromal structure replacing adipose tissue [3].

Final differentiation of the acini is dependent upon the availability of prolactin. Prolactin is produced by the anterior pituitary but its release is ordinarily inhibited by the presence of prolactin-inhibiting factor (PIF) from the hypothalamus. Apparently, during pregnancy the high levels of estrogen and progesterone block the release of PIF and thus allow for secretion of prolactin [7].

Prolactin levels peak around the time of delivery and then fall rapidly. This raises two questions: Why isn't milk produced before delivery? And, how is milk then produced after delivery if lactation is dependent upon prolactin availability?

Apparently the high levels of estrogen and progesterone inhibit milk secretion by the acini, so that only colostrum, a thin, watery fluid, is secreted during pregnancy. It is only after delivery of the placenta and the resultant decrease in estrogen and progesterone levels, that the acini can produce milk.

The previous explanation shows that initial post-partum milk secretion is not dependent upon the presence of prolactin. However, continued and copious milk secretion does require prolactin and so a second mechanism is needed to ensure prolactin release. Suckling or mechanical stimulation of the nipple results in hypothalamic inhibition of PIF allowing for prolactin release. The frequency and magnitude of prolactin secretion is directly related to the frequency and magnitude of suckling [7]. Thus, prolactin secretion during lactation is transient.

There is one last step involved in lactation. A second response to nipple stimulation is the release of oxytocin from the posterior pituitary into the blood. It causes the smooth muscle of the acini and ductal network to contract. This forces milk out of the acini and through the ducts to the lactiferous sinuses. The milk is then able to be expressed through the nipple by the infant's suckling. The movement of the milk from the acini to the ducts is called milk letdown.

While further prolactin release is dependent upon suckling, oxytocin release is not. Other stimuli such as a baby's cry or an awareness that feeding time is approaching can result in hypothalamic release of oxytocin and consequently, milk letdown. Thus, these two hormones play entirely separate roles in lactation and although they may be released simultaneously, they can also be secreted and released independently.

PSYCHOLOGIC FACTORS. The mechanical, sensory nerve stimulation of the nipple during lactation and its resultant physiologic response is the same as with sexual stimulation and response. Often women report experiencing an orgasm while breastfeeding. They may feel embarrassed and wonder if they are abnormal. A simple explanation will probably reassure them of their normal, physiologic response to this preconditioned, pleasurable experience.

CONTRACEPTION AND LACTATION. Many women erroneously believe that lactation is an effective contraceptive. While there is a period of infertility following delivery, it is very short term. There seems to be about four to five weeks of pituitary insensitivity to LH-RH as well as lack of ovarian response to gonadotropins during this time [3]. In addition, there may be a short-term hypothalamic suppression of LH-RH along with PIF suppression. About 40–75 percent of nursing mothers will begin to menstruate and most likely ovulate while they are still breastfeeding [7]. Thus, contraception will be needed prior to resuming sexual activity, unless, of course, pregnancy is again desired.

DISCONTINUING LACTATION. In order for the epithelial cells to continue secreting milk, the lumen of the acini and the cells themselves must be continuously emptied. Therefore, lactation is discontinued simply by ceasing to empty the breasts. Once breastfeeding is stopped, pressure from the milk in the engorged lumen interferes with further function of the epithelial cells. In addition, lack of suckling results in decreasing levels of prolactin. The hypothalamus resumes PIF secretion further inhibiting prolactin release. After a few days the fluid engorgement and swelling in the breasts will be absorbed and the breasts will be said to have "dried up" [4].

The Pelvic Organs

In Sexual Function. As you have already noted or may wish to review, many of the internal and external genitals contain varying amounts of erectile tissue (labia, clitoris, bulbourethral glands, vagina, and uterus). Most of these structures receive their blood from branches of the internal iliac artery and most are innervated by branches from the hypogastric plexus, the pudendal nerve or both. This common blood supply and innervation of the pelvic erectile tissues allows them to respond to sexual stimulation as a unit.

Details of female sexual physiology are not yet completely known. However, it is generally presumed that female sexual response occurs in a sequence very similar to that of the male which has been more clearly validated. You will find neurophysiology described here. Descriptive details of sexual response can be found in chapter 22.

Initially the autonomic nervous system receives input which originated either from an erotic thought or idea or from sexual stimulation of the genitals. In the latter event, a nerve impulse travels via the pudendal (sensory) nerve to the spinal cord and up to the hypothalamus. From here input to the ANS results in parasympathetic response and a local arteriole dilation in the vulva occurs. There is a resultant vasocongestion of the tissue which is noted as swelling and a deepening skin color. Within the vagina, the interstitial fluid from the vasocongestion begins to seep or "sweat" through the walls resulting in a lubricating effect. Contrary to common thought, Bartholin and cervical glands are not responsible for vaginal lubrication during intercourse.

As sexual (clitoral) stimulation continues, three things happen. First, a message is sent to the cortex and the woman becomes consciously aware of the sensations of genital stimulation and consequent tissue response. Second, the ANS response becomes more generalized and produces respiratory, cardiovascular and other parasympathetic responses. Third, the continued sensory input will eventually initiate a motor nerve response from the spinal reflex center. There is a resultant sympathetic neural discharge which produces the genital contractions and other genital and systemic changes associated with orgasm [6]. Tissue edema will slowly resolve as it is dependent upon reabsorption of the excess interstitial fluid by the circulatory system.

As noted with sexual response of the breast, psychologic factors become an important part of genital sexual response. Physical sensations are monitored through the hypothalamus and thus put into contact with virtually all other parts of the brain. Past experience, attitudes, and beliefs all become a part of a woman's interpretation of sexual sensations whether they are experienced by her as pleasurable and desirable or in a more negative way. Orgasmic response originates at the spinal reflex center. It can be helped or hindered by higher centers in the brain. Thus sexual response is dependent on psychologic as well as physical factors.

In Reproductive Function. Female fertility is ensured by regular, cyclical changes in all of the organs of reproduction. These cycles of fertility are generally referred to collectively as the menstrual cycle. Since it is a visible signal of reproductive changes, menstruation is studied and charted by scientists and by the women who experience it.

A menstrual cycle starts with the onset of menstrual flow. As it continues, specific internal and external changes occur in the woman's body, especially in relation to the genital organs. Approximately twenty-eight days later, the cycle ends. The reappearance of menstrual flow defines day one of a new menstrual cycle. Detailed definitions and descriptions of cycle length and flow variability are found in chapter 9.

Menstruation is the sloughing and shedding of the built-up endometrium. Despite all of the concern and attention focused on it, it is not the singularly most important event of the menstrual cycle. Instead, fertility depends upon the completion of a complex series of cyclic events.

There are three major components of the cyclical events of fertility. Menstruation signals the beginning of a new cycle for each of them. These three events which begin with the onset of menstruation include:

1. New ovarian follicles and eggs begin to mature.
2. As soon as endometrial sloughing begins, rebuilding of the new endometrium is begun.
3. The levels of hormones (FSH, LH, and estrogen) begin slowly to rise and direct the events of this new cycle.

Briefly summarized, fertility is dependent upon a sequence of many events. First, the ovaries must be able to cyclically develop a mature follicle which will, at the right time, burst and release the egg. Shortly after ovulation, the egg must be fertilized by sperm and then nourished and kept alive until it can implant in the endometrium. Thus, concurrent with follicle growth, the endometrium must be prepared so as to be optimum for implantation should the other preceding events have transpired. Pregnancy then continues until delivery at term, nine months later. However, failure at any of the steps will mean that the endometrium must be discarded and rebuilt.

These various steps and stages of fertility are controlled and directed by the cyclic interplay of the hormones of reproduction. In many ways, the tissue changes are reflections of the hormonal changes in the hypothalamic-pituitary-ovarian axis. Specifically, the hormones include LH-RH, FSH, LH, estrogen, and progesterone. Each of these hormones control and are controlled by the others. (Table 3-1.) In many cases we still do not understand the many interrelationships of these hormones [1]. In addition, prostaglandins and a fluid secreted by the Fallopian tubes play important roles in the process of reproduction.

Because the cycles of ovarian, uterine, and hormonal changes are concurrent and interdependent, it is helpful to "see" them in that configuration. A stage-by-stage comparison is provided so that each cycle may be seen separately as well as within the context of the whole. The outline of the presentation is as follows:

1. *Menstruation* (Beginning of new cycle)
    First Stage or growth stage
        proliferative (uterus)—uterine endometrium grows
        follicular (ovary)—ovarian follicles grow
2. *Ovulation* (Beginning of second stage of cycle)
    Second stage or secretory stage
        secretory (uterus)—endometrium begins secretory activity
        luteal (ovary)—corpus luteum forms and secretes progesterone

MORE ABOUT HORMONES

Extensive research continues in the area of hormones and reproduction. More knowledge is needed to deal with the contrasting concerns of fertility and contraception as well as with pathology. As mentioned before, much of the information is still speculative. The numerous knowledge gaps often make this information seem confusing and difficult. At the same time, with a little persistence, the material is fascinating and exciting. We have summarized a very small bit of some of the more accepted studies in endocrinologic research.

The Menstrual Cycle.

Stage 1 (days one to thirteen in a twenty-eight-day cycle)

Day	Hormones	Ovary (follicular stage)	Uterus (proliferative stage)
1	1. *Hypothalamus*—LH-RH begins to increase. 2. *Anterior pituitary*—FSH & LH levels begin to rise. 3. *Ovary*—Follicle growth begins and estrogen levels begin to rise about day four.	Growth of several new follicles begins. As pituitary hormones begin to rise, both thecal and interstitial cells of the follicle are stimulated, thus estrogen levels gradually begin to increase.	MENSTRUATION—As endometrium sloughs off leaving a denuded basal layer, regrowth is immediately initiated to replenish and cover the areas.
4 ↓ 13	1. *Hypothalamus*—A positive feedback exists with estrogen so that as estrogen levels rise, the secretion of LH-RH is increased. 2. *Anterior pituitary*—In response to LH-RH, gonadotropin secretion continues to increase. 3. *Ovary*—Estrogen secretion continues to increase in response to gonadotropins. Follicle continues to mature.	Many of the follicles which began to develop will regress. A few others continue growth, and one will grow to maturation. Production and secretion of estrogen from the thecal cells of the maturing follicles continues to increase.	Endometrial growth (or proliferation) proceeds as follows: In the presence of estrogen, matrix cells increase, endometrial glands grow in length, and there is an especially rapid growth of the coiled arteries and their venous network. (In fact, it is thought that the reason these arteries are so coiled and tortuous is that they grow much faster than the surrounding matrix. With no support, they "coil back" on themselves.)

NOTE: There are also changes in other estrogen-sensitive tissues of the body throughout the cycle. As ovulation nears, columnar cells in the Fallopian tubes begin to secrete, and cilia and muscle activity increases. The fimbriae of the tubes are positioned over the ovary to be in optimum placement for receiving the egg. Cyclic changes are also noted in the cells of the vaginal walls.

No matter what length a woman's menstrual cycle may be, ovulation occurs approximately fourteen days before menstruation. In a twenty-one-day cycle, ovulation would occur on day seven. Variations in cycle length will most likely occur in the proliferative/follicular stage rather than in the secretory/luteal stage [3].

Stage 2 (days fourteen to twenty-eight in a twenty-eight-day cycle)

Day	Hormones	Ovary (luteal stage)	Uterus (secretory stage)
14	1. *Hypothalamus*—High estrogen level seems to increase hypothalamic sensitivity—Increased LH-RH output. 2. *Anterior pituitary*—Sudden surge of LH and FSH occurs in response to LH-RH. 3. *Ovary*—LH causes thinning of follicle cells in preparation for release of egg. Estrogen continues to be secreted. At this time evidence indicates that prostaglandin $F_{2\alpha}$ increases smooth muscle contractility of ovary causing the mechanical rupture of the follicle [3].	OVULATION—Rupture of follicle and release of ova to abdominal cavity occurs within a burst of fluid.	Cervical mucus exhibits ferning (if the mucus is dried on a slide and then examined with a microscope the pattern resembles fronds of a fern.) (See Figure 14-3.)
15	1. *Hypothalamus*—LH-RH levels begin to decline due to coexisting negative feedback with estrogen. 2. *Anterior pituitary*—LH is instrumental in bringing about functioning of corpus luteum. However, estrogen also has a negative feedback effect on FSH and LH and so secretion begins to decline despite high levels of LH-RH.	The vacated follicle is transformed into a yellow structure called the corpus luteum. This structure is an active endocrine gland which secretes progesterone.	Endometrium now begins to grow very rapidly. The *coiled arteries* send out many branches near the surface. This forms a maternal basis of blood supply for a placenta should fertilization and implantation occur. The *endometrial glands* begin to secrete a nutrient-rich mucus to nourish the egg. *Myometrial* activity is reduced by progesterone. *Cervical* secretions become viscous and more opaque, acting as a "plug."

Day	Hormones	Ovary	Uterus
	3. *Ovary*—The corpus luteum secretes high levels of progesterone and estrogen, further stimulating endometrial growth. However, progesterone has an antagonistic effect on LH, thereby contributing to disintegration of the corpus luteum. Prostaglandins may also be involved with failure of the corpus luteum but details are not yet clear [3].		Finally three events occur: 1) the coiled arteries become so twisted they create something of a tourniquet effect on themselves, thereby creating ischemic areas in parts of the endometrium. 2) Prostaglandin $F_{2\alpha}$ is secreted by the ischemic areas, stimulating myometrial contraction [1]. 3) Endometrial matrix begins to regress with decreasing supplies of estrogen and progesterone. This increases the tortuousness of the coiled arteries since it means their tissue support is lessened. Very quickly, the endometrium begins to slough and bleeding appears as . . .
28	1. *Hypothalamus*—LH-RH levels low. 2. *Anterior pituitary*—FSH and LH levels low. 3. *Ovary*—Estrogen and progesterone reach lowest levels.	As FSH and LH levels are decreased, corpus luteum support is reduced and the structure begins to disintegrate.	
1	1. *Hypothalamus*—LH-RH begins to rise.	New follicle growth begins.	MENSTRUATION

NOTE: Should the egg be fertilized (preferably while it is still in the upper two-thirds of the tube) the above sequence is, of course, changed. The tube secretes a fluid which aids in capacitation of the sperm, nourishes the blastocyst and also supplies nutrients to the morulla until implantation [4]. With implantation, changes occur to maintain the corpus luteum's secretion of progesterone and estrogen until the placenta can begin to secrete HCG. The continued hormone supply supports the endometrium and, brings about its further development, preparing it to become the decidua of pregnancy.

Figure 3-27 illustrates the events that have been outlined.

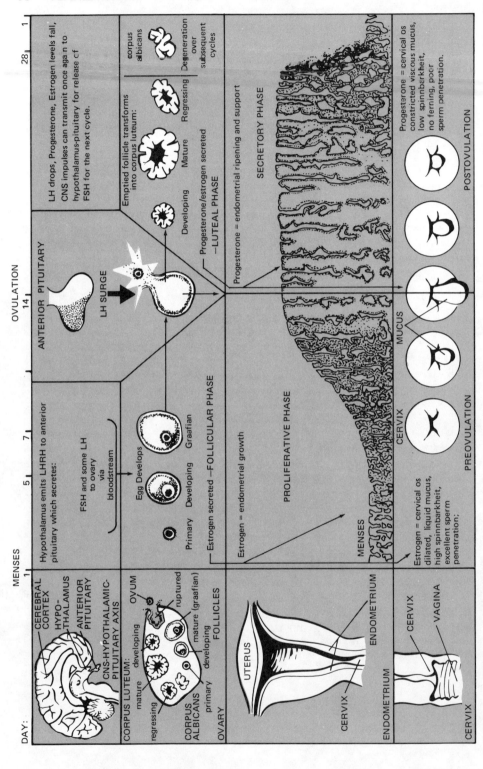

Figure 3-27. Schematic representation of events of the menstrual cycle.

Hormones from the hypothalamus and pituitary are secreted in short bursts or spurts instead of in a steady rate. Higher levels of these hormones are achieved by increasing the frequency and/or amplitude of "spurts." Thus, the levels of these hormones can change very rapidly [1]. This is how the midcycle LH surge is able to be accomplished.

While the hypothalamus may be the master coordinator for the body, the message which it sends out is rough. The pituitary acts as an encoder and interpretor, refining the message which is delivered to the target organ. Information available to the pituitary is what determines its action. For example, estrogen works on a negative feedback system with the pituitary. Once a specific blood level of estrogen is available, the pituitary will stop secreting FSH and LH despite the presence of LH-RH from the hypothalamus [3].

The hypothalamus seems to work on both a positive and negative feedback with estrogen. That is, as estrogen levels rise, hypothalamic sensitivity seems to increase, and it releases more LH-RH. However, once a specific level of estrogen is available, LH-RH production declines. In addition, the absence of estrogen will result in higher levels of LH-RH [1].

The hypothalamus is thought by some to be the initiator of puberty. One hypothesis is that throughout childhood, the hypothalamus grows increasingly sensitive to estrogen. This causes LH-RH levels to gradually increase resulting in a rise in gonadotropin levels. The corresponding rise in estrogen produces the pubertal changes, menarche, and finally ovulation. This system then supposedly reverses itself at menopause. Many researchers feel that evidence is available to refute these ideas, although the theory does have possibilities [1, 3].

The action of *FSH* on the ovary to bring about maturation of the follicle has already been described. More specifically, FSH acts on the granulosa cells to increase production of follicular fluid, stimulates the secretion of an enzyme needed for steroid production, and combines its efforts with estradiol to form LH receptors on the follicle cells [3]. Thus, it has many roles in preparing for ovulation.

LH is released by the anterior pituitary with FSH but initially more slowly. As estrogen reaches a peak causing a rapid burst of LH-RH, there is a consequent burst of LH secreted. LH exerts a specific action on the follicle cells preparing them to burst and release the egg. It also leutinizes the thecal cells, transforming them into the corpus luteum, and acts with FSH to bring about the production of estrogen.

Progesterone is produced in small amounts by the granulosa cells of the preovulatory follicle and by the thecal cells after ovulation [4]. Since high progesterone levels are dependent upon establishment of the corpus luteum, it is not surprising to find that they are low both in prepubertal and postmenopausal women. In pregnancy the placenta secretes increased levels of progesterone.

It was mentioned on page 67 that the cyclic decline in progesterone levels is due to its antagonistic effect on LH. It seems that progesterone increases the conversion of estradiol to estriol while simultaneously inhibiting the formation of oxidation products. These oxidation products, however, are needed for the continued stimulation of LH release. The resultant decline in LH causes disintegration of the corpus luteum [4].

Progesterone acts to decrease smooth muscle contractility. This has some effect in keeping the endometrium intact, especially if pregnancy occurs. The reduced activity of the tubes allows for the needed retention time of the fertilized egg.

Details of "why" are unknown [4].

Some suggest that declining progesterone levels from an aging placenta play a role in initiating labor by allowing for gradually increased myometrial activity [1]. Others contest this, suggesting factors such as prostaglandins or changing estrogen/progesterone balance as being responsible for the onset of labor. To date, why labor begins is unknown.

Estrogen is actually a collective term. To date, there have been twenty-five different estrogens identified [1]. Along with progesterone, they are considered the female sex hormones because of their characteristic effects on the human body. However, most of these estrogens seem unimportant, with the exception of three. (Table 3-2.)

The most important estrogens include estradiol, estrone, and estriol. Estriol is weak and actually only a by-product of excretion. Urine estriol levels are used as an indirect measure of the amount of estrogen available. Estrone is a more potent compound. It is secreted by the adrenal cortex, the brain, fatty tissue, and other structures. It is the major circulating estrogen prior to puberty and after menopause. The strongest of the estrogens is estradiol. It is manufactured by the ovarian follicle and the placenta and is the estrogen which is generally being referred to in a discussion involving a woman's reproductive years.

Estrogens are manufactured by a series of enzyme conversions and follow one of two pathways (simplified):

1. Acetate→ cholesterol→ pregnenolone→ progesterone→ 17 hydroxyprogesterone→ androstenedione + testosterone→ estrone + estrodiol 17β.

2. Acetate→ cholesterol→ pregnenolone→ 17 hydroxyprogesterone→ dihydroepiandrosterone→ androstenedione + testosterone→ estrone + estrodial 17β.

As can be seen, both of these routes are connected at various stages and in both, the final step is preceded by androgens. Note that the step from androgen to estrogens is irreversible while estrone to estradiol can be reversed.

Because estrogens are stored in fatty tissue (as well as being able to be converted by these tissues) any excessive weight gain or loss, or sudden increase in exercise may result in a change in the hypothalamic-pituitary-ovarian axis, and the woman may experience a physiologic amenorrhea. The high estrogen levels found in an excessively overweight female may cause her to experience a delayed menarche, while a slightly obese woman may have an early menarche [3]. For a more detailed explanation, see chapter 7.

Testosterone is produced by the stroma and interstitial cells of the ovary under the influence of LH. It has the same effect on the body of women as it does on men. That is, it maintains sex drive, hair growth, the tendency toward acne, and, during puberty, bone and muscle growth. It is known as the male sex hormone and is found in much greater concentrations in the male.

Prostaglandins exert only a local effect and for only a very short time. They are not stored, but are very rapidly synthesized from fatty acids when needed. In reproductive physiology the two most important prostaglandins are E_2 and $F_2\alpha$. They seem to exert an antagonistic effect on each other, producing smooth muscle relaxation (E_2) or contractility ($F_2\alpha$). The result is that they exert a variety of actions and are known to be involved with the processes of ovulation, corpus luteum function, and menstruation.

TABLE 3-2.   *Effects of Female Sex Steroids.*

Effects of Estrogen

1. Growth of ovaries and follicles
2. Growth and maintenance of the smooth muscle and epithelial linings of the entire reproductive tract
   Also: a. Oviducts: increased motility and ciliary activity
   b. Uterus: increased motility, secretion of abundant, clear cervical mucous
   c. Vagina: increased "cornification" (layering of epithelial cells)
3. Growth of external genitalia
4. Growth of breasts (particularly ducts)
5. Development of female body configuration: narrow shoulders, broad hips, converging thighs, diverging arms
6. Stimulation of fluid sebaceous gland secretions ("anti-acne")
7. Pattern of pubic hair (actual growth of pubic and axillary hair is androgen-stimulated)
8. Stimulation of protein anabolism and closure of the epiphyses (? due to stimulation of adrenal androgens)
9. Sex drive and behavior (? role of androgens)
10. Reduction of blood cholesterol
11. Vascular effects (deficiency → "hot flashes")
12. Feedback effect on hypothalamus and anterior pituitary

Effects of Progesterone

1. Stimulation of secretion by endometrium; also induces thick, sticky, cervical secretions
2. Stimulation of growth of myometrium
3. Decrease in motility of oviducts and uterus
4. Decrease in vaginal "cornification"
5. Stimulation of breast growth (particularly glandular tissue)
6. Inhibition of effect of prolactin on the breasts
7. Elevation of body temperature
8. Feedback effects on hypothalamus and anterior pituitary

Reprinted with permission from McGraw-Hill, Inc., *from* A. J. Vander, J. H. Sherman, and D. S. Luciano, *Human Physiology* (1975) p. 447.

Prostaglandins influence ovulation in three different ways:

1. They play an undefined role in regulation of hypothalamic–pituitary secretion of FSH and LH.

2. They are involved in the initiation, maintenance and dissolution of the corpus luteum.

3. They are responsible for the mechanical expulsion of the ovum from the follicle [3].

Many of the details involved are unclear at this time. However, it is known that through their vasoconstriction/vasodilation effect, prostaglandins seem to first favor the blood supply to the corpus luteum and then to decrease it. Their effect on smooth muscle contraction causes the LH primed follicle to burst and release the egg, that is, ovulation. It has been observed that if indomethacin, a prostaglandin inhibitor, is given just prior to ovulation, the ovum will not be expelled. However, all of the clinical parameters of ovulation will occur, including rising progesterone levels, increased basal body temperature, changes in the cervical mucus and the endometrium, and formation of the corpus luteum. If the woman is taking normal doses of aspirin, a weaker prostaglandin inhibitor, this effect does not occur [3].

Prostaglandin effect on smooth muscle is an important element in transporting the ovum through the tube. These hormones are responsible for the uterine contractions which mechanically help to expel the endometrium during menstruation as well as the cramping of dysmenorrhea. They play a role in labor contractions and some researchers suggest that prostaglandins may be a factor in toxemia of pregnancy [3].

Prostaglandins in semen may enhance sperm entry into the uterus. However, if an IUD is in place, the prostaglandin release by the endometrium prevents implantation. (Studies have shown that implantation will occur with an IUD in place if prostaglandin inhibitors are given. However, fertilization is less likely to occur if the IUD is impregnated with copper, since copper is toxic to the sperm) [3].

Clearly there is much more information available than has been summarized here. In addition, new knowledge is available on a regular basis. It is hoped that the reader will continue to seek it out for a continued, clearer understanding of how a woman's body functions.

ANATOMY REFERENCES

1. Ahmed A: Atlas of the Ultrastructure of Human Breast Diseases. New York, Churchill Livingstone, 1978
2. Anderson JE: Grants Atlas of Anatomy, 7th ed. Baltimore, Williams and Wilkins, 1978
3. Bates B: A Guide to Physical Examination. Philadelphia, J. B. Lippincott, 1974
4. Benson RC: Handbook of Obstetrics and Gynecology, 5th ed. Los Altos, CA, Lange Medical Publishers, 1974
5. Burn JH: The Autonomic Nervous System, 5th ed. Philadelphia, J. B. Lippincott, 1975
6. Gardner E: Fundamentals of Neurology, 6th ed. Philadelphia, W. B. Saunders, 1976
7. Haagensen CD: Diseases of the Breast, 2nd ed. Philadelphia, W. B. Saunders, 1971
8. Kistner RW: Gynecology: Principles and Practice, 3rd ed. Chicago, Yearbook Medical Publishers, 1979
9. Martin LL: Health Care of Women. Philadelphia, J. B. Lippincott, 1978
10. McDivitt RW and Ellis JT: Diseases of the breast. *In* Bronson JG and Gall EA (eds): Concepts of Disease: A Textbook of Human Pathology. New York, Macmillan, 1971
11. Netter TH: The Ciba Collection of Medical Illustrations, Volume 2, Reproductive System. Ciba Pharmaceutical Co., 1965
12. Novak ER, Jones GS, Jones HW: Textbook of Gynecology, 9th ed. Baltimore, Williams and Wilkins, 1975
13. Pansky B, House EL: Review of Gross Anatomy. New York, Macmillan, 1975
14. Prichard JA, MacDonald PC: William's Obstetrics, 16th ed. New York, Appleton-Century-Crofts, 1980
15. Ross J, Wilson K: Foundations of Anatomy and Physiology, 4th ed. New York, Longman, 1973
16. The Breast Cancer Digest. Bethesda, National Cancer Institute, NIH Pub. #80-1691, December 1979
17. Vander AJ, Sherman JH, Luciano DS: Human Physiology: The Mechanisms of Body Functions. New York, McGraw-Hill, 1975

PHYSIOLOGY REFERENCES

1. Bidlingmaier F, Knorr D: Oestrogens: Physiological and Clinical Aspects. Basel, Switzerland, S. Karger, 1978
2. Haagensen CD: Diseases of the Breast, 2nd ed. Philadelphia, W. B. Saunders, 1971
3. Hafez ESE: Human Reproduction: Conception and Contraception, 2nd ed. Hagerstown, MD, Harper and Row, 1980
4. Kistner RW: Gynecology: Principles and Practice, 3rd ed. Chicago, Yearbook Medical Publishers, Inc., 1979
5. Pritchard JA, MacDonald PC: William's Obstetrics, 16th ed. New York, Appleton-Century-Crofts, 1980
6. Sloane E: Biology of Women. New York, John Wiley and Sons, 1980
7. Speroff L, Glass RH, Kase NG: Clinical Gynecologic Endocrinology and Infertility. Baltimore, Williams and Wilkins, 1973
8. Stedman's Medical Dictionary, 23rd ed. Baltimore, Williams and Wilkins, 1976
9. Vander AJ, Sherman JH, Luciano DS: Human Physiology: The Mechanisms of Body Functions. New York, McGraw-Hill, 1970

Section II

INFANCY AND CHILDHOOD

4

Physical Development: Infancy Through Childhood

From conception through puberty the physical growth and development of humans is continuous and rapid. It does not occur at a constant rate nor does it always parallel the published "averages." In a very general way, height and weight slowly increase in a somewhat constant ratio until full growth is reached sometime around puberty.

From a closer perspective, the endocrine system maintains the responsibility for growth, maturation, metabolic processes, reproduction, and integration of the body's response to stress. These hormones will initiate associated body responses whether they are manufactured internally or received exogenously. Thus, many of the rapid physical changes which occur pre- and postnatally are a reflection of the changes in circulating hormone levels.

Our current knowledge of endocrine functioning during childhood is limited. However, we do know that estrogens, and to a lesser extent progesterone, are chiefly responsible for the growth and development of primary and secondary female sexual characteristics. Less well known is that estrogens also play an active developmental role throughout infancy and childhood exerting their influence on many other body systems as well.

This chapter focuses on these normal growth changes from birth to puberty. Scipien uses the following terms to describe the different periods of childhood [7]:

Newborn	=	birth to 1 week
Neonate	=	birth to 1 month
Infant	=	1-12 months
Childhood		
Toddler	=	1-3 years
Preschooler	=	3-5 years
School Age	=	6-12 years
Adolescent	=	13-19 years

NEONATE

Hormones

During pregnancy, urine and plasma estrogen levels of the mother become increasingly higher. Although some of this rise can be accounted for by a slight increase in maternal ovarian production, most of it is derived from the placenta.

However, the placenta is not able to complete steroid synthesis on its own and must depend upon precursors supplied by fetal metabolism. Likewise, the fetus is unable to completely synthesize estrogen by itself and is dependent on placental help. This cooperative effort is called the fetoplacental unit [2].

The placenta releases enormous amounts of estrogen into both maternal and fetal circulations; the ratio being about 10:1. The fetus then rapidly metabolizes and inactivates this estrogen, possibly in an effort to protect itself from the potent effects of estrogen. Eventually, the metabolized estrogens are excreted into the maternal circulation mostly in the form of estriol. In fact, most of the estriol excreted by the mother during pregnancy is from the fetus; about one-half of the estrone and estradiol in her plasma is also from the placenta [2].

The rising maternal estrogen level is a good indicator of the well-being of the fetus. An immediate fall in maternal estrogens follows placental expulsion or fetal death or both. Low maternal estrogen values may indicate a fetal or placental problem. It is interesting to note that circadian rhythms of maternal plasma estrogen levels may be detected by the third trimester. These are possibly reflective of the fetus' own, already established rhythms [2].

Studies have shown that the levels of active estrogens which enter fetal circulation are almost one hundred times higher than those found in healthy, nonpregnant adult women. Bidlingmaier reports a study by Tulchinsky which showed that the amount of free plasma estradiol is higher in the newborn than at any other period of development [2]. Since the fetus cannot inactivate such a great quantity of estrogen, there are some feminization effects at birth whether the baby is a boy or girl. It is not understood why these effects are so limited given the amount of estrogen present, but it is clear that many of the rapid changes in the neonatal period are due to the presence and then withdrawal of these high estrogen levels.

Breasts

The newborn, whether male or female, often has enlarged, puffy breasts. A white milk-like fluid commonly referred to as "witch's milk" may be secreted. This estrogen-related condition is transient and will disappear in a few days. Subsequently the breasts will be flat with a light pigmentation of the nipple and areola.

Vulva

The newborn's vulva often shows the results of high estrogen exposure. The labia are large and puffy with the labia minora often protruding beyond the labia majora. In fact, the labia majora are actually still the fetal labioscrotal swelling and do not develop into distinct structures until late childhood [9].

The protusion of the labia minora is often even more marked in a premature baby, although the reason is not known. The labia are symmetrical and easily separated. Often a dark, pigmented border will outline the anterior surface of the labia majora. The skin of the labia minora is pink and moist. Both the edema and pigmentation will disappear within the first week.

Clitoris

The clitoris is usually only a few mm long although hypertrophy in response to placental hormones is normal. However, care must be taken to distinguish between hypertrophy and ambiguous genitalia. Thus, it is important to also locate the urinary meatus which is very small and may be difficult to find.

Bartholin's and Skene's glands are not ordinarily palpable in the newborn. The vaginal introitus is easily identified and appears reddened at birth. This is not a sign of inflammation, but of hormone response. The hymen is thick with a central opening of about 0.5 cm. This begins to thin as soon as estrogen levels are reduced.

Vagina

The vagina is approximately 4 cm long and has a slightly acid pH. As estrogen stimulation is withdrawn, the pH becomes neutral and then alkaline within just a few days. Some lactobacilli are present in the vaginal flora. Smears of the hypertrophied vaginal walls show a mature well-developed epithelium. This estrogen effect will not appear again until puberty.

Fluid secreted by the cervical glands may accumulate behind an imperforate hymen although this rarely occurs. The resultant bulge or swelling on the perineum is called a hydrocolpos. A similar but blue-colored swelling, due to blood in the vagina, is called a hematocolpos.

Whether this blood is retained by an imperforate hymen or appears at the introitus as vaginal bleeding, it is called pseudomenstruation. It results when the baby's highly developed endometrium is no longer supported by placental hormones and begins to slough just as it will again in response to cyclic hormone production in another decade. Pseudomenstruation may occur transiently up to one month after birth.

Uterus

Within the first few postnatal weeks, the newborn's uterus will involute and lose up to one-half of its birth weight. The cervix is one-half to two-thirds longer than the fundus. Uterine and cervical glands at birth may be well-developed, but after estrogen levels are lowered they become simple, tubular structures. Uterine size, weight, and glandular structure will not substantially change until they receive adequate estrogen stimulation around puberty. (These uterine changes are seen in Figure 3-14.)

Ovary

The ovary follows a somewhat different pattern than the other reproductive structures. It shows a rapid postnatal growth and doubles its birthweight by the time the baby is six months old [5]. Growth then ceases until two years before menarche, although some developmental changes continue throughout childhood. The newborn ovary is not palpable as it is located in the false pelvis at the pelvic brim and, of course, is very small.

The ovarian cortex of the newborn contains one to two million primordial follicles [8]. Thus, it is much thicker than it will be by puberty. Within the cortex, numerous primordial ova surrounded by a single layer of cells exist as primary follicles. The continuous development of these follicles to various degrees short of maturation accounts for the increasing numbers of cystic and atretic follicular structures seen on the ovary from birth onward.

INFANCY TO MID SCHOOL AGE

Hormones

Most of the prenatal estrogen effects which are present at birth disappear by the end of the neonatal time period. However, this does not mean that estrogen is not present in the female's body during childhood or that changes other than height and weight do not occur.

From about age two weeks to seven years, female estrone (secreted by the adrenal cortex) values remain low and are about the same level as those found in males. Estradiol (secreted by the ovary) follows a different course. About the second week, estradiol levels begin to rise until they finally peak about the third or fourth month. These peak levels are far above upper normal values for prepubertal females. They then decline and between ages three to seven, estrone levels are higher than estradiol levels [2].

It seems that FSH levels also increase following birth, rise to a peak about the second to third month and slowly begin to fall after the fourth month. There is simultaneous follicular growth in the ovaries including some luteinization of the theca interna. This activity is most marked about the fourth month. It seems that the estradiol production in female infants is a normal physiologic response to gonadotropin presence.

The physiologic explanation and significance of this hormone activity is not understood. One suggestion is that high levels of steroids during the last trimester of intrauterine life may suppress pituitary function. The rapid fall in steroid level resulting from birth removes this inhibition. Gonadotropins are subsequently secreted, the ovarian follicles are stimulated, and estradiol is produced. Lack of ovulation may be due to insufficient FSH, LH, cellular sensitivity, or other causes [2].

Breasts

Female breasts from infancy through the prepubertal years are composed mainly of fatty tissue. A few incomplete, branching ducts can be found as well as minimal stroma. In fact, the presence of gland tissue and/or more complete stroma or duct development may be an early indication of pathology.

Vulva

The external genitals of the toddler are small but are in proportion to each other and the perineum. The labia minora are flat while the labia majora seem puffy. However, if this "puffiness" is out of proportion or looks inflamed, it should be investigated for pathology such as vaginitis or perineal skin infections. (See chapter 6.) By the time school age is reached, the labia may be asymmetrical. This is apparently a normal growth occurrence and usually does not last. The mons remains flat until the pre-menarche years. The redness of the vaginal introitus persists during childhood.

Vagina

By this time, the vagina is approximately 5cm long, the walls are thin and show only basal and parabasal cells on cytology smears. There are no mature epithelial cells. The pH remains neutral to alkaline.

Uterus

The uterus remains in its postneonatal, involuted state throughout childhood. There is some minimal myometrial growth after about age five. Cervix and fundus length ratio is approximately 1:1 by mid-childhood and prepubertal years. (See Figure 3-14.)

Ovary

During infancy and childhood the ovaries gradually begin to taper and take on the almond shape of the adult. The ovarian surface appears smooth and gray. Cystic and atretic structures continue to increase. As a result of the growth of the pelvic cavity, their position becomes lower and they enter the true pelvis although they remain nonpalpable.

Transition

Other changes throughout the body occur during childhood. Bone, muscle, organ size and functions, body mass, and brain development with resultant neurological maturation are only a few of the phenomena which we take for granted in a normally growing child. Suddenly, around age eight or nine this growth will become very rapid in many parts of the body, signaling the approach of puberty and finally, adulthood. These changes are discussed in chapter 7.

REFERENCES

1. Alexander HM, Brown MS: Pediatric History Taking and Physical Diagnosis for Nurses, 2nd ed. New York, McGraw-Hill, 1979
2. Bidlingmaier F, Knorr D: Oestrogens, Physiological and Clinical Aspects. Basel, Switzerland, S. Karger, 1978
3. Falkner F, Tanner JM (eds): Human Growth, Vol. 2. New York, Plenum Press, 1978
4. Kistner RW: Gynecology: Principles and Practice, 3rd ed. Chicago, Yearbook Medical Publishers, 1979
5. Lowry GH: Growth and Development of Children, 7th ed. Chicago, Yearbook Medical Publishers, 1978
6. Parson CL, Jr.: Van Leuwen's Newborn Medicine, 2nd ed. Chicago, Yearbook Medical Publishers, 1979
7. Scipien CM et al: Comprehensive Pediatric Nursing, 2nd ed. New York, McGraw-Hill, 1979
8. Speroff L, Glass RH, Kase NG: Clinical Gynecologic Endocrinology and Infertility, 2nd ed. Baltimore, Williams and Wilkins, 1978
9. Tanner JM: Growth at Adolescence, 3rd ed. Oxford, England, Blackwell Scientific Publications, 1962
10. Vander AJ, Sherman JH, Luciano DS: Human Physiology: The Mechanisms of Body Functions, 2nd ed. New York, McGraw-Hill, 1975

5

Beginnings of Psychosocial Growth:
Infancy Through Childhood

If a comprehensive understanding of a given individual is desired, every aspect of that individual's life would have to be reviewed in its entirety. The starting place for this review would be with that person's conception and would continue to the present moment. It would include all of the available social, cultural, economic, and environmental resources. Consideration must be given for all of the thoughts, emotions, feelings, attitudes, interpretations, understandings, and reactions which the person had experienced. All of these psychosocial factors would be viewed in the context of the individual's physical and genetic structures. Finally, it would take into account the person's ability to cognitively coordinate this information, draw conclusions, and make meaningful, future-directed decisions.

The contemplation of this task helps one to realize the complexity of the psychosocial growth process. The structuring of an identity is dynamic and ongoing. Each person is a combination of what has already been developed as well as the goals toward which that person is striving. At any point an individual's maturity must be measured for that age even though they are in the process of reaching toward further maturation.

Other than by educated guessing, we cannot know what the future will bring. To enhance our "guessing" we look at human history from an individual as well as a collective perspective. This approach helps us to define factors which contribute to the growth of an identity.

Through searching and researching, psychologists and sociologists have provided us with a multitude of developmental theories and explanations. The variety of different perspectives and approaches helps us to realize and appreciate the richness and diversity which characterizes each human. In addition, the theories give us a framework for anticipating, guiding and enriching the personality development of a child. With these thoughts as a basis, this chapter will consider the contributions of prenatal and birth influences, cognitive growth, and psychosocial elements to the development of an identity.

PRENATAL CONTRIBUTIONS

Almost all of the theories of human development suggest that the basis of an individual's behavior and personality is formed very early. Most theorists suggest that identity formation begins at birth. Some suggest that prenatal experiences also play an important role in influencing early personality development [1, 3].

As described in chapter 2, a zygote must receive at least one X chromosome to ensure viability. Additional X or Y chromosomes, hormones, and the response of the developing body determine the sex of the fetus. Thus, gender, a major influence in each person's life, is established at conception and immediately begins to affect the development of other body tissues.

There are a host of additional factors which influence prenatal development. Factors contributed by the fetus include genetic structure, blood-incompatibility with the mother, and endocrine problems. Maternal influences on fetal development include nutrition, drugs, smoking, use of alcohol, infections, trauma, tumors (especially endocrine), and many other health-related maternal considerations. In addition, the healthy or defective status of the placenta will affect fetal growth. Any of these influences may interfere with normal brain, gender, or general development and, in turn, later affect psychosocial patterns.

Well before birth, a new life exhibits both reflex and spontaneous movement and the maintenance of life functions. It has the ability to see and hear. The mother knows that the baby within her establishes patterns of quiet and activity. It will respond to an environmental change or stimulus, sometimes with a sharp kick. The activities and responses of the newborn clearly represent continuations rather than beginnings of functions and behaviors.

In the past people believed that the mother's activities or thoughts during her pregnancy would influence the child's direction in life. For example, if the family wanted to raise a musician, they would expose the mother to music during her pregnancy. It was also felt that if a mother-to-be was gloomy and depressed, she would produce a child with a stormy disposition and vice versa, a happy woman would produce a happy child. Even into the early 1900s, many physicians in the United States believed that "pronounced impressions made upon the mind of a pregnant mother predisposes to bodily defects and birthmarks in the child" [3].

Most of these prenatal influence "theories" have finally been discarded with credit for maternal influence transferred to the postnatal period. Many people, however, feel that we have been too zealous in our discrediting of the effects of prenatal factors on the fetus. They say that we do not yet understand the mental capability of the fetus and so should not discard possibilities of prenatal influence [7].

Reese includes a description of a research study done by Spelt in 1948 which reported the successful conditioning of certain behavioral responses (i.e., increased heart rate) of human fetuses in utero. Although the design of the study is complicated and results are difficult to interpret, it has been suggested that further research would probably again demonstrate the presence of conditioned responses [11].

More recently technology has given documented evidence of embryo response by six weeks to the placement of a hand on the mother's abdomen. Throughout the pregnancy, the fetus responds to noise, movement, and touch. Body postural changes and various leg and arm movement suggest practice of movements later needed for crawling and walking. Facial expressions change and at times a fetus appears to be crying [1, 9]. Whether all of these "behaviors" are just reflexes or instead evidence of early intelligence and response to environmental stimuli is, of course, as difficult to "prove" as is Spelt's conditioning.

Ferreira maintains that "the infant brings into the world its prenatal experiences" which may become the core of the child's first reaction patterns and personality characteristics. He speaks of an interaction between the fetus and mother [3]. It has been suggested that babies can feel pain immediately following birth and so it seems reasonable to assume that they can feel pain before birth [1]. An additional important question is whether a fetus interprets or attaches meaning to any prenatal experiences.

Does this mean that the fetus is capable of primitive learning? Is this conditioned response merely a reflex pattern? In either case, what does this mean in terms of later personality development? We do not know. One thing that is certain is that scientific examination of early postnatal capabilities has produced a reexamination of beliefs about intrauterine life. The result has been a multitude of changes in prenatal care and delivery methods.

BIRTH EXPERIENCES

Any mother, father, or delivery room attendant will tell you that each baby arrives with a unique personality. Given a relatively drug-free labor and delivery, each infant interacts with its new environment in a very individualized manner from the minute of birth. We do not know the origin of these already individual personality patterns.

We know that labor and the birth process differs with each delivery. The initial handling and holding by birth attendants is a different experience for each infant. Do these first interactions with other human beings and the extrauterine world begin to form our personality patterns? Some people think they do.

Dr. Leboyer described birth as being a traumatic event which our modern delivery methods have made even more difficult. His suggested birthing method is to keep the lighting dim and the room warm and quiet, approximating as closely as possible the uterine environment [1].

Following birth the infant is placed on the mother's abdomen and the umbilical cord left intact for at least ten minutes. This allows for optimum oxygenation of blood without external stimulation or suctioning of the infant. Once the cord is cut, the father immerses the baby in a bathtub of warm water. The baby's response is one of relaxation and "playing" in its bath. Finally, breastfeeding may be initiated while the mother is still on the delivery table. Immediate interaction of the parents with the baby is encouraged [1].

The central idea of Leboyer's methods is that of viewing the birth process from the infant's perspective. He felt that the birth ordeal, followed by the overpowering sensory overload of bright lights, cold air, loud noises, and rough handling must be a terrifying experience for the newborn. Since a newborn does not yet have a way to cope with this trauma, one wonders what the long-term effects might be. In any case it seemed to Leboyer that a more humanitarian approach to delivery was needed in which the child would be introduced to its new environment in stages.

Whether Leboyer's method approximates intrauterine life is not as important as the attention it has drawn to the treatment of the mother and infant during the birth process. In the past, labor and delivery techniques bordered on being abusive. More currently, needs and wishes of the family unit have priority over those of the health care providers.

Childbirth education accomplishes at least two things. The first purpose is to lower the risk of trauma to the infant by reducing maternal need for analgesic drugs during labor. The second is to facilitate a more "natural" birth by reducing the mother's fear and allowing her to work with the labor process. In addition, the parents' involvement in the birth of the child is said to establish bonding and parent–child interaction. The events of birth then may be seen as contributing both physical and emotional factors to influence psychosocial growth.

Studies have shown that socializing begins from the moment of birth. Attendants handle babies differently. Female infants are treated and held with more gentleness and talked to more soothingly than are male infants. The baby is wrapped in a pink or blue blanket and carried to the nursery where the color coding signals further "appropriate" socializing. Other input and attention to the baby will be dependent on several factors such as the physical status of both the mother and the baby, the hospital's rules, and the baby's responsiveness and demands [7, 8].

It is relatively easy to see how physical factors such as trauma or oxygen deprivation will affect development in an ongoing way, but what about the social experiences associated with birth? Are they recorded in the infant's brain? Is there a personal, psychological reaction to the experiences of birth? Do the simple responses and actions of the baby represent primitive beginnings of psychologic behavior patterns which are then reinforced by those who care for the child? We do not know, but some current research suggests these ideas [1, 4, 10].

Higher brain centers are largely undeveloped by birth. Although all of the neurons exist, they will undergo a great deal of development and reorganization before adulthood [4]. Does this mean then, that these first, early experiences are either not retained or have no impact on later development? Or does it perhaps mean the reverse? Perhaps natal experiences have the potential to redirect or change neural connections and cell divisions. If this is so, perhaps birth experiences provide the most important influence on psychosocial growth in life.

We do not know the effect of these experiences nor their permanence. Yet we do have evidence that there is a continuity to the child's developmental experiences. As a consequence, we should keep these ideas in mind and use them to guide our teaching and practice, but retain an overall perspective regarding their implications.

COGNITIVE GROWTH

During the first eighteen months of extrauterine life, the human brain grows at a tremendous rate, in fact, faster than at any other time of life. Growth slows during childhood until another, less drastic growth spurt occurs at the beginning of adolescence. Further physical development of the brain ceases by adulthood, although cognitive and emotional development continues throughout life.

During infancy, brain development is very involved. It includes the appearance of glial cells, further development of already existing neurons, and the growth and development of axons as well as the appearance of the myelin sheath which covers them. Synaptic connections are established and chemical neurotransmitters become available to aid neural connections. Overall reorganization of the various cellular components also occurs.

The growth and development of these higher brain centers is exhibited externally in two ways. First, muscle control becomes more differentiated and reflexes give way to conscious control of movement. Second, the individual demonstrates the ability to use increasingly complex cognitive skills, learning abilities, and language.

Cognitive capability is the ability to understand, interpret, retain, process, and utilize information. The acquisition of language enhances these capabilities since, through communication, the individual is better able to acquire new or extend old concepts. Cognitive growth is dependent on both physical maturation and psychosocial information.

Jean Piaget, a developmental psychologist, spent the greater part of his life studying human learning. He believed that mental development begins at birth and possibly sooner. He has described intellectual behavior at any age as evolving directly from previous levels of understanding and proceeding as a function of the interaction of the individual with the environment.

Piaget's theory of learning includes an additional, broader perspective. He believes that collectively, human learning develops on the same basis as does individual learning; that is, people are both at their own level of mental development and also at the stage of learning which their society has reached. Thus an individual is both helped and hindered by the knowledge level of society.

Piaget described four major stages of human learning which are somewhat parallel to the biologic growth and differentiation of the brain. While the age range for each individual's progress through these stages will vary, the sequence does not change [12]. Thus, an individual experiences mental growth in a way that is both a unique and shared human experience.

According to Piaget, as people move through infancy and childhood, they actively *assimilate* new information and make *accommodations* (based on that information) either in themselves or in their environment. Learning is inherently interesting and exciting and so it is self-perpetuated by even the very young infant. Thus, a baby who is bored will fuss and cry as a result of feeling a need for stimulation.

Piaget's four stages of learning are summarized very briefly as follows:

The first stage of learning is the *sensorimotor stage.* It lasts from birth to approximately two years. During this time learning seems to be primarily that of acquiring motor skills. While cognitive activities are seen, the individual does not actually "think" conceptually, that is, by forming ideas.

The *preoperational stage* follows the sensorimotor stage and ranges from approximately two to seven years. Language is acquired and developed during this time. It is important to note that verbal skills do not mark the beginning of intelligence. Instead, word or thought symbols increase thinking ability by adding range and speed to already existent thought processes. Thoughts are still influenced and controlled by perceptions, even though actions can be internalized by symbols.

Conceptions which exist at this time are egocentric. Children are not capable of taking on the role or viewpoint of other people. In fact, they cannot really question their own thoughts. Rather they think that their own thoughts are the only ones possible.

Preoperational concepts are communicative. Children's activities become increasingly social during this time. They begin to play together and enjoy games with rules. Communication and socialization are interdependent, and so language and communication skills become increasingly complex.

Concrete operations characterize the mental activities of children between the ages of seven to eleven or twelve years. During this time, the child begins to use logical thought processes in order to solve problems. Decision-making is no longer limited by perceptions. Language becomes more complex. There is increased social interaction with increasing language abilities. True cooperation and competition with others appear during this time. The individual begins to share information and see the viewpoint of others as well as seek validation for personal thoughts and ideas.

During concrete operations, the individual cannot yet solve problems which are completely abstract and verbal. These more complex thought operations appear during the fourth stage, *formal operations*. This final stage of learning evolves about the same time as adolescence and makes adult thought capabilities possible.

Piaget wrote that conceptual growth is best understood by realizing that thinking ability grows increasingly more complex in an ongoing way. Movement from stage to stage does not suddenly just happen. An individual in the early sensorimotor period is very different by the end of that stage. An infant at the end of that stage is much more like the child in the preoperational stage. Thus, there is a gradual transition through the stages rather than the sudden appearance of dramatic landmarks. Piaget also felt that conceptual growth is fundamental to growth of psychosocial patterns [12].

Cognitive ability is clearly a needed asset in complex societies. Those who are born with mental defects are not able to attain the potential which our society values. Conversely, intelligent people seem able, many times, to overcome adverse problems and situations and lead successful lives. Perhaps it is not terribly important to decide whether cognitive growth is equal or basic to other components of identity. It seems more useful to appreciate the value of each human mind and nurture the growth of each intelligence as an enriching part of a fuller personal identity.

PSYCHOLOGICAL GROWTH

Very soon after birth, an infant learns to behave in ways that will ensure the satisfaction of needs and elicit care and attention from others. These behaviors become more sophisticated and complicated as the child grows and are determined in part by experience, perceptions, attitudes, and cognitive ability. However, behavior patterns are also formed as a result of active choice by the person.

Erik Erikson provides a framework for understanding the process of personality development. He suggests that identity formation occurs throughout life and involves a progressive series of steps which he organizes into eight stages. As one grows a crisis is encountered in each of the stages. (Crisis is used in the developmental sense meaning a turning point rather than a time of catastrophe.) The successful resolution of each crisis contributes to further growth of previously mastered tasks. It also provides a springboard for making the shift in perspective needed to enable one to go on to the next stage.

Of the eight stages which Erikson describes, four occur during infancy and childhood. Although psychosocial growth continues throughout life, he believes that the basis for successful, later development is established during childhood. Thus, emotional growth during childhood becomes an extremely important process. Briefly summarized, Erikson describes early psychosocial growth as follows:

Stage 1: *Trust vs. Mistrust:* The task of infancy involves developing a balanced sense of trust and mistrust. As the caregiver provides needed satisfaction the child begins to trust others, as well as self. The ability to trust both self and others is fundamental to the rest of psychosocial development.

Successful mastery of this stage is not just accomplishing the ability to trust. Rather it is learning to achieve a balance between the two extremes of trust and mistrust. For example, the six-month-old infant's fear of strangers is as important to understand and respect as is the trust exhibited at other ages. A healthy sense of mistrust provides the individual with a protective coping mechanism.

Stage 2: *Autonomy vs. Self-Doubt:* As the infant reaches the early toddler stage of physical growth, the second of Erikson's stages is approached. The task of this stage is to achieve a balance between autonomy and shame and doubt. The child's demand for freedom of will becomes very strong.

Sometimes the independence which is demanded is more than the child can handle. Punishment or discipline teaches the need to restrain demands for independence. The child soon translates this into a feeling of shame when a failure occurs. A healthy balance between the two extremes of this stage results in a sense of self-certainty instead of a sense of self-doubt.

Stage 3: *Initiative vs. Guilt:* During the preschool years the third step of personality growth is mastered, and a balance between initiative and guilt is attained. Initiative differs from autonomy in that it is a desire to explore and try new things rather than being a demand for the right to express one's will. Many new roles are attempted and discarded as if the child is experimenting with the possibilities in life. In doing this, the child learns to take realistic, moderate risks.

The desire to explore new areas may bring with it a sense of rivalry with one who may already occupy that territory. An example may be that of a female child who feels that her mother is a rival in her bid for her father's attention. If her difficulty with sorting out this situation is handled poorly, the child may develop a strong, rigid sense of guilt.

Stage 4: *Industry vs. Inferiority:* The fourth and last stage of childhood psychosocial growth parallels the school-age years. The task of this stage is to develop a sense of industry or capability with "work" to be balanced against a sense of inferiority. The balance here maintains a sense of perspective of one's own capabilities and accomplishments. Without this balance the person is left with the feeling of either great inadequacy or of false capability. The individual thus begins to prepare for a competency with a chosen life work.

These four stages represent the psychologic tasks which Erikson feels must be mastered during childhood. If mastery of one stage is not accomplished, the individual is not as well equipped to master the next step. One can go back at any time in life and master a previously unfinished task. Progress is then made through the other stages in sequence, strengthening each of them in the process [2].

When working with children, it is important to keep a balanced perspective in mind. While the focus is on developing a sense of trust, autonomy, initiative, and industry, one must also learn the realistic limitations the world and oneself places on these ideals. In addition, if they occur, a child can successfully overcome psychological problems. Nurses can help in that process by providing care, intervention, and redirection, using these psychological tasks as guides or directives.

The remaining four stages of psychosocial growth occur during adolescence or adulthood. They are discussed elsewhere in this book, if the reader desires this information. In addition, Erikson's *Childhood and Society* clearly outlines these stages and gives a much more complete description of them.

SOCIAL GROWTH

We know that with adequate nutrition, oxygen, and protection from harm, human physical growth will continue. However, there is another equally important element essential for human growth. A human infant who is not held, talked to, and touched by other humans will not thrive. In fact, some will die. Visual and tactile stimulation supplied by other humans is a necessity for normal physical, psychosocial and cognitive growth and development [10].

As with prenatal experiences, we do not know how early postnatal social experiences are understood and interpreted in the infant mind. We do know that throughout life, human physical and psychological health is related to being cared about by significant others. The intensity of individual need varies in situations and from person to person. There is also a need for reciprocal caring or someone to care about. Humans are very social creatures.

At birth our dependence and appearance will elicit, in most cases, the social help, care, and attention we need. Adults want to sooth a crying infant or cuddle and play with a smiling, happy baby. As we grow, in order to retain needed social attention, we must learn to interact with our social environment in an acceptable way. In turn, our social environment becomes very involved with teaching us further acceptable behaviors. Thus, society takes on a responsibility for socializing its younger members.

The socialization process is accomplished both formally and informally. Informal groups include parents or guardians, peers, siblings and extended families. Formal groups such as health care providers, churches, schools, and various clubs and community organizations become involved with our socialization as we grow through childhood. In other words, all of those who are responsible for, or in some way interact or are involved with a child help direct that child toward adulthood.

Havighurst describes two major aspects of social development. First, *social learning* includes all of the behaviors and "ways of life" a child must learn in order to become recognized as part of any group. The second, the development of *social loyalties*, involves the development of feelings of allegiance and participation in various groups. These two aspects of socialization are interrelated and occur simultaneously [5]. They represent internalization of the knowledge and commitments which give to each of us the form of civilized members of society.

The socialization of a child begins at birth in the delivery room. As the infant grows, parents or caregivers teach acceptable ways of eating, drinking, and behaving. Later they teach the child how to walk, talk, and interact with them and with other people. All of these social behaviors must be within acceptable limits for the child to be given membership status in the larger groups of society.

Teachers, siblings, and peer groups give additional input and define and teach roles which that particular society considers acceptable for any given person. Factors which are used to match a person and a role include sex, race, and socioeconomic status. These factors represent major influences in determining the accomplishment of a person's potential, even though they are bestowed without choice.

Another product of socialization is the development of a self-concept. Zander writes that "self-conceptions emerge from social interactions with other people." One's self-concepts then in turn influence one's behavior [13]. In part, a self-concept is the perception of how well one fulfills one's designated role, plus the approval society gives to fulfillment of that role.

When a person is accepted by a group, that person is in turn expected to be loyal and demonstrate an allegiance to that group and to participate in its activities. In order to retain membership in any social group, people must give up some personal freedom and goals. They must conform to group requirements and work toward the accomplishment of group goals.

This task is a difficult one for the child. The child is expected to join groups that may not be desired (such as school). The child is then expected to participate in that group's activities. Next, the child must learn to stratify group loyalties and make decisions regarding allegiance to these various groups. Does one owe primary loyalty to one's siblings, peer groups, school, or parents? The available social network helps the child to develop these values and make these decisions. Nurses can help to make that a feasible and growth-enhancing process for the child.

FEMALE PSYCHOSOCIAL GROWTH

All of the factors involved with shaping an individual identity take a somewhat different perspective when considered from either a male or female viewpoint. That is, gender has a great impact in determining life choices and opportunities for an individual, as well as affecting self-concept and confidence. John Money states that gender is the core of identity [8].

A female newborn is wrapped in a pink blanket and marked by a pink name card over her crib in the nursery. The world responds by teaching her that she must be held and handled more gently. She is dressed in delicate, lacy clothes and her cries receive quick response.

As she grows, she is taught to walk and talk like a "little lady." She plays games of hopscotch or jump rope with her friends, instead of football with her brothers. If she does play more competitive sports, she must play by "girls' rules." When not playing, she learns to sit with her legs crossed or at least to keep her knees together.

Female children are often not encouraged to find a solution to their problems. Daddy, not Mommy, is usually the one to help with broken toys or difficult homework. Competition with other female children becomes necessary to retain the adult help which is needed for survival and accomplishment in life.

This is all too often the pattern of psychosocial growth provided for female children in our society. It does not direct the child toward accomplishment of goals which have been outlined as necessary for a healthy, well-adjusted personality. It puts them into the conflict position of deciding between learning and fulfilling their female role versus learning and fulfilling their human potential.

A female child can still identify with her peers while simultaneously developing her cognitive skills. It is important for female children to accomplish psychological tasks and learn to be autonomous as well as trusting, to take risks in life, and to develop a sense of competency about work they have chosen to do. As health care providers, nurses are in a unique position to encourage and foster the healthy psychologic growth of women.

REFERENCES

1. Berezin N: The Gentle Birth Book. New York, Simon and Schuster, 1980
2. Erikson EH: Childhood and Society. New York, W.W. Norton, 1963
3. Ferreira AJ: Prenatal Environment. Springfield, IL, Charles C. Thomas Publishers, 1969
4. Freiberg K: Human Development. North Scituate, MA, Duxbury Press, 1979
5. Havighurst RJ, Neugarten BL: Society and Education, 2nd ed. Boston, Allyn and Bacon, 1962
6. Maslow AH: Toward a Psychology of Being, 2nd ed. New York, D. Van Nostrand Co., 1968
7. Mims FH, Swenson M: Sexuality: A Nursing Perspective. New York, McGraw-Hill, 1980
8. Money J, Tucker P: Sexual Signatures: On Being a Man or a Woman. Boston, Little, Brown, and Co., 1975
9. Nilsson L: A Child Is Born. New York, Delacorte Press, 1977
10. Osofsky JD (ed): Handbook of Infant Development. New York, John Wiley and Sons, 1979
11. Reese HW, Lipsitt LP: Experimental Child Psychology. New York, Academic Press, 1970
12. Wadsworth BJ: Piaget's Theory of Cognitive Growth. New York, David McKay Co., Inc., 1971
13. Zander JW: Sociology, 4th ed. New York, John Wiley and Sons, 1979

6

Health Issues of Childhood

Rose M. Mays

   Nurses can be found interacting with children and their families over the entire span of childhood and in varying states of health. But our pediatric population remains sadly neglected when it comes to assessment and interventions relative to the reproductive system. Normal reproductive functioning is often taken for granted until the onset of menarche. Education regarding body functioning and sexuality is likewise frequently postponed until adolescence. Health care providers must become more aware of the needs of children and intervene appropriately to promote their gynecologic and sexual health.

   The following chapter includes a discussion of gynecologic issues pertinent to children from infancy to puberty. Three major areas are presented. The first section, "Educational Issues," is written from the perspective that the primary role of the nurse in this area is to assist parents in educating their children about sex and sexuality. However, it is recognized that there are times when the nurse will impart instruction directly to the child. The portion on "Assessment" describes the gynecologic exam of the child and offers suggestions for individualizing the procedure based on the child's age and level of wellness. The last part, "Health Issues," discusses health problems seen commonly in female children.

EDUCATIONAL ISSUES

   Health care with respect to the reproductive tract begins with sound instruction related to the child's sex and sexuality. The education of children about sexual functioning and sexuality is an area which encompasses many controversial issues. Questions often raised include: when does one begin such instruction, how is it done, and more important, who are the persons best prepared to do it? Despite differences of opinion on these matters, it cannot be denied that children need to have clear, factual, age-appropriate information and ongoing adult guidance on sexual matters so that they may grow and develop into responsible, sexually fulfilled adults.

Conveying Attitudes About Sexuality

   To date, there is no definitive guide about what to teach about sex because of differing cultural, religious and family values. However, most experts agree that parents are the most influential educators of children regarding sexual issues. Sex education entails more than conveying factual information. Also conveyed are attitudes about sexuality. Whether aware or not, parents begin communicating such attitudes from infancy on, beginning perhaps with their reaction to the child's exploration of her genitals in the bath or during a diaper change. Children are quick to note embarrassment or hesitancy on the part of adults. Although one may be verbally saying intercourse and the birth process are natural occurrences, something very different may be communicated nonverbally.

The Young Child

Children vary in the type of information and guidance needed according to their individual development. Table 6-1 presents an overview of children's sexual needs and interests. Very young children receive mostly subtle cues about sex from the behavior of parents and little direct verbal information. As they become increasingly able to command language, direct questions are asked of parents. This questioning and curiosity typically begins about two and one-half to three years of age and includes such questions as "Where do babies come from?" and "What are breasts for?" The need to establish gender identity and gender role during this period also precipitates much curiosity about sex differences.

Preschoolers need their questions answered promptly in a simple but honest manner. Young children are able to assimilate only small amounts of information at one time; therefore, explanation should be kept short and repetition anticipated. In determining the detail of the explanation, it is best to have a relaxed conversation with the child and listen carefully to discern exactly what she is asking. A three year old genuinely does not know where babies come from when she asks that question and a response of "from Mommy" is sufficient. In successive years the explanation can expand to entail the father's role in conception, growth of the fetus and details of the birth process, depending on the child's needs and level of development. The use of correct terminology is advocated to prevent confusion for the child in later years.

Preschoolers are also learning about sex from observation and direct activity. Parents of the same sex are role models for children. Female children are acutely aware of their mother's and other women's role behaviors so that by age seven, male and female roles are understood to be dichotomous. Part of this awareness includes curiosity and concern about sex differences. Children may peep at their naked parents or engage in subtle sexual games with playmates (like "playing doctor") in which the genitals are exposed. Parental handling of these situations, of course, is highly individualized. The goal is to not instill guilt or anxiety, since this curiosity is normal and necessary for healthy formation of gender roles.

Table 6-1. *Overview of Children's Sexual Interests and Behaviors from Birth to Six Years.*

Age	Interests and behaviors
Birth to eighteen months	When clothes are off, handles genitals. Fusses to be changed when wet or soiled. No verbal distinction between boys and girls.
Two years	May be unable to function in strange bathrooms. Distinguishes boys from girls by clothes and style of haircut. Conscious of own sex organs and may handle them when clothes are off. Interested in watching others in bathroom or when they are undressed. Later distinguishes boys from girls by different postures when urinating (may not verbalize this). Beginning of interest in physiological differences between the sexes. Inquires about mother's breasts.
Three years	Verbally expresses interest in physiological differences between the sexes and in different postures for urination. Girls may make one or two experimental attempts to urinate standing up. Has desire to look at or touch adults, especially mother's breasts. Expresses a general interest in babies and wants the family to have one. Asks questions about babies: Where do they come from; where are they before they are born? May not understand the answer that babies grow inside the mother.
Four to five years	May play the game of "show" either exposing genitals or urinating before another child outside. Questions how babies get out of the mother's "stomach." Marked interest in anatomical difference between sexes begins to decline. Interested in parents' babyhood; in having a baby brother or sister; and in having a baby herself when she grows up. Later questions how babies got in the mother's "stomach."
Six years	Asks factual questions about having a baby; does it hurt? May have a beginning interest in the part the father plays in reproduction.

Adapted from "Comparative Growth Sequences," pp. 272-275 in *Infant and Child In the Culture of Today*, Revised edition by Arnold Gesell, M.D., Frances L. Ilg, M.D. and Louise Bates Ames, Ph.D. Copyright © 1974 by Gesell Institute of Child Development. Reprinted by permission of Harper & Row, Publishers, Inc.

The School Age Child

The school age years have been characterized as a latency period with respect to sex because the child becomes more guarded about revealing her inner self to adults. However, sexual feelings, awareness, and curiosity are present in the young school-age child as evidenced by masturbation, telling off-color jokes and stories, and reading sexually explicit magazines. School-age children are eager for all types of information and sexual data is of no exception.

This eagerness has prompted many educators to initiate formal classes into the curriculum of schools to ensure that children receive accurate and uniform information about sex. Some states have passed legislation mandating sex education in the context of family living courses in the public schools.

Sex education in schools, of course, is a controversial issue, with those in opposition feeling that the family or church, or both, should be the educators on such matters. If such instruction is instituted in schools, it should be done with the philosophy that the school is not the principal source of the child's education. Curriculum should be planned in collaboration with parents with special attention given to values to be transmitted as well as the biology of puberty and reproduction.

Role of the Nurse

The primary role of the nurse is to provide support and guidance to parents as they educate their children about sex. Some parents are quite uncomfortable conveying information of a sexual nature to their children. They may lack the necessary knowledge or communication skills to undertake the task or may be unclear about their own values and consequently communicate mixed messages.

In counseling with parents who express concern or hesitancy about their role as educators, one should express acceptance of their feelings but also communicate the importance of the child's needs. Often the problem is one of lack of information. The parents may themselves be unclear about reproductive and body functioning facts or they may not understand the child's developmental needs. The nurse can readily fill in these information gaps in a supportive, accepting manner. Books such as Salk's *What Every Child Would Like His Parents to Know* can supplement such instruction [7]. For those parents with difficulty in communicating, there are several children's books available to facilitate the process. *Where do Babies Come From?—A Book for Children and Their Parents* by Sheffield, for instance, tells of conception and the birth process directly, yet beautifully [8]. Pamphlets or texts should always be reviewed before recommending them to parents.

Often the parent will present the nurse with a specific problem situation and ask for advice. For example, "My mother-in-law thinks my preschool age children (male and female) shouldn't bathe together. What do you think?" Domestic nudity, of course, is another controversial subject. Regardless of one's personal view, a candid answer should be given. The nurse should guide the parent in considering the many aspects of the situation and assist in clarifying values and feelings.

ASSESSMENT

Although often omitted, a careful appraisal of the reproductive system should be included in the nursing assessment of every child. Frequently children do not recognize symptoms to be abnormal nor are their parents aware of the presence of warning signs due to the increased independence of the child in hygiene and toileting. Knowledge of anatomy, physiology and developmental norms, coupled with comfort in exploring sexual issues, are prerequisites for such a nursing assessment. Refer to chapter 4 for a summary of anatomy and physiology of the developing female reproductive tract.

The Newborn Infant

Assessment of the reproductive system of a newborn infant is embodied in the total appraisal of the child. The assessment is usually done in the first day of life and includes consideration of prenatal history followed by inspection and palpation of the genitalia and breasts for congenital anomalies and disease. The full-term newborn female characteristically has enlarged labia minora and breasts, resulting from the placental hormones. Leukorrhea, pseudomenstruation and breast secretions may also be manifestations of high prenatal hormone levels. Vaginal bleeding occurring in the neonate is normal. However, it should not occur at any other time in a child's life prior to menarche. As the levels of hormones drop, there is a slow regression of the structures to their normal size as well as a cessation of discharges. This process is completed by six to eight weeks of age.

Ambiguous genitalia is a congenital condition of the newborn which merits prompt and immediate medical referral. There are several etiologies and variations of this condition. The nurse should be supportive of the family while the medical personnel attempt to make a gender designation.

If possible, a nursing assessment should be conducted with the parent(s) present. This is an ideal opportunity for discussion and teaching about physical norms and expected changes in the newborn period and for eliciting concerns. It is expected that an open, informative approach in the neonatal period will lay the foundation for future discussions related to the child's reproductive development and sexuality.

The Well Child

In eliciting the objective data of a nursing assessment which is part of a health maintenance encounter, the nurse should explore the following areas with respect to the reproductive system:

History
1. Did the mother take DES (diethylstilbesterol) while the child was in utero?
2. Have there been any previous infections or surgeries of the genital tract?

Habits (which may predispose to disease)
1. What is child's routine of cleansing herself after a bowel movement? (May

ask child to demonstrate her wiping technique.)
2. Does the child use harsh soaps or bubble bath for bathing?
Present signs and symptoms
1. Is there vaginal discharge?
2. Is there vulvar pruritis?
Sexuality and development
1. What has child asked about sex?
2. What does she know?
3. How comfortable are parents in discussing sexual issues with the child?
4. To what extent have they discussed such issues?
5. Does the child have any signs of sexual development?

During assessment the nurse should inspect the external genitalia. An internal exam with endoscope is indicated only for a specific complaint and is usually done by a physician or nurse practitioner. As with other aspects of a physical assessment, the child should be apprised of the procedure beforehand. A brief explanation such as, "Now I want you to lie back and spread your legs apart so I can look at your bottom," spoken matter-of-factly is usually sufficient for cooperation. It may also be helpful to position the child with her knees apart and feet touching for maximal relaxation. The very young child can be positioned on her mother's lap for the exam. A child as young as a toddler can help hold the labia apart.

A brief inspection of the external genitalia includes noting the color and structure of the labia minora and majora. Also noted is the presence of vaginal discharge, state of perineal hygiene, presence of pubic hair and any lesions. The breasts are observed and palpated for precocious development.

Table 6-2. *Sequence of Sexual Maturation in Females During Puberty*

Stage	Pubic hair	Breasts
1	Absent	Areola lightly pigmented, chest appears flat
2	Sparse, lightly pigmented, straight; appears on inner border of labia	Breast and nipple elevated as small mound (breast buds); areola diameter increased
3	Darker, beginning to curl, increased amount	Breast and areola enlarged and contour continuous
4	Coarse, curly, and more abundant	Areola and nipple form secondary mound
5	Adult distribution of inverted triangle with spread to thighs	Mature contour; nipple and areola darkly pigmented and part of breast contour

Adapted from J. M. Tanner, *Growth at Adolescence*, 2nd ed. (Oxford, England, Blackwell Scientific Publications, 1962).

Finally, the child's sexual maturation is assessed. The onset, rate and completion of developmental changes that occur in puberty are highly variable among children but the *sequence* of the changes is the same. The Tanner method of assessing sexual maturation (Table 6-2) is an economical and simple procedure which can easily be incorporated into the exam. A pictorial representation of the descriptions is found in Figures 6-1 and 6-2. The sequence and variability of events is shown in Figure 6-3 and chapter 7 describes pubertal growth.

To determine a sexual maturity rating (SMR) or Tanner stage, breast changes and pubic hair are critically observed, then compared to the standards. This assessment procedure can be used by nurses to judge the normality of growth and development as well as serve as a basis for counseling children and their parents about pubertal changes.

The Ill Child

An assessment of a child with a complaint of the reproductive system focuses on the presenting symptomatology and integrates this information into a holistic assessment of the child. Following the history of the presenting concern and background, a thorough physical exam is indicated. Both the child and her accompanying parent should be instructed as to how the exam will proceed (usually a general exam precedes the gynecological assessment), what will be done and what their role will be. As in infancy, the external genitalia can be viewed with the child supine on her mother's lap. Older children may recline in the lithotomy position or use stirrups if available.

It must be remembered that a child's primary fear relative to an exam is of pain or body mutilation, not of embarrassment as with the adolescent. Therefore, it is important to be honest and calm, and repeat explanations to gain trust.

If the chief concern and history dictate the need, an internal or pelvic exam will be done. Practitioners vary in their choice of instruments for visualization of the internal structures. The following have been cited for such use in medical and advanced nursing references: otoscope with a nasal speculum, vaginoscope (a modified Kelly cystoscope) and Huffman–Graves virginal speculum. Permitting the child to experience the sensation of the vaginoscope first on her hands, then inner thigh and labia while simultaneously describing the instrument as "slippery, funny and cool" has gained good cooperation by some [2]. Collection of samples of vaginal discharge can be accomplished relatively painlessly with a saline-moistened (not dry) cotton swab or plastic eye dropper. Various types of analyses and preparations of the samples are discussed in chapter 16.

The knee-chest position has been found to be particularly valuable for inspecting the internal structures using no instrumentation [3]. Basically, the child is asked to rest on her abdomen with her buttocks in the air. Her head is rested to one side atop her folded arms with her remaining weight being supported by her knees bent six to eight inches apart. A key factor to the success of the procedure is the relaxation of the child. If no instrumentation is to be used, she is reassured that nothing will be put inside her. She is told to take several deep breaths while simultaneously concentrating on letting her abdomen sag downward. An assis-

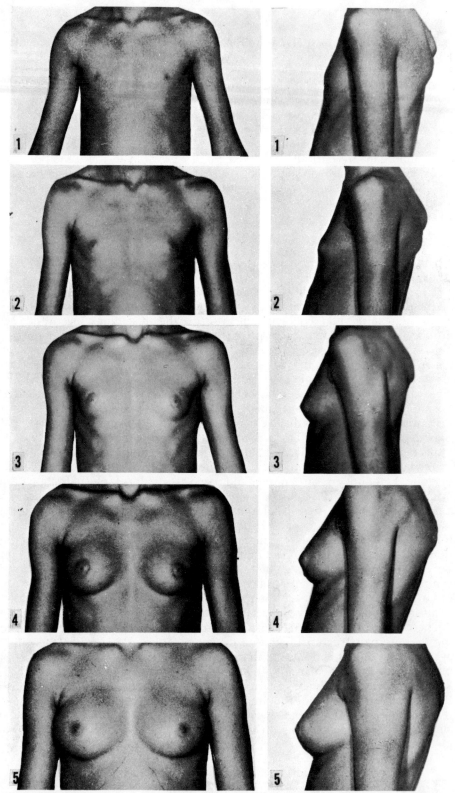

*Figure 6-1. Breast development during puberty. Used with permission of J. M. Tanner from **Growth at Adolescence, ed 2.** Oxford, England, Blackwell Scientific Publications, 1962.*

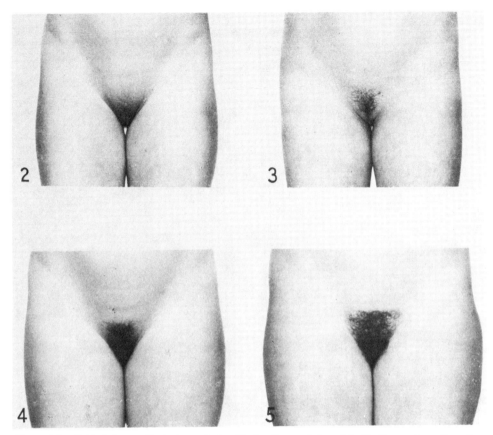

Figure 6-2. Pubic hair growth during puberty. Used with permission of J. M. Tanner from **Growth at Adolescence, ed 2.** *Oxford, England, Blackwell Scientific Publications, 1962.*

tant holding the buttocks apart while pressing laterally and upward permits maximal visualization of the vagina and cervix for foreign bodies, discharge or other abnormalities. Illumination can be provided with an otoscope or penlight. (Figure 6-4.) The final portion of the exam is rectoabdominal palpation. It is normal to be able to palpate only the uterus—not the ovaries in a prepubertal female.

HEALTH ISSUES

The discussion of health issues found in the final section of this chapter is by no means extensive or inclusive. The more common ones which the nurse may see or be asked to comment about in her role as community resource are included here.

Labial Adhesions

Adhesions of the labia are commonly seen in females of two to six years of age. The cause of this inflammatory condition is unknown, but is thought to be due to trauma or irritation of the hypoestrogenic tissues which results in their fibrous union.

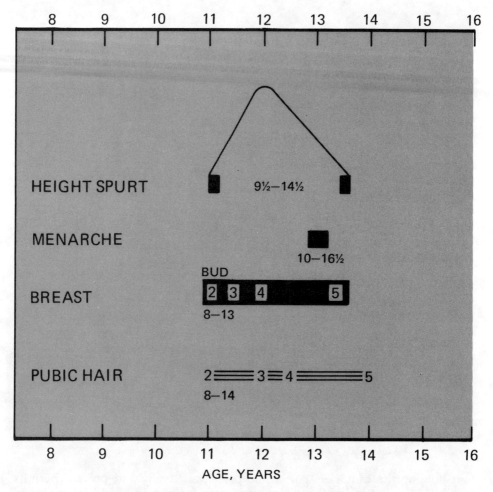

*Figure 6-3. Diagram of sequence of events at adolescence in girls. An average girl is represented: the range of ages within which some of the events may occur is given by the figures placed directly below them. Used with the permission of J. M. Tanner from **Growth at Adolescence, ed 2**. Oxford, England, Blackwell Scientific Publications, 1962.*

Mothers frequently are the first to discover the condition and are quite concerned because the vagina may appear to be absent. Health care personnel unfamiliar with the condition may also initially confuse it with an imperforate hymen or ambigious genitalia. The condition is self-limiting, resolving spontaneously with the onset of puberty and its accompanying increase in estrogen. Usually no treatment is indicated other than reassuring the mother–daughter dyad.

If, however, the fusion results in obstruction of the urinary meatus or vaginal orifice so that flow of secretions is inhibited, an estrogen cream or ointment is indicated to induce separation. Premarin®, or dienestrol, is the preparation of choice and is applied to the adhesions once or twice daily for two to three weeks.

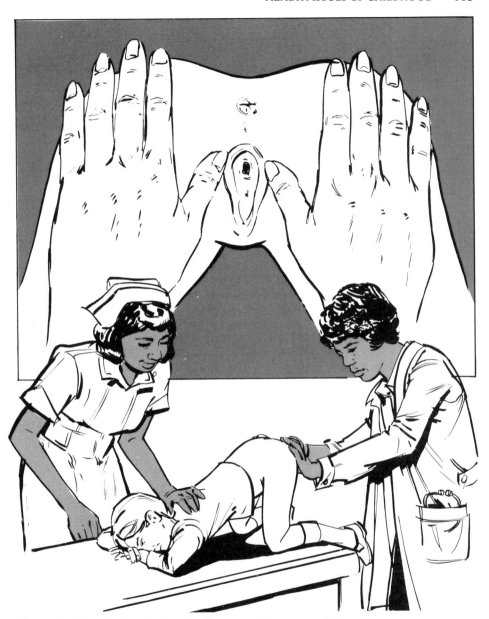

Figure 6-4.   Use of the knee-chest position for a gynecologic exam of a child.

This preparation is used no longer than three weeks because of systemic absorption resulting in breast tenderness and darkening of the vulva. These side effects are reversible when the preparation is discontinued. Forceful separation of the adhesions is not recommended. This is painful to the child and the associated trauma may stimulate further formation of adhesions.

Vulvovaginitis

Vulvovaginitis is an inflammation of the vulva and lower one-third of the vagina. It is probably the most common gynecological problem seen in prepubertal females. The young child's vulva and vagina are particularly susceptible to inflammation due to the absence of pubic hair and the vagina's nonacidic pH and thin, atrophic epithelium. These risk factors, combined with trauma, irritation or microbial contamination, readily create the condition. Symptoms are individual and may include varying amounts of discharge, redness and swelling of the vulva, and pruritis. Following the resolution of the inflammatory process, labial adhesions may appear.

Eighty percent of the cases of vulvovaginitis are termed nonspecific in etiology. Most are probably the result of poor perineal hygiene. Improper wiping and direct contamination of the genitalia with hands soiled from toileting can introduce microorganisms into the defenseless vagina. Pinworm infestation has been implicated in some cases of vulvovaginitis. Harsh soaps, bubble baths and mechanical irritants such as tight-fitting, nonabsorbent underclothing or foreign bodies in the vagina may also be predisposing to vulvovaginitis.

Treatment of nonspecific vulvovaginitis is primarily aimed at removing the source of trauma, irritation and/or contamination. Perineal hygiene is stressed, with concomitant application of corn starch or talc to the vulva. White cotton underpants are recommended. If present, foreign bodies are removed.

Parasitic and bacterial infections are treated according to their etiology. For acute or persistent cases (those lasting more than four weeks despite local measures) a course of broad spectrum antibiotic therapy may be given locally or orally. Estrogen cream may also be applied to the area for two to three weeks to lower the pH. Vulvovaginitis of a specific etiology is found in twenty percent of children seen. Since these conditions are presented in chapter 16 (Lower Reproductive Tract Disorders), only a brief discussion of the ways in which they characteristically vary in childhood is presented.

Gonorrhea in a child should always prompt the provider to consider sexual assault. It is unlikely that gonorrhea will be present without a prior sexual contact. A child with gonorrhea should be asked tactfully if she has ever experienced sex or been forced into a sexual situation and then should be examined carefully for signs of assault. In children the infection is usually limited to the lower reproductive tract. *Trichomonas* is rarely seen in children before the onset of puberty. *Candidiasis* or *monilia* also is infrequently seen in the child under nine years of age unless she is diabetic, receiving prolonged antibiotic therapy, or a neonate. *Pneumococcus* and *Group A or B hemolytic streptococcus* may also be cultured from the vaginal tract. Pharmacological agents used to treat a specific vulvovaginitis are similar to those recommended for adults. If concomitant trauma or irritation are present, measures are instituted to relieve or eliminate their source.

Precocious Puberty

Sexual maturation before age eight in females is termed precocious puberty. It can occur any time during childhood with menarche having been documented in children as young as one year and pregnancy observed as early as age five-and-one-half years. Precocious puberty can be further categorized as true precocious puberty and pseudo-precocious puberty.

True precocious puberty is the result of the early activation of the hypothalamic-pituitary-ovarian axis. This activation can result in complete maturation of the gonads and appearance of secondary sex characteristics. The cause of true precocious puberty is unknown in more than eight percent of the cases. However, since approximately twenty percent of the cases are the result of cerebral disorders such as brain tumors, postinfectious encephalitis, and neurofibromatosis, an extensive medical evaluation is indicated.

In *pseudo-precocious puberty* there is appearance of secondary sex characteristics but no increase in gonadotropin release by the pituitary. This development of breasts, pubic and axillary hair results when there is increased production of sex hormones by the gonads or adrenals. Pseudo-precocious puberty can be due to ovarian tumors, adrenal tumors or adrenal hyperplasia, and exogenous hormones.

It is possible to have isolated premature development of the breasts without any other signs of puberty. This condition is termed *premature thelarche* and is seen most commonly in females age one-and-one-half to four years. Pubic and axillary hair can also appear before age eight with no other signs of puberty. *Premature andrenarche* or *pubarce* are the terms used to describe these manifestations. Both of these conditions are usually benign and often the result of end-organ sensitivity to estrogen or androgen. However, since these changes may indicate the beginning of precocious puberty, the child should be carefully evaluated and followed closely to detect other signs of puberty or organic disease.

If an organic cause is found for precocious puberty, it should be treated promptly. However, the large majority of the cases are termed constitutional or idiopathic. These children continue on their early course of maturation but are seen frequently for ongoing medical evaluation to exclude the possibility of disease.

Support to the family and child with constitutional precocious puberty is of paramount importance. Parents must be reassured that their daughter's psychosocial maturity is not congruent with her physical maturity and that experiences, relationships and clothing should remain consistent with her chronologic age. Due to premature epiphyseal closure, these females often are shorter in height than their peers when they reach adolescence.

Families should be told of this potential outcome. In interpreting precocious development to the child, it is best to stress the normality of the situation. She should understand that her growth is normal but early, and that all of her peers will eventually experience similar changes. Education about menses, of course, will have to be initiated at an earlier age.

Sexual Assault

Sexual assault of children, a criminal phenomenon that is significantly under-recognized and under-reported, is estimated to account for a substantial portion of child abuse. Females are reported to be victims twice as frequently as males. There is tremendous variability in assault cases depending on the relationship of the offender to the child, the nature of the assault, and the family's reaction to the event—as well as other factors. Assessment, intervention and long-term follow-up require skill and a multidisciplinary approach. Several metropolitan areas have developed comprehensive programs for the assault victim and her family [1,5,6]. These programs typically offer in-depth physical and emotional assessment of the child and her family, treatment for physical trauma, referral to appropriate authorities, and counseling until the crisis is resolved. Where possible, such programs should be utilized as referral sources.

Recognition of sexual assault in children requires understanding the variability of cases and their presentation. Offenders have in the past been stereotyped as demented, older men who are not previously known to the victim. While such a description may be accurate in some instances, offenders are found in all age groups, are usually *not* insane, *not* under the influence of drugs, *not* retarded, and are frequently known by the child.

The behavior of an offender is a complex and multidetermined phenomenon. Motivational intent ranges from a genuine caring and need to be sexually close to the child to frank exploitation and abuse. These persons often benefit from professional help if identified and referred.

Many instances of sexual assault that come to the attention of professionals do so because the child tells about the experience. Sometimes an adult will make the discovery and consequently seek assistance. Frequently these are situations in which the offender was a stranger and/or the encounter was traumatic to the child. Many more instances of assault are not readily recognized by health care providers because they have become part of the child's lifestyle. She may have been pressured into the sexual relationship and into later secrecy by an admired adult who may even be a relative. Under such circumstances the sexual victimization may have occurred over an extended period of time.

Health care providers can help to identify victimized children by being alert to the possibility of sexual abuse when vulvovaginitis, venereal disease, foreign body or traumatic lesions of the genitalia are found in little children. Also, assault should be considered as a possible underlying cause of vague somatic complaints and behavior problems such as crying without provocation, or frequent bathing.

The interview of a child who has been assaulted sexually is conducted to collect information about the assault and to assess her ability to cope with the event. It is important to ascertain early under what circumstances the family is seeking help. Knowledge of who reported the event, the time it occurred, the suspected offender and the family's reaction will influence the direction of the interview.

Sgroi suggests keeping in mind the following points when interviewing the child for facts about the incident: 1) interview the child alone to obtain an independent version of the event; 2) approach the child in a relaxed, nonjudgmental manner, preferably establishing a relationship before discussing the assault; 3) identify the level of understanding and terms the child uses for body organs and functions and use these terms when appropriate; and 4) do not overly interrogate the child about the identity of the offender [1].

Interviewing techniques may include open-ended questioning, asking the child to draw a picture of the event and role-playing or acting out the assault. The prepubertal female has little awareness of the sexual significance of the event and her primary concern is usually of physical harm, especially if force was used. She may also fear punishment or feel guilt depending on her parent's reaction. The interviewer must be alert to the child's *affective* presentation of the facts and offer reassurance appropriately. Parents should be cautioned to refrain from overreacting to the event.

Family dynamics are also noted throughout the encounter. How does the family support the child? What are relationships like? For instance, in some cases of father–daughter incest, the mother may be torn between being loyal to both her husband and daughter and therefore be of little support to the child. Or some families may view the discovery of abuse as a crisis which significantly disrupts family functioning. In such situations nurses should be alert to the need for long-term supportive counseling as well as crisis intervention strategies for families. If a comprehensive victim counseling program is not available, the nurse may consider referral to a community mental health center or family counseling agency.

A comprehensive physical examination is conducted to collect objective data about the assault. In addition to an assessment of all body systems, the following activities are included in the exam:

1. inspection of the external genitalia and rectum for evidence of trauma (bruises, lacerations, bleeding) and disease;
2. inspection of the rectum, vagina and urethra for foreign bodies; and
3. collection of specimens from the throat, anus, vagina and urethra to detect sperm and gonorrhea.

Many instances of assault do not involve penile penetration; therefore, a lack of sperm in the vagina or of traumatic lesions should not lull the examiner into concluding assault did not occur.

Any child age five and under being examined for assault is also to be considered at risk for battering and neglect and examined thoroughly for other bodily trauma and developmental delays. Initial and follow-up blood tests for syphilis are also indicated for victims. Prophylactic antibiotics for gonorrhea are given if penetration has occurred orally, rectally or vaginally.

Careful documentation of the interview and exam is imperative since sexual assault of children is a crime and must be reported to the local authorities. Nurses working with such children and their families typically collaborate with social workers or counseling professionals who have the skill and opportunity to do in-depth assessments and intensive interventions. In instances of incest, for example, long-term counseling may be indicated since family relationships are usually chronically disturbed. Also, if the child's future welfare is at risk, arrangements frequently must be made to remove the child from the situation and ongoing evaluation provided. Sexual assault is a form of child abuse. Hopefully, its early recognition by alert health professionals will help lessen the drastic toll on the emotional lives of children.

REFERENCES

1. Burgess AW, Groth AN, Holstrom LL, Sgroi SM: Sexual Assault of Children and Adolescents. Lexington, MA, Lexington Books, 1978
2. Capraro V: Gynecologic examination in children and adolescents. Pediatric Clinics of North America, 19, August 1972
3. Emans SJ, Goldstein DP: The gynecologic examination of the prepubertal child with vulvovaginitis: Use of the knee-chest position. Pediatrics, 65, April 1980

4. Falkner F, Tanner JM (eds): Human Growth, Vol. 2. New York, Plenum Press, 1978
5. Giarretto H: Humanistic treatment of father-daughter incest. *In* Helfer RE, Kempe CH (eds): Child Abuse and Neglect: The Family and Community. Cambridge, MA, Ballinger, 1976
6. Gorline LL, Ray MM: Examining and caring for the child who has been sexually assaulted. Maternal Child Nursing, 4, March/April 1979
7. Salk L: What Every Child Would Like His Parents to Know. New York, David McKay, 1973
8. Sheffield M: Where Do Babies Come From? A Book for Children and Their Parents. New York, Alfred A. Knopf, 1977
9. Tanner JM: Growth at Adolescence 2nd ed. Oxford, England, Blackwell Scientific Publications, 1962

ADDITIONAL RESOURCES

Alexander MM, Brown MS: Pediatric History Taking and Physical Diagnosis for Nurses. New York, McGraw-Hill, 1979
Hockleman RA, Blatman S, Brunell PA, Friedman SB, Seidal HM: Principles of Pediatrics: Health Care of the Young. New York, McGraw-Hill, 1978
Pomeroy WB: Your Child and Sex: A Guide for Parents. New York, Delacorte, 1974
Preston H: How to Teach Your Children About Sex. Chatsworth, CA, Books for Better Living, 1974
Rybicki LL: Preparing parents to teach their children about human sexuality. Maternal Child Nursing, 1, May/June 1976
Stone J, Church J: Childhood and Adolescence: A Psychology of the Growing Person. New York, Random House, 1979
Summit R, Kryso J: Sexual abuse of children: A clinical spectrum. American Journal of Orthopsychiatry, 48, April 1978, pp. 237-251
Terrell ME: Identifying the sexually abused child in a medical setting. Health and Social Work, 2, November 1977, pp. 113-130
Vaughn VC, McKay JR, Behrmon RE: Nelson's Textbook of Pediatrics. Philadelphia, W. B. Saunders, 1979

Section III

PUBERTY AND ADOLESCENCE

7

Physical Growth and Pubertal Changes

Some time toward the end of the school-age years, children begin to grow more rapidly. This growth involves almost all parts of the body; however, the onset, timing, and speed of growth of the different body parts vary among systems and organs as well as among individuals. Important factors that determine when a system or organ will begin this growth spurt are the individual's sex, genetic structure, and environmental factors, including fulfillment of physical and psychological needs.

This growth spurt almost seems like the "magic beanstalk" in one of the child's fairytales. It seems as if overnight they shoot up to a great height. There is, in fact, a sudden growth spurt, but it doesn't come unannounced. The changes that occur are actually emphasized continuations of growth which had been in progress all along. Finally, there is a spurt toward maturity as a result of the ongoing hormonal interplay.

This time period is usually referred to as puberty. The associated early and late changes are called pre- and postpubertal or pubescent changes. Puberty means to acquire the ability to reproduce. For women then, this would occur when cyclic ovulation has been established. Historically, this was thought to happen at the time of menarche and so the two events were closely linked in people's minds.

Recent research has established that, in fact, women do not usually ovulate until well after menarche. Regular, cyclic ovulation often does not become established until late adolescence or the early twenties when most of the other growth changes are complete. Thus, the terminology referring to this stage of growth has become inexact and confusing.

In an attempt to maintain clarity, we will use the following references. *Puberty* means the acquisition of the ability to reproduce. It can only be determined in retrospect. *Pubertal growth* is that which occurs during the time of rising estrogen levels. Since this growth occurs throughout the adolescent years, one can also refer to pubertal growth as the physical changes of adolescence.

W. A. Marshall summarizes the principal manifestations of puberty as follows:
1. The adolescent growth spurt. This is an acceleration, followed by a decelera-

111

tion of growth in most skeletal dimensions and in several internal organs.

2. The development of the gonads.

3. The development of the secondary reproductive organs and the secondary sex characteristics.

4. Changes in body composition mainly from changes in the quantity and distribution of fat in association with growth of the skeleton and musculature.

5. Development of the circulatory and respiratory systems leading, particularly in males, to an increase in strength and endurance [6].

This chapter will focus on the development of the gonads and secondary sex characteristics of young women. Many of these pubertal growth events will be referred to in relation to menarche, one of the visual signposts of approaching sexual maturity.

HORMONES

The hypothalamus plays a central role in coordinating peripheral and central nervous system information as well as endocrine system function. It also seems to carry the responsibility of initiating and controlling maturation of body systems including reproduction. As blood levels of gonadotropins rise, the gonads begin increasing their production of the sex hormones.

Thus, around age eight, before there are any visible signs of the approach of puberty, there will be a rise in FSH levels. The resultant increased follicle stimulation produces an immediate slight rise in estrogen levels. This continues until about age ten or eleven (or one and one-half years prior to menarche), when there is a sudden sharp rise in FSH and then in estrogen production. These estrogen levels may also show cyclic fluctuations about this time. More specifically, estrone increase is gradual and parallel to the increase of other adrenal steroids, while estradiol rises sharply, reflecting increased ovarian activity.

Ovulation does not occur until the level of estradiol exceeds a specific, high threshold needed to stimulate pituitary release of LH. Below this threshold, estrogen levels are sufficient to build up the endometrium but are not enough to trigger the LH surge. Once the endometrium has been sufficiently established, any transient fall in estrogen levels will result in anovulatory bleeding.

Because of the ability of fatty tissue to store and convert estrogens, an excessively overweight female may have highly elevated blood estrogen levels. This, in turn, suppresses the release of FSH. Thus estradiol production will be minimal, endometrial buildup scanty, and menarche may be delayed. A female who is slightly overweight may have blood estrogen levels raised just enough to stimulate endometrial growth and early menarche [5].

Menarche, the first menstrual period, is usually anovulatory. The subsequent early menstrual periods are also frequently anovulatory and irregular. Coming full circle then, we find this ovarian, uterine, and pituitary interplay reflected in the blood levels of estrogen. For a few years following menarche, they are lower than the estrogen levels of an adult woman who has established regular, cyclic ovulation.

There is an additional factor which promotes irregularity of early menstrual cycles. Even when estrogen production is sufficient to induce ovulation, it is questionable whether a functional corpus luteum is able to be established [1]. Thus, the progesterone and estrogen needed to complete the secretory phase may not be available during these early menstrual cycles, thereby allowing early (or late) endometrial sloughing. This also accounts for the lower estrogen levels generally found before regular, cyclic functioning is attained.

This overall process of fluctuating hormone levels and body responses continues until finally, regular cyclic ovulation and menstruation are established. For many women this process will not be complete until they are in their twenties [1].

BREASTS

The first outward sign of approaching puberty for the female appears in the breasts and is referred to as thelarche. This is derived from the Greek "thele" meaning nipple, and "arche" meaning beginning. Breast development actually proceeds through five stages, with the first stage being the neonatal changes. Sometime around age eight or nine, the nipples become elevated and Stage II is entered. Stage III is marked by a protuberance or "budding" of the areola. In Stage IV, there is an obvious increase in breast size and the typical cone shape develops. This happens about the same time as menarche. Stage V is the completion of breast development until adult proportions are reached [10]. (See Figure 6-1.)

Along with these outward changes, the internal stroma, support structures and duct and gland systems of the breasts are also developing. (Figure 7-1.) Progesterone is needed to complete duct and acini growth, thus breast development continues until ovulation and corpus luteum development is better established. Prolactin also plays a role in breast development but the details are not understood at this time.

PUBIC AND AXILLARY HAIR

Shortly after breast development begins, pubic hair begins to appear, usually first on the labia and then extends to the mons. The growth of pubic and axillary hair also occurs in five stages. During Stage II (in Stage I, there is no hair) the hair is sparse, soft, and downy, fulfilling the literal meaning of the word pubescent. This growth of hair precedes menarche by approximately one year. In Stage III, the hair begins to darken. Stage IV is when the characteristic female triangle pattern of pubic hair distribution is defined. Stage V includes the extension of hair growth onto the thighs, assuming the final adult distribution. Axillary hair growth starts approximately one year after pubic hair growth begins [10]. See Figure 6-2 and Table 6-1.

VULVA

Fat deposits enlarge the mons and the labia; however, their proportion to the perineum during the pubertal growth process is maintained. The labia majora having finally completed development from the labial-scrotal stage, become pigmented, symmetrical, and puffy. The skin begins to look wrinkled and hair

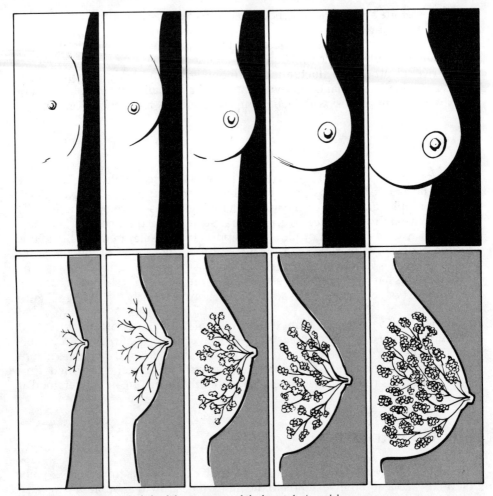

Figure 7-1.   Development of glandular structures of the breast during adolescence.

appears. The labia minora are smaller, pink and moist. Clitoral size increases somewhat and the urethral "mound" enlarges. The hymenal opening increases in size.

VAGINA

In response to the increasing estrogen levels, the vaginal epithelium gradually becomes layered, and superficial and intermediate epithelial cells appear. In fact, cytology studies of vaginal epithelium will give the first clinical indication that pubertal growth has started [6]. The pH begins to increase in acidity and a white, milky vaginal discharge may appear. This is in response to the growing activity of the cervical glands, and changing vaginal flora.

The vagina grows to about 10–11 cm in length and becomes more elastic. The introitus loses its red appearance and takes on the color of the surrounding skin.

UTERUS

The uterus is a major target organ for estrogen. Therefore, in response to rising estrogen levels, it begins a rapid growth until it finally reaches its adult measurements. In addition, the ratio of cervix to uterine body length is reversed and becomes 1:3. (See Figure 3-14.)

Early uterine growth is mainly of the myometrium. Just prior to menarche, the endometrium begins to proliferate. However, until ovulation and corpus luteum formation is established, the secretory stage of the endometrium is not reached.

Once this proliferative endometrium has become established, its continual maintenance is dependent upon adequate estrogen supply. Thus, an irregular or too heavy endometrial build-up or a transient drop in estrogen will result in endometrial sloughing. By this process menarche commonly occurs somewhere between ages ten to sixteen in the United States [2]. Menstrual periods often do not become ovulatory until one, two, or even several years later.

The cervical canal enlarges, and the growing cervical glands begin to secrete a clear, thready mucus. These secretions become copious just before menarche and will show ferning in response to the estrogen stimulation [6].

OVARIES

One result of the enlarging pelvic bone structure is that the ovaries (as well as the other reproductive organs) end up in the true pelvis and in their adult location posterior-lateral to the uterus. About two years before menarche, the ovaries begin to grow, reaching a weight of about 6gm at menarche. During the pubertal years, the final adult proportions and characteristic almond shape are assumed.

By the time puberty is reached, only about 300,000 follicles remain. Many atretic and cystic structures are present as a result of the minimal but continuous ovarian activity during childhood. As the gonadotropic hormones continue to rise, a greater number of follicles than during childhood begin to develop simultaneously. This, in turn, means that more theca cells are stimulated to produce estrodial. The end product is, of course, a greater blood level of estrogen.

Eventually there is enough estrogen available to trigger the LH surge and ovulation occurs. In one study, ovulatory cycles were still irregular in 20 percent of the participating women up to five years following menarche [1]. The amount of time needed to establish regular ovulatory cycles varies from woman to woman.

GENERAL BODY CHANGES

Pubertal skeletal and muscle growth does not seem to correlate with reproductive system growth. In fact, Falkner and Tanner point out that growth is truly an individual process. Averages may help summarize knowledge but they cannot predict individual changes. For example, while many women first begin breast development and then axillary and pubic hair growth follows, for others this hair growth will be completed before breast growth is initiated [2]. The variations are due to individual organ sensitivity, genetic directions, the variability of available estrogens, and, as previously mentioned, such external factors as nutrition and fulfillment of emotional needs.

All of these internal changes as well as external changes in shape and body ratio must be adjusted to and accepted by the growing woman. As her breasts, hips, and thighs begin to take on the female "curves" of adulthood, she begins to experience herself differently. The old, familiar body has been replaced, and the new one may seem clumsy (the body trunk grows more than the legs, thereby changing the ratio of trunk to leg size) and may do unexpected things, such as menstruate. Adulthood may seem a questionable attainment. Clearly these physical changes give a basis for and add to the psychosocial growth which occurs during adolescence.

REFERENCES

1. Bidlingmaier F, Knorr D: Oestrogens: Physiological and Clinical Aspects. Basel, Switzerland, S. Karger, 1978
2. Falkner F, Tanner JM (eds): Human Growth, Vol. 2. New York, Plenum Press, 1978
3. Hafez ESE: Human Reproduction: Conception and Contraception, 2nd ed. Hagerstown, MD, Harper and Row, 1980
4. Kistner RW: Gynecology: Principles and Practice, 3rd ed. Chicago, Yearbook Medical Publishers, 1979
5. Lowry GH: Growth and Development of Children, 7th ed. Chicago, Yearbook Medical Publishers, 1978
6. Marshall WA: Puberty. In Falkner F, Tanner JM (eds): Human Growth, Vol. 2, Postnatal Growth. New York, Plenum Press, 1978
7. Netter F: Ciba Collection of Medical Illustrations: Volume 2, The Reproductive System. New York, Color Press, 1965
8. Scipien CM et al: Comprehensive Pediatric Nursing, 2nd ed. New York, McGraw-Hill, 1979
9. Speroff L, Glass RG, Kase NG: Clinical Gynecologic Endocrinology and Infertility, 2nd ed. Baltimore, Williams and Wilkins, 1978
10. Tanner JM: Growth at Adolescence, 3rd ed. Oxford, England, Blackwell Scientific Publications, 1962
11. Vander AJ, Sherman JH, Luciano DS: Human Physiology: The Mechanisms of Body Functions, 2nd ed. New York, McGraw-Hill, 1975

8

Psychosocial Growth—Identity Consolidation

Historically, childhood ended early, sometimes as early as the age of six or seven. Because of society's limited resources, children were expected to assume adult responsibilities immediately and contribute to their family's and culture's struggle for survival. Education and issues of psychological development were not even considerations for most.

As societies grew more sophisticated and complex, they created a demand for the individuals within them to develop more and more complicated skills and knowledge. Further societal growth and maintenance depended upon the education and personal development of its citizens. Thus society granted a time period for its members to acquire the necessary skills of adulthood. This transition of growth from child to adult is called adolescence.

DEVELOPMENTAL TASKS

The word adolescence comes from the Latin *adolescere* and means "to grow up." [12] It spans the teenage years and ends at our culturally-established date of maturity, eighteen years old. Adolescence roughly parallels puberty and pre-pubertal growth. In the United States it is considered a psychosocial developmental stage.

As most parents and adolescents know, this can be a very difficult time period. Erikson describes these years as turbulent and demanding. During this time the individual is expected to formulate and consolidate an adult identity. Conflicts arise around the many life decisions that must be made. Confusion is created by multiple changes in societal and self expectations as well as in body structure and functioning [1].

The female must use these years to establish a basis for a mature personality both as a woman and as an individual. She must learn how to combine or separate these roles as the occasion demands. She must pull together her childhood knowledge about women and about herself to form a unique, adult "me." In summary, the adolescent female begins to think of herself as being in an adult female role and to make decisions about life from this perspective.

COMPONENTS OF IDENTITY

The adult identity an adolescent must formulate has many components or roles. These components include a cultural identity, social identity, career or professional identity, gender or sexual identity, and a personal identity. Overall, these various roles interact and interrelate to define an individual from both a self and societal perspective.

Cultural identity is defined by the country and community to which the person belongs. Conformity of one's behavior to group expectations is an implied obligation of citizenship of any community. Adolescents must learn the behavior which is expected of an adult in that society and then act accordingly. In turn, they are accepted as an American or French or English citizen, and then even further defined by the region of the country from which they come.

The role of women varies from one society to another. While expectations for them are similar in most western societies, they differ in subtle ways from one country to another. In some cultures women assume leadership roles while in others, including the United States, women assume more secondary positions. The adolescent female must learn what is acceptable behavior for her according to her society, sort out her personal values and expectations, compromise where she feels she must and can, and assume her own, personal version of a woman citizen of that culture.

Social identity is the economic and social position that individuals assume within their own community. In the United States people are grouped according to upper, middle, or lower income status. Often this designation takes on a "class" connotation which may help or hinder identity formation, but in either case does shape it.

The adolescent female learns quickly that others hold stereotyped expectations of behavior from women of high, middle, or lower socioeconomic status. These prejudices often revolve around values regarding sexuality, family, children, and career choices. She must learn either to mentally incorporate or reject these societal expectations of her, and to behave accordingly.

Career and professional identity implies that we are known by what we do. In other words, people are known to be or designated as being housewives, factory workers, teachers, lawyers, nurses, or whatever title fits the work they do. Adolescents must decide not only who they are, but also who and what they want to be.

Female adolescents in our society often feel frustrated and limited by the career choices our culture sanctions for women. Although changes are slowly being made and a wider career choice is available to female adolescents, they still must deal with many difficulties if they choose to enter a traditionally male field. At times an adolescent female may feel she must choose between developing as a woman or developing her career potential, rather than expecting her growth in both of these areas to be a simultaneous process.

Gender or sexual identity involves the growing definition of oneself as a male or female. As the familiar childlike body begins to take on adult configurations, adolescents are forced to decide what that sex role means. They then begin to demonstrate by their actions what it means to them to be an adult man or woman. Yorburg defines sexual identity as the image of the self as a male or female with the central focus being beliefs held about how one "ought to think, act, or feel" because of being male or female. [13].

A female must sift through all of the values, beliefs, and experiences from childhood which taught her what she currently knows about being a woman. She must take information from peers, from respected adult women, and from society, sort through it and then accept what "fits" for her. Changes within her body force her to consider her reproductive potential. She must make decisions about sexual and reproductive behaviors which will begin to define much of her adult life.

Personal identity is the structuring of an intimate self-knowledge. It contains thoughts and secrets known only to oneself. It is the "me" central to all of the rest of identity. During adolescence a young woman will struggle with how her own values and beliefs conform to or contradict those held by her family, friends, and society. This process will establish her uniqueness as well as create contradictions that may be difficult for her to resolve.

ASPECTS OF IDENTITY CONSOLIDATION

Many decisions relevant to a lifetime must be made about each of these identity subunits. The overlapping and interacting of these role areas further compounds the difficulty of the decision-making process. Lack of experience adds to the difficulty of making a choice about something that may have far-reaching implications and possibly unexpected repercussions.

Childhood experiences provide input for adolescent decision-making. Additional input for the consolidation of identity comes from a variety of resources within the individual. These include cognitive growth, body image, self-esteem, values, and competency. A third source that helps in the shaping of identity is one's social structures and resources.

Many other elements become involved in identity formation, of course. Those just listed assume major importance in female identity consolidation and so they will be included in this discussion. Childhood contributions are not included since they are discussed in chapter 5.

Cognitive Growth

According to Piaget the capability for using mature thought processes develops sometime around eleven to fifteen years of age. The individual attains the ability to formulate hypotheses and consider all of the available alternatives when solving problems [11]. The result is that an adolescent begins to understand the world from a whole new perspective. Insights change and grow and former beliefs and values are reexamined and tested. Ideas are then retained or discarded.

This new mental ability is both exciting and confusing. Important decisions about various aspects of one's identity are waiting to be made. It is fun to consider different possibilities and even try them out to some extent. However, it is one thing to "see" all of the alternatives and quite another thing to know the implications of choosing any one of them.

The adolescent measures life choices against "right" and "wrong" ideals. Lacking experience with the realities life brings, compromise is a difficult and often unacceptable alternative. Therefore, recognizing the differences between what seems best and what is more realistic for one's own unique situation is often not in an adolescent's repertoire. Indirect guidance in the use of developing cognitive skills is needed by the adolescent.

Growing females begin to hypothesize what womanhood will mean to them. Available information is limited. To start with, they have not yet had any personal experience of being an adult woman. Yet they cannot wait to gain experience before some critical choices must be made. Input can be gained from available role models (mother, teachers, other adult women whom they know), from friends, school, reading, church, and television. Since some of their critical decision-making revolves around areas such as sexuality, sexual experimentation, and contraception, it is important that they have responsible, accurate, nonjudgmental information as readily available as possible to make informed choices for themselves.

Body Image

Adolescent growth brings with it a need to reaccept and familiarize oneself with a new, changed body. Changing proportions of limbs and torso make the person feel awkward and clumsy. Hair growth and distribution, body contours, voice differences, and genital changes make it difficult to even recognize oneself.

Growing females must learn to be comfortable with new body contours of developing breasts and hips. As much as growing women look forward to these changes, they also feel embarrassed and exposed when they happen. Menstrual periods give evidence of a feminine ability to reproduce and indicate that "I am a normal woman." They also bring worries about cramps, stained underwear, odor, and being caught "unprepared." There are many pros and cons about this new, changing body.

The adolescent demand for perfection and for meeting an ideal standard sets up a different situation in terms of body image. The slightest flaw, whether imagined or real, is perceived as being of immense proportions. Anything that falls short of this standard of perfection is unacceptable to her and, she assumes, to anyone else. The emphasis within our society on movie star beauty and poise underscores the "correctness" of the adolescent's position. She may be devastated by a misplaced comment, a misunderstanding, or by the fact that she is developing sooner than, later than, or differently from her peers. Learning to accept, appreciate, and "love" her body as a part of her "self" is a major adolescent task.

As she grows, the young woman will find that her body again becomes predictable. She becomes acquainted and comfortable with this new, adult form. Her expectations conform with reality and she accepts her new self. She also learns to appreciate and enjoy her new femininity. The values she holds in regard to her body become a part of her gender identity.

Self-esteem

Hamachek describes self-esteem as being "one's belief about his relative value and ultimate worth" [3]. It is a combination of how well we think we measure up in comparison with others and how well we think we measure up to a self-established ideal. One's perception and one's values become the vital elements in self-esteem.

Self-esteem, which is developed during childhood, may be reinforced or changed during adolescence. As the individual's perception of the world and self changes, one's self-esteem may be adjusted in view of new information, new thinking abilities, and a new body shape. Input from others may serve to strengthen or weaken this developing self-esteem.

At adolescence a female will measure her growing femininity and sexuality against that of her friends. She will take into consideration the values she sees her mother and other close adult women hold about themselves. She will learn the value and worth that society hold for her sex. By sifting through this information she will form for herself a concept of her own worth as a woman. This, in turn, will serve as a basis for her overall regard for herself as a human being.

Values

Many adolescent decisions are made from the standpoint of the internal value system that has been developed. The components of identity may be formed around a set of values rather than clear facts and accurate information. All too often the values that direct adolescent decision-making are not clear even to the one who holds them.

Values influence the formation of such things as self-esteem or body image. In turn, these concepts influence career choices, gender identity, and personal and social identity. For women especially, it may be important to learn to separate one's own value system from that of others. Then decisions about these areas may more accurately reflect what is important to the woman rather than what she thinks ought to be important for her.

L. Rath outlined a seven-step formula for clarifying one's own values. These steps fall into three major categories including prizing, choosing, and acting on one's own belief system. One way these seven steps can be used is having the individual answer the following seven questions after first taking a position on an issue of concern.

1. Are you *proud* of (do you prize or cherish) your position?
2. Have you *publicly affirmed* your position?
3. Have you chosen your position from *alternatives?*
4. Have you chosen your position after *thoughtful consideration* of the pros and cons and consequences?
5. Have you chosen your position *freely?*
6. Have you *acted* on or done anything about your beliefs?
7. Have you acted with *repetition,* pattern or consistency on this issue? [7]

A process such as this may help a young woman clarify her ideas rather than tell her what to do. It will give her guidance without taking away the independence and control she is trying to develop (and will protect). It also provides a way for her to ask for additional guidance or to talk it through without "losing face" or being embarrassed. It respects her dignity by showing confidence in her ability to think through an idea. Whatever process is used, adolescence is an ideal time to begin to teach a woman to understand herself and her actions by looking at the values she holds about herself and other women.

Competency

Everyone can think of friends or acquaintances whom they would describe as competent. Whether these people are nurses, physicians, accountants, sales-clerks, or babysitters, they project a sense of sureness and capability. What's more, their efforts prove to be worthy of that description, and so they earn trust and respect from others.

When trying to explain what that person's competency consists of, one usually starts by describing a person's mastery of a skill. Thinking further about it one realizes that this is only one aspect. Self-assurance, confidence, and endorsement by others also seem to be terms that are used to describe an individual who projects a sense of competency.

From a psychosocial perspective, the competent person may be seen as someone with a well-integrated personality. Elements involved in this integration include self-acceptance, an internal sense of control over life's events, a sense of self-efficacy, interpersonal trust, adequate ego strength, and active coping abilities. The person also seems to have a sense of freedom about and acceptance of responsibility for her own life. Such people are actively involved in planning the direction they wish their life to take [10].

Competency is developed both by the individual and by the society in which the individual lives. During adolescence the fierce need to succeed in sports, school, peer groups, or some other defined skill represents the individual urgency to develop an internal sense of capability [1]. In addition, societal approval directs, reinforces, and encourages further development of this competence [9].

An example helps to interpret these ideas. If a society were to reserve only mothering roles for its women, it would not recognize a sense of competency in the female who begins to develop her skill in mathematics. No matter how great her potential she would be considered a deviant until she either gives up the math as a primary career or simultaneously masters her designated mothering role.

In other words, accommodation would have to come either from the woman, her society, or both if she is to reconcile the inner and outer pressures demanding her to fulfill one or both of her designated potentials. Ideally, society would support the person's development who would in turn contribute to that society's development. Accommodation would have to come from both. More commonly, accommodation within the person is what is chosen.

Competency is further developed each time the individual encounters and must deal with a new situation. According to Tyler this development occurs in three phases. In the first phase, *search and organize*, the individual establishes the alternatives that are available. Next, the person *implements* an approach to her goal. The third phase, *culminate, conclude, and redefine*, involves completion and evaluation of the situation [10]. In some ways, a competent person is one who uses a problem-solving approach to life, who is able to seek and set goals, work out and implement strategies to attain them and then enjoy success, suffer failure and build from both. Identity consolidation during adolescence is shaped by the person's sense of competency. It includes that which was developed during childhood. In addition, the adolescent's increased ability for problem-solving, successful interactions, and societal approval contribute to the further development of competency. This cycle can also occur in reverse as shown in Figure 8-1.

It is important to recognize that this cycle can be entered or exited at any point. Changes in society's or the individual's perspective can interrupt the equation although the individual still must struggle for mastery. Optimum chances for developing a competent personality occur when both society and the adolescent

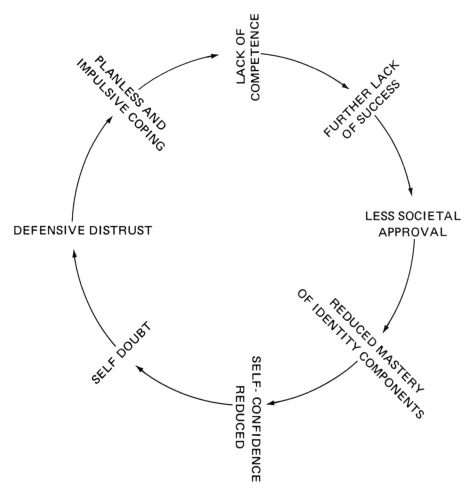

Figure 8.1.   Schematic representation of lack of competency and its interference with personality development.

are working together toward development of individual potential in a form that can serve both the individual and society.

Social Structures and Resources

Development of the various components of identity is a psychosocial process. This means that part of the process of establishing an adult identity involves factors outside the adolescent. That is, one's peer groups, family, adult role models, community structures such as schools, churches, clubs, and government and political agencies will take part in building one's identity. Society and social resources provide the adolescent a chance to sound out, compare, and further develop ideas. They then are given approval or disapproval by their society.

The female will observe how adult women in her society accept or reject their designated roles. Their attitudes toward such things as their own sexuality or career choices will make an impression on her vision of herself as an adult woman. Their acceptance of her as a peer builds her self-confidence and self-esteem. She learns from them what her society considers acceptable behaviors for adult women and how to incorporate them into her repertoire.

The values that a society places on its women are reflected by the resources it grants to the development of their potential. It is reflected by the esteem it holds for the contributions of its female members. It is also reflected by the public positions and placements it holds open and makes available for women to fill (i.e., professions, politics, policy formation). These societal values are adopted and perpetuated by the members of the society, including its women. Thus it is essential that society include roles for women which will encourage the development of their potential and thereby the healthy development of their personalities.

Society plays a vital role in accomplishing the task of identity consolidation of its young female members. In many societies, including the United States, a second-best attitude is extended toward women. Expectations and opportunities to develop their potential are of a lower status than those reserved for men. This situation creates a confusing predicament for the adolescent female. Why would anyone want to accept a predetermined lower status? How can one passively accept a secondary status? Yet in order to identify successfully with the female component of her society, she must accept that she will not fully succeed by her society's standards. However, societal pressure to conform is so strong that the majority of women continue to insist that this position is logical and valid and urge its adoption by developing adolescents.

DISCUSSION

Each of us uses resources and materials from others, from our environment, and from ourselves to develop a product we call "me." We then look to our own reactions and to those of others for feedback and decide whether to accept or reject various directions of the developing components of this growing self. The parts of personality which were developed in childhood are then reexamined during adolescence. In view of many sudden changes within the self and in societal expectations, these earlier developed components of personality are understood in a new way [2].

These ideas become very important when one attempts to understand adolescent females. They must overcome their initial embarrassment of physical prepubertal changes and develop a sense of comfort with and pride in their female bodies. They must reconcile these changes with a growing sense of their own sexuality. Decisions about sexual activity, contraception, drugs, alcohol use, pregnancy, career, and marriage become involved with day-to-day choices of how to dress, whom to date, and whom to choose to tell your secrets to. All of this becomes the adolescent's growing definition of herself as an adult woman.

As has been shown, these choices are made on the basis of individual experience and societal input mediated through self-esteem, body image, general beliefs and values, cognitive growth, and competency. How all of these factors interact can be demonstrated by using an example of one female adolescent problem.

The female adolescent who is not sexually active is in the minority. It is the norm for an adolescent couple to have a sexual relationship. Yet, few of the young women involved use contraception. They intellectually know that they are risking pregnancy, parental wrath and other attendant problems, but that doesn't seem to make any difference even if contraception is readily available. Reasons which they give are "it won't happen to me," "that makes it seem planned," and "I'm embarrassed. [8]" These answers and other forms of conduct are not consistent with the idea that as adolescents develop the ability for formal thought processes, they will consider all of the alternatives.

To be able to generate and consider alternatives does not mean they *will* consider alternatives. Additional factors become involved. The first and last of these adolescent "reasons" for not using contraceptives, seem to suggest that a poor or inadequate body image may be a factor in this situation. The second answer seems to relate to a confused value system. A third factor which may be involved in all three answers has to do with the development of competence.

As noted earlier, the socialization of women in our culture teaches them to be passive and accepting of what life brings rather than actively involved in shaping their lives. To decide to be sexually active and then to choose and use contraception is very active planning and acceptance of responsibility for one's own behavior. No matter how much biology is known, it is very difficult to take such action when it goes against a well-integrated and socially reinforced belief system which says that one must do otherwise to succeed as a woman.

One of the most common remarks adults make about adolescents is "I cannot understand them." Yet to study and understand someone usually implies that they are in a stable, steady state and thus able to be understood. The adult people whom we do understand have a stable identity that they have developed. The problem with adolescence is that it is a transition stage, a phase of rapid change, at times from one day to the next. We demand that these people stand still and let us understand them when, in fact, they cannot. Until we build a flexible framework that can incorporate this change process, we will continue to have difficulty understanding adolescents. Until then, perhaps our best approach is to learn about and try to understand the context, components, and molding elements of adolescent change. With this understanding we can provide direction, information, role modeling, and above all, support for them to develop their own personal sense of a competent identity.

REFERENCES

1. Erikson EH: Identity: Youth and Crisis. New York, W. W. Norton, 1968
2. Erikson EH: Dimensions of a New Identity. New York, W. W. Norton, 1974
3. Hamachek DE: Encounters with the Self. New York, Holt, Reinhart, and Winston, 1971
4. Havighurst RJ, Bowman PH, et al: Growing up in River City. New York, John Wiley and Sons, 1972
5. Mims FH, Swenson M: Sexuality: A Nursing Perspective. New York, McGraw-Hill, 1980
6. Pengelley ET: Sex and Human Life, 2nd ed. Reading, MA, Addison Wesley, 1978
7. Raths L, Harmin M, Simon S: Values and Teaching. Columbus, OH, Charles C. Merrill, 1966

8. Sorenson RC: The Sorenson Report: Adolescent Sexuality in Contemporary America. New York, World Publishing Company, 1973
9. Tyler F: Adolescent competence: A different point of view. Virginia Medical Monthly, Vol. 100, October 1973, pp. 919-926
10. Tyler F: Psychosocial competence differences among adolescents on entering group counseling. Psychological Reports, Vol. 44, 1979, pp. 811-822
11. Wadsworth BJ: Piaget's Theory of Cognitive Development. New York, David McKay, 1971
12. Webster's Seventh New Collegiate Dictionary. Springfield, MA, G and C Mirriam Co., 1963
13. Yorburg B: Sexual Identity. New York, John Wiley and Sons, 1974

Section IV

ADULT WOMAN—CHILDBEARING YEARS

9

Physical Status of the Reproductive Years

L. COLETTE JONES

Throughout the childbearing years, the primary and secondary sex organs change anatomically and physiologically. These changes are a result of the normal maturation and aging processes as well as of childbearing. This chapter will identify the changes that occur in the reproductive organs during the childbearing years.

THE MENSTRUAL CYCLE

The events of the menstrual cycle and menstruation vary greatly from one woman to another. In addition, many women note changes in their own menstrual pattern from time to time. These changes include variations in cycle length, duration of flow, and intensity of flow.

Cycle Length

Cycle length refers to the number of days between the start of one cycle (menstrual period) to the onset of the next cycle. The textbook twenty-eight day cycle is a statistical average and characterizes only about 10–15 percent of all women's cycle length [5]. A normal cycle length may last anywhere from twenty-one to forty-five days [7].

Factors that determine cycle length include genetics, nutrition, weight gain or loss as well as overall proportion of body fat, exercise, drugs, emotions, illness, and possibly climate [5]. This list helps make it clear why menstrual cycles vary from one woman to another and why a woman's cycles are considered normal for her if they are regular. A regular cycle length is one that does not vary by more than five days [5].

Menstrual bleeding may last anywhere from four to six days, although some women may have normal menstrual periods which last two or eight days [10]. Again, regularity of pattern is what determines normality.

Menstrual irregularity may occur as a result of aging. For about five years following menarche, cycles may vary greatly both in length and duration. Then almost in a mirror-image effect, similar cycle changes again may occur for about five or six years prior to menopause. The period of time when a woman may experience most cycle regularity, barring all other interfering factors, would be around age thirty-five [5].

Regardless of the age at menarche, it takes a period of time to establish a so-called normal pattern of menstruation. Studies of a large number of women who recorded their menstrual cycles over many years show that there is a great variability in the length of the cycles following menarche. Vollman found that the length of the first cycle after menarche in thirty-nine adolescents ranged from 11 to 211 days. The average cycle length was 45.6 days. In 50 percent of these females, the cycle was thirty-four days or longer. This variability decreases as women mature; but it appears to take an average of twenty cycles after menarche for a stable pattern to emerge in each individual [13].

In a study involving 656 women, Vollman found that the average cycle length dropped from 35.1 days at age twelve to a low of 27.1 days at age forty-three. It then rose to 51.9 days at age fifty-five. Although there is some information lost when statistical averages are used, nearly all women experience the described changes throughout the childbearing years but each individual's experience may differ considerably from the norms described here [13].

Menstrual Flow

Other sources of variability in the menstrual cycle are the duration and character of menses and amount of flow. The normal menses usually lasts from three to seven days but periods of one or nine days are considered within normal range if a pattern is consistent for an individual [15].

The amount of total *menstrual* flow varies from 30 to 112 ml. One tampon or pad absorbs 20 to 30 ml when saturated. A total *blood* loss of 30 to 60 ml during a menstrual period is average [14]. Blood loss is considered heavy to abnormal if it exceeds 80 ml [5].

Obviously, the duration and amount of flow is a poor indicator of blood loss. Since it accounts for about only forty percent of menstrual fluid, it helps to know what, in addition to blood, accounts for total menstrual volume. The remaining 60 percent of the flow is a combination of leukocytes, desquamated epithelium, cervical mucus, vaginal cells, and bacteria.

The usual pattern in early adulthood is a heavier flow the first two days and then the amount slowly decreases and stops. After thirty years of age, some women note a day or two of spotting before a heavier flow that tapers off gradually. Women in the mid to late forties may experience heavy menses prior to the climacteric [8].

Normal menstrual discharge is less viscous than blood and usually does not clot. This facilitates its passage from the uterus. Although menstrual blood can clot within the endometrial cavity, most clots are readily lysed by fibrinolytic enzymes. Thus menstrual bleeding generally leaves the uterine cavity as a fluid. However, with heavy bleeding all uterine clots may not be lysed and therefore will be intact when they leave the cervix.

Additional Factors

Variations in cycle length, duration of menses, and amount of flow occur because of the very complex relationships of the hypothalamic-pituitary-ovarian axis and the variations in end organ response as described in chapter 3. In addition, thyroid dysfunction, malnutrition, pelvic inflammatory disease, fibroid tumors, certain drugs, (i.e., phenothiazines, anticoagulants, thiazide diuretics) may change the character or pattern of the menses. Most women with IUD's find their periods heavier and longer while those who take birth control pills usually have a lighter flow. Deviations from the individual's normal pattern should be investigated to rule out a serious underlying cause. However, once abnormalities are ruled out, women may need education and reassurance about normal variability in menstruation. Although the twenty-eight day cycle with five days of flow does occur, a variance from this pattern is just as likely and just as normal. As Paula Weidiger observes:

Because so much of the process of menstruation and menopause is hidden (physically, culturally, and psychologically), changes in bleeding patterns of any sort often trigger anxiety. We long for a nonexistent regularity [14].

THE REPRODUCTIVE ORGANS

Breasts

Functionally the breasts are accessory to the reproductive system because of milk secretion, but structurally they are closely related to the integument. Each breast weighs an average of 150 to 211 gm, but may increase to between 400 to 500 gm during lactation. The left breast is usually slightly larger then the right. In response to the menstrual cycle the breasts may feel more lumpy and congested prior to menstruation.

After childbirth and lactation, breasts may not return to the nulliparous state. About the age of thirty-five there is a very gradual reduction in the size of the functional lobes. Adipose tissue is laid down as the glandular tissue regresses until about the age of forty-five. With increasing age, the lobular structures are lost and replaced by dense, hyalinized tissue.

External Genitalia

In the reproductive years, the mons pubis is formed by fatty tissue under the skin and is well covered with hair in an inverted triangular shape. Pubic hair varies from coarse and crinkly in black women to fine and sparse in Oriental women. During the late reproductive years, hair begins to thicken, become coarser, and may turn gray. The fat pad of the mons decreases.

The labia majora extend from the lateral boundaries of the vulva and vary in shape, size, and structure with height, weight, age, parity, and pelvic architecture of the individual. Hair covers their surfaces, particularly the lateral and anterior. During intercourse, the labia majora flatten and become somewhat elevated as they become congested with blood. In the late reproductive years, they also lose subcutaneous fat and the hair becomes sparse.

The skin on the labia minora is smooth and pigmented in adulthood. They become engorged and bright red in color during sexual excitement. Following childbirth, they are less regular in appearance. In the later childbearing years, they tend to flatten and become less distinct. They regress less than do the labia majora, thus they become more prominent just as in childhood.

As the focus of sensation with sexual excitement, the clitoris assumes a psychological as well as physical significance during adulthood. Clitoral excitation leading to orgasm may be derived from a variety of stimuli. Stimulation may be brought about by means of penile, manual, oral, or mechanical contact either directly to the clitoris or indirectly by vaginal penetration. Finally, clitoral erection and orgasm may result from psychological stimulation including thoughts, fantasies, and erotic materials. The meaning and interpretation of psychological stimuli is, of course, related to the woman's past and present experiences.

The pelvic girdle of large and powerful muscles and fascia supports the genitourinary organs. Western culture provides little opportunity for exercising these muscles (such as in squatting). With pregnancies and the aging process, these muscles and fascia become more relaxed. Herniation into the vagina from the rectum (rectocele) and from the bladder (cystocele), or prolapse of the uterus into the vagina may occur. Improved obstetrical care and better nutrition have decreased the incidence and severity of these problems but surgical repair may be necessary. Some urinary problems of the childbearing years are due to or aggravated by pelvic relaxation.

Internal Reproductive Organs

After puberty and during the early reproductive years, the *vaginal walls* have many deep folds or rugae. The rich blood supply promotes a deep pink color. The pH is acid and many nonpathogenic organisms such as Döderlein bacillus are present. Streptococci, coliforms, cornybacteria and fungi may be present without symptoms. With increasing age and decreasing estrogenic stimulation, the rugae in the vagina smooth out, the color of the vagina and cervix becomes paler and the pH becomes less acidic.

The *uterus* is a target organ of estrogen in the childbearing years. Throughout 400–500 cycles it is prepared for pregnancy as a result of ovarian hormones. If pregnancy does not occur, the menstrual cycle is completed with the menses. The uterus has a greater capacity for growth than any other organ in the body so that it may contain and expel a full-term infant.

The nulliparous uterus weighs 30–40gm, is 7–9cm in length, 6–7cm in width, and has an anteroposterior diameter of 4cm. Following childbirth, the uterus weighs about 42gm which is slightly larger than in a nulliparous woman. The cavity of the uterus has a depth of approximately 6cm and a capacity of 4–8ml. It remains slightly larger after childbirth [4].

About 75 percent of the thickness of the uterine wall is in the myometrium or muscle layers. During pregnancy, this layer becomes enormously enlarged to accommodate the fetus. It is primarily through the orderly contraction of the myometrium that the infant is delivered.

The *cervix* opens into the vagina through the external os. After childbirth the os remains wider and the opening less regular in shape. The squamocolumnar junction lies at or near the level of the external os in many women, although it may as readily be found higher in the cervical canal. It is at this transitional zone that the majority of cervical malignancies begin. Thus it is essential that a Pap smear contain cells taken from this area. For additional information see chapter 16 (Lower Reproductive Tract Disorders) and chapter 23 (Gynecologic Exam).

The epithelium of the *Fallopian tubes* responds to the hormones of the menstrual cycle. The columnar secretory cells increase in size and function at the time of ovulation. The type of secretion is not fully known but it undoubtedly facilitates movement of the ovum and its growth if it is fertilized.

The integrity of the tube is vital to fertility. Infections and subsequent scarring may close the very small lumen permanently. Fertilized ova may implant too soon and result in a tubal pregnancy.

PHYSICAL CHANGES IN PREGNANCY

Pregnancy causes many major changes in the body. The reproductive organs exhibit the most obvious changes. However, changes occur in the integument, respiratory, cardiovascular, renal, metabolic, and musculoskeletal systems.

The *uterus* grows to accommodate the fetus, placenta, and other tissues until it reaches the xiphoid process in the ninth month. Changes in uterine consistency occur early. Softening of the isthmus, known as Hegar's sign, is noted on bimanual examination as early as six weeks after the last menses. By the second month, the cervix also softens and by term the os may admit a fingertip. The corpus also softens as the fetus grows. These changes are all useful in an early diagnosis of pregnancy.

The *endocervical epithelium* proliferates and often everts, producing a visible red area around the os which may be mistaken for an erosion. Thick, clear, odorless mucus is also produced by the endocervix throughout pregnancy and forms a mucous plug in the os that protects the fetus from infection.

The *vagina*, as do all pelvic organs, becomes more vascular. It may assume a deep violet color known as Chadwick's sign. The *vulva* also becomes more vascular. In some women both vulva and vagina are prone to varicosities due to congestion. These may disappear after delivery. The *ovaries* enlarge in response to the progesterone produced by the corpus luteum and placenta while other tissues within the pelvis such as the ligaments also hypertrophy.

The *breasts* undergo several changes. The areolae enlarge and become pigmented. There is a general growth of ductile elements as the breasts prepare for lactation. Tingling and fullness of the breasts is a very early sign of pregnancy for some women. A supportive brassiere in a larger size may be needed.

Generalized *pigment changes* are common and are more pronounced in women with darker skin. It is surmised that these changes are due to an increase of melanin stimulating hormone (MSH) from the pituitary. A line of increased pigment forms between the umbilicus and the symphysis pubis called the linea nigra. Patches of increased pigmentation on the cheeks and nose are seen in some women and are known as chloasma or the mask of pregnancy. Preexisting nevi or other lesions may become more pigmented in pregnancy. All these changes resolve to some extent after delivery although the linea nigra and enlarged areola remain to some extent, particularly in darker skinned women.

Another *integumentary* change which may occur is striae or stretch marks on the abdomen, breasts, and thighs. The etiology is not entirely known but they are probably caused by changes in the subcutaneous tissues. They will be pink during pregnancy but become permanent white streaks after delivery.

Cardiovascular changes occur that are related to the increased blood volume and increased demand of the growing fetus. Physiologic systolic cardiac murmurs are frequently heard because of increased flow and decreased viscosity of the blood. Although the red cell mass increases somewhat, with the increased volume a relative "anemia" in pregnancy is normal. The hemoglobin at twenty-four to thirty-two weeks drops to 12.1gm on the average. White blood cells and several clotting factors also increase. Toward term, the heart rotates somewhat due to the encroachment of the uterus.

The *respiratory rate* is often increased and mild dyspnea on exertion is seen as term approaches. The general hyperemia of the body is noted in the mucous membranes of the respiratory system. Nasal stuffiness and blocked eustachian tubes are common complaints.

The *metabolic rate* increases gradually until it is 25 percent above the nonpregnant state. The pituitary and thyroid increase in both weight and function.

The *musculoskeletal system* responds to the enlarged uterus with an increased pelvic tilt and increased dorsal kyphosis and cervical lordosis. Joints in the pelvis become more movable. Backache is common because of the postural changes.

The *urinary system* is greatly affected by pregnancy. There is relaxation and dilation of the ureters. Some degree of hydronephrosis is normal due to the pressure of the uterus on the ureters. Minor trauma to the bladder commonly occurs in labor and delivery. Without complications such as urinary tract infections, all of these changes normally resolve within four to six weeks after delivery.

The physical status of a woman radically changes throughout normal pregnancy, labor, and delivery. The genitourinary system undergoes the most extreme changes. Most women suffer no irreversible physical effects but the nulliparous physical state is never regained.

The childbearing years are the longest phase in most women's lives. Reproductive capacity matures, then very gradually regresses. The rhythm of the menstrual cycle is a major influence both physiologically and psychosocially. Many women in the twenty to forty-nine age group utilize health care services primarily in relation to reproductive system needs. Entry of women into the health care system for gynecological services provides nurses an opportunity to do teaching and counseling for women as well as for their families.

REFERENCES

1. Blaustein A: Pathology of the Female Genital Tract. New York, Springer-Verlag, 1977
2. Erikson EH: Childhood and Society, 2nd ed. New York, W. W. Norton, 1963
3. Frame PS, Carson SJ: A critical review of periodic health screening using specific screening criteria, part I. Journal of Family Practice, Vol. 2 No. I, 1975
4. Goss CM (ed): Gray's Anatomy, 29th American edition. Philadelphia, Lea and Febiger, 1973
5. Hafez ESE: Human Reproduction: Conception and Contraception, 2nd ed. Hagerstown, MD, Harper and Row, 1980
6. Hall JH, Zwemer JD: Prospective Medicine. Indianapolis, IN, Methodist Hospital of Indiana, 1979
7. Kistner RW: Gynecology: Principles and Practice, 3rd ed. Chicago, Yearbook Medical Publishers, Inc., 1979
8. Martin LL: Health Care of Women. Philadelphia, J. B. Lippincott, 1978
9. Phillip EE, Barnes J, Newton M: Scientific Foundations of Obstetrics and Gynecology. Chicago, Yearbook Medical Publishers, Inc., 1977
10. Pritchard JA, MacDonald PC: William's Obstetrics, 16th ed. New York, Appleton-Century-Crofts, 1980
11. Romney SL et al: Gynecology and Obstetrics: The Health Care of Women. New York, McGraw-Hill, 1975
12. Speroff L, Glass RH, Kase NG: Clinical Gynecologic Endocrinology and Infertility, 2nd ed. Baltimore, Williams and Wilkins, 1978
13. Vollman RF: The Menstrual Cycle. Philadelphia, W. B. Saunders, 1977
14. Weidiger P: Menstruation and Menopause: The Physiology and Psychology, The Myth and the Reality. New York, Alfred A. Knopf, 1976
15. Ziegel E, Van Blarcom CC: Obstetric Nursing, 6th ed. New York, Macmillan Co., 1972

10

Psychosocial Growth of Young Adulthood

ETHEL HALE NAUGLE

Young women who stand on the threshold of adulthood are faced with a bewildering array of complex interrelationships in the psychological, social, and cultural spheres. The criteria for mature personality has been defined as the ability to integrate experiences into a stable identity, use knowledge and skills effectively, relate to others in a significant and sensitive manner, assume responsibility, and develop and maintain a life direction that will lead to self-fulfillment [19]. Each adult must meet challenges and choose paths in unexplored areas of life, including sex, love, careers, family, and social groups.

Out of wavering adolescent yearnings must come a definitive sexual identity, an occupation to provide sustenance (physical and emotional), and satisfactory love and social relationships. Women must decide whether or not to marry, select a mate, and decide when, if ever, to have children. They must choose a vocation commensurate with their abilities, interests, and economic reality, and must manage living arrangements and solve economic problems. In sum, they must assume responsibility for their own lives.

A woman's values serve as a major directive in making these life choices and assuming her responsibilities. There are two important factors involved in the values that she holds. She is influenced by her historical past and by her culture. Major components of these factors include myths, religion, and psychology.

HISTORICAL PERSPECTIVES OF FEMALE BEHAVIOR

Throughout history, women have been set apart from their fathers, brothers, and husbands, not only because of their different anatomy, but also because of the beliefs that people held. From earliest times, women were thought to possess some dark, mysterious force. If a man bled, he was hurt, or ill. Conversely, blood issued from a woman's body every month, yet she was not ill.

Myths grew and were told and retold. Here was this strange creature—woman. It was she who brought evil into the world. Pandora pried the lid off a secret chest and let out the miseries to bedevil man. Eve munched on a forbidden apple, generously offered a bite to her mate, and as a result God threw both of them out of Paradise. Delilah sheared off Samson's locks and robbed him of his power. Women accused of witchcraft and consorting with the devil were hunted during the middle ages and burned at the stake [16]. So from earliest times, woman was portrayed as a weak, deceitful creature who could bring great harm to man. In spite of this, she was also worshipped because of her powers as a goddess of fertility, the giver of life [11]. Women seemed to possess some power over life that men did not have. While she could seduce and destroy him, she could also bring forth new life.

If myth set the stage, religion wrote the play. The first act starts with Paul and his letters to the Corinthians emphasizing woman's rightful place, subject to man, under his domination. The early Church fathers continued Paul's teachings. Woman was different; she had her place as a submissive and obedient servant to her master. First, she owed allegiance to God, then to father, then to husband, and finally to her son. Not only was she different, but around her there hovered that odor—that taint of evil. As Tertullian, an early churchman put it, woman was, if awakened to her nature, "junua diaboli," "the devil's door." [6]

In the next act, psychology enters: Freud, Adler, Jung, Erikson, and others who focused on personality development. Freud, prowling the labyrinths of the inner world, decided that woman suffered from envy. She envied man not his role, but his penis!

Freud postulated that stages of development occur psychologically. The growing person passes through successive psychological stages of development just as with physical development. These stages are related to instinctive centers rather than to conscious ones. Adler saw the individual as striving to overcome his helpless beginning and gain superiority. Jung believed in a collective unconscious, a collection of myths which form the genetic heritage of all human beings. In all of these frameworks, the focus was on the individual's development of personality.

According to Erikson, the healthy personality masters the environment, exhibits a unity of personality, and perceives the world and self in perspective. In early adult stages, the person begins to nurture and guide the next generation. The healthy personality finally arrives at a meaningful old age in which wisdom and integrity, rather than despair, are the results of mastering each of the successive stages of life in a satisfactory fashion. Thus, Erikson moved beyond Freud to see a continuing process of development during the life cycle [8].

Many psychologists focused their efforts on understanding how learning takes place. Their approach took different perspectives. One group, the Behaviorists, studied changes in behavior as demonstrations of learning. Others measured learning by changes in perception, attention span, thought development, and motivation. Yet another perspective is suggested by Murray Bowen who explains individual behavior as being molded by the family system. For example, he believes that in families of persons who suffer from schizophrenia a faulty type of learning can be identified and traced back through the family tree [4].

All of these mythical, religious, and psychological perspectives contribute to ideas we form about ourselves. While we may intellectually reject a myth or idea, we may still incorporate the attitude it generates. Whether or not we individually accept these ideas, we still must cope with society's acceptance of them.

Traditional beliefs that woman is evil, unclean, magical, and inferior have long influenced her self-esteem as well as her position in society. Until the myths can be separated from reality, women will have to struggle with them in order to fulfill their potential.

CURRENT PERSPECTIVES OF FEMALE BEHAVIOR

Currently there is an interest in developing a more realistic explanation of the differences between male and female behaviors. Some areas of investigation include the effect of socialization. Other aspects focus more on physical processes, such as the role of hormones and the structure and function of the brain. Further understandings of adult psychological development will also aid in explaining female behavior.

Dr. Paul MacLean offers his description of the human brain. He conceives it as being three separate structures operating as a unit he calls the triune brain. He says, "The three sub-brains might be regarded as biological computers, each with its own special form of subjectivity, intelligence, time measuring, memory, motor and other functions" [14]. (Figure 10-1.)

The most primitive structure (or reptilian brain) programs instinctual forms of behavior—those based on ancestral memories and learning. In animals, this "alligator brain" dictates stereotyped sex-mating behavior. For example, the copulatory act can be triggered in tom turkeys by a phantom—the dummy head of a hen turkey. Other dummy-induced behaviors are aggressive display, fighting, and flight-following reactions [14].

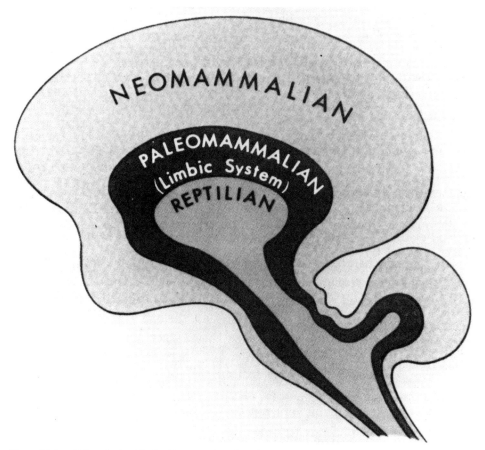

Figure 10-1.   Triune brain. Used with permission of Paul D. MacLean from A Triune Concept of Brain and Behavior. Toronto, Canada, University of Toronto Press, 1973.

The second brain, which is called limbic, meaning "forming a border around," is described by Dr. MacLean as "Nature's attempt to provide the reptilian brain with a 'thinking cap.' " Within this limbic system are centers of emotional feelings and behaviors that assure self-preservation. Here also are located feelings related to sociability, procreation, and preservation of the species [14].

The last and most complicated brain is the neocortex, which in humans culminates in reading, writing, and arithmetic skills. It, along with the other two brains, receives sensations, images, and chemicals from many other stations located throughout the body. Secretions from the hormone systems act to trigger many complex activities of growth and development.

Does this mean then that the rush of hormones generated at puberty spark activity in the limbic system or within the "alligator brain?" Is the giggling, the endless preening of hair, the phonitis of the pubescent female merely a form of courting behavior, stereotyped and programmed in the primitive center? Perhaps so, but no one has yet proved it in regard to humans.

Many studies of women have been conducted in an attempt to find links between behavior and hormone levels. Few women would argue that mood changes do occur during the monthly cycle. However, it is wise to be cautious in assigning such changes to the power outage of one hormone.

John Money states that hormones are only one of the influences on the brain. Other factors including olfactory, visual or tactile stimuli also affect behavior [16]. Thus, it seems that many complex interactions including physical, psychological, and cultural elements contribute to these mood changes. It is unlikely that a woman is the pawn of her hormones—being pushed, pulled, and tormented by mysterious surges and fadings.

Few writers have examined the impact of television or the pervasive themes of advertising on directing and defining women's roles. A casual perusal of magazines and television ads will show one theme, repeated endlessly. Every task should be *easy*, completed quickly. From jiffy patterns to minute steak, the woman is instructed that she should make as little effort as possible. A woman is seldom encouraged by the media to learn and develop difficult skills. Why is it that so many women with good intellectual potential accomplish so little as measured by our society's standards?

The message is relayed that the only plausible roles for women are the perfect lover, wife, mother, and hostess. These roles are said to be accomplished on an instinctual level requiring minimal thought. Within the framework of the triune brain, it is almost as if women have never developed the neocortex. Whatever the reference point, women in our society have not traditionally been actively encouraged to develop intellectual skills.

Adult Issues and Decisions

Time brings change in many ways, including societal attitudes and values. In our society this is beginning to be reflected in a wider choice of possibilities for women to develop their potential. These choices revolve around career, family issues, sexuality, and community commitments.

Career. Psychologists postulate that in our culture females are put into a "Catch

22″ position. They are taught from birth to be nice. Passive/dependent behavior is rewarded, while independence and aggressiveness are discouraged. Dependency is not a quality that leads to achievement, yet women are then criticized for not achieving [5].

Bardwick characterizes this passivity as helpless choicelessness. She suggests that it may be a coping mechanism in response to cultural expectations [2]. Hyde wrote that many women who were successful attributed their success to causes outside their own efforts, such as to luck or ease of task. They apparently did not give credit to their own effort and ability [11].

Traditionally, women who have worked outside the home have chosen careers as nurses, teachers, or secretaries. Careers in law, medicine, or politics have been considered to be for men. The value a society places on a career is reflected in wages, self-esteem, and respect. In our society, male-dominated careers are highly valued while women's careers fall much lower on the value scale.

Careers designated as acceptable for women have traditionally been extensions of the nurturing role that was expected of them. The idea this presents is that if a woman is going to work she should at least retain her femininity. The aggressiveness and intellectual discipline needed to succeed in the male careers were thought to be incompatible with characteristics associated with femininity [5]. These ideas still prevail in our society [17].

Another difficulty for women trying to succeed in male careers is a scarcity of role models. Studies indicate that a factor leading to success is direction from a mentor. As women strive for and reach highly valued positions, they increase their own confidence. The demonstration of their competence provides a role model for others to follow [18].

Family Choices. At some point a woman will decide whether or not to get married and whether or not to have children. In the past, marriage and family were not so much choice as expectation. A woman's domain became house and children. As compensation for assuming these responsibilities she would receive companionship, financial support, and sexual fulfillment. For her, there was no need for higher education or career development.

Today, with increasing economic pressures on the family, the choice of staying home or working becomes a moot point. Most women in America will work, either because of economic necessity or to provide their children with what are considered niceties—music lessons, swimming pool membership, or college education. This stark reality is frequently ignored by parents, by counselors, and by college advisors. Thus, while men have accepted that they will spend the major portion of their lives working outside the home, women have not been prepared to deal with this reality.

In trying to come to terms with family and career decisions, women will grapple with issues such as these: Will this career mesh with my mate's? Will it afford me the option of having children, home, and family, or does it demand all of my time and energy? If it demands a high degree of competence (as do the physical sciences) and is competitive with males, will it limit my choices for marriage partners? Often, the balance is tipped in favor of a less demanding job or career which will be more readily adaptable to home and family life. In addition, it will fit more closely with the expectations of society.

Reality soon jars young women who believe that it is easy to have children and to work. Popular magazines as well as scientific journals have devoted much space to the motherhood–career conflict, but few address the crux of that problem. There are monumental difficulties in arranging for satisfactory child care. In addition, combining career and family requires a dual commitment with extraordinary effort expended over a very long period of time.

A woman who works often retains the full measure of her home and child care responsibilities. She frequently becomes dissatisfied with her accomplishments in both areas and spends much of her precious store of energy trying to do the impossible, that is, to be in two places at one time. Conflicts between fulfilling her role as wife, as mother and as career person may threaten at times to engulf any conscientious woman.

Although many women who juggle career and family responsibilities become overwhelmed at times, research shows that they also claim the highest level of life satisfaction. Baruch and Barnett's study shows, in fact, that women's satisfaction with life seems related to job prestige rather than husband and children. Those who reported most dissatisfaction were single women holding low prestige jobs and married women without children or career [3]. Apparently women who hold a variety of responsibilities also find creative ways to cope.

Partners who decide to share in wage earning are beginning to realize that they must also share more fully in the tasks of householding and child care. Such task-sharing requires a willingness to sacrifice some measure of individuality in order to serve mutual goals. In such sharing, the woman who gives up some of her traditional responsibility for running the home must learn to be appreciative and uncritical of her partner's efforts. All too often, a sincere attempt to help is squelched by criticism that the chore was not done "properly" (i.e., "my way").

A legitimate concern of working mothers revolves around the safety, dependability, and quality of child care. There aren't enough grandmothers or neighborhood babysitters around who fit these qualifications. This problem has mushroomed as more and more women have been economically forced to go to work. Licensing of low-cost day care centers and cooperative nursery schools is needed.

Many women today are choosing an alternate lifestyle to that of marriage and family. The woman who remains single may be envied for some of her freedom and carefree life. While it may be true that she is unhampered by family responsibilities, it is also true that she must look elsewhere to fulfill her needs for love and companionship. She must also provide for her own financial needs, both present and future.

Sexuality. A woman's sexuality is her female behavior. While some define this as a drive to reproduce, it actually encompasses a much broader meaning. Sexuality is expressed in the way a woman walks, talks, dresses, and relates to others. These relationships, whether with males or other females, may be of a physical or emotional nature.

Physical expressions of sexuality may be of a heterosexual, homosexual or bisexual nature. Some women may choose to remain or will become sexually autonomous or celibate. Many speculations exist regarding one's sexual preference. These include prenatal influences, hormonal causes, early parenting, or childhood and adolescent experiences. In addition, societal judgments are imposed as to which orientation is right or wrong.

Despite all the research and arguments, no one has yet been able to determine a conclusive cause for human variations in sexual preference. What does seem to be agreed upon is that there are two components to genital sex. There is both emotional and physical involvement.

Regarding physical sexual response, Masters and Johnson report that:

> When a man or woman is orgasmic, he or she is responding to sexual stimuli with the same basic physiologic response patterns regardless of whether the stimulative technique is masturbation, partner manipulation, fellatio/cunnilingus, vaginal or rectal coitus—and also regardless of whether the sexual partner is of the same or opposite gender [15].

The emotional needs of a woman will be met within a sexual relationship that is consistent with her individual psychological makeup. Thus, it becomes meaningless to judge and to place expectations on other peoples' right to choose sexual orientation.

For all women the sexual drive continues throughout life; however, initial choices or forms of expressing sexuality may change. Changes may result for a variety of reasons, including separation from a partner (death, war, illness, divorce), disability of self or partner (disease, impairment of sexual function, injury or loss of body parts), or change in emotional needs or status. Adjustments to these changes may be made within the existing relationship, by forming a new relationship, or by rejection of any primary sexual relationship. Whether homosexual, bisexual or heterosexual, all women may find themselves, at some time, confronted with these issues.

Community Commitment. During the early adult years, a woman's major focus is often on beginning the development of a family or career or both. Community involvement is likely to be restricted to activities that complement her focus. She may assume leadership roles in scouting and 4-H activities, PTA, church and Sunday school. Time is also spent participating in women's and homemakers' clubs, car pooling, and cooperative babysitting arrangements. These and other activities support community need as well as provide for personal development, whether the direction is career or family.

As families grow up and careers become more established, women find that more time is available to them. They begin to reach out in many different directions to satisfy their need for self-growth. These directions assume different forms.

One form of this "reaching out" is in additional community involvement. Some women find satisfaction through volunteer activities in institutions such as hospitals and charitable organizations. Other women prefer receiving wages for their working time, either because of economic need or for personal satisfaction. Finally, some women become actively involved in political or professional organizations. Whatever form the social activity takes, it is almost as if the woman is returning to society some of its investment in her.

WOMEN AND THE FUTURE

In the past, challenges and adult responsibilities women faced were predetermined and defined by society. Roles society designated for women were clear, although limited and not always desired. The women's movement increased the awareness of these limitations and of the hidden dissatisfaction of many women with the status quo. Women began to make it clear that they resented being considered inately inferior.

One of the results of the group effort of the women's movement is that women now have a wider range of possibilities from which to determine and define their own lives. However, transition is often accompanied by problems. Although more choices are available, career planning is a skill that must be learned. Old familiar roles at least represent security, whereas new, untried domains may be threatening and uncertain. Women who want to advance, particulary in professional fields, will find few role models or mentors available to help. Finally, some women choosing a more traditional role feel guilty because they are not "developing" their potential [18].

Another outcome of the women's movement has been the polarization of two groups. One group prefers to maintain the traditional roles previously determined by society. They fear that change will disrupt the family unit and undermine our social structure. The other group feels that the family unit is strengthened by recognition of women's equality. The idea is that a woman who feels good about herself and her accomplishments will instill these same characteristics in her children [17].

The differences between the traditional and the newly emerging groups represent more than a simple philosophical conflict. The issues have far-reaching political ramifications in terms of economics, education, health care, career advancement, and other social matters. Thus, these concerns are vitally important to all.

Many women seem to be unwilling to acknowledge that the women's movement has touched their lives. They maintain this tunnel vision despite their right to vote, pursue a college education, receive more equal wages, and compete for professional positions. Others grow complacent about women's progress towards equality, feeling that their small "enlightened" group is representative of the whole. Unless women recognize the need for continued group action toward fuller recognition of their equal status, they may find that they support efforts that will destroy their own self-esteem [17].

Many of the developmental issues facing young adult women are currently unknown or poorly defined. It is hoped that continued research of these developmental patterns will provide frameworks of approach for purposes of education and intervention. In the mean time, it is important for nurses to be aware of concerns that women confront, both personally and socially, the conflicts created by these concerns, and the transitions that they will experience. Education, support, role modeling, and reassurance are useful nursing interventions for managing the confusion that this stage of life may bring.

REFERENCES

1. Astin H, Suniewick N, Dweck S: Women: A Bibliography on Their Education and Careers. Washington, DC, Human Services Press, 1971
2. Bardwick JM: Psychology of Women: A Study of Bio-cultural Conflicts. New York, Harper and Row, 1971
3. Bourne LE, Jr., Ekstrand BR: Psychology, Its Principles and Meanings. New York, Holt, Reinhart, and Winston, 1973

4. Bowen M: Family Therapy in Clinical Practice. New York, Jason Aronson, 1978
5. Broverman IK: Sex role stereotypes and clinical judgments of mental health. Journal of Consulting Clinical Psychology, 34, February 1970
6. Campbell J: The Masks of God: Creative Mythology. New York, Viking Press, 1970
7. Craig GJ: Human Development. Englewood Cliffs, NJ, Prentice-Hall, 1976
8. Erikson EH: Childhood and Society, 2nd ed. New York, W. W. Norton, 1963
9. Freiberg KL: Human Development. North Scituate, MA, Duxbury Press, 1979
10. Hill WF: Learning, A Survey of Psychological Interpretations. Scranton, PA, Chandler Publishing Co., 1971
11. Hyde JS, Rosenberg RG: The Psychology of Women: Half the Human Experience, 2nd ed. Lexington, MA, D. C. Heath, 1980
12. Kundsin RB: Women and Success: The Anatomy of Achievement. New York, William Morrow, 1974
13. Maccoby EE, Jacklin CN: The Psychology of Sex Difference. Stanford, CA, Stanford University Press, 1974
14. MacLean PD: A Triune Concept of Brain and Behavior (Chapter One). Toronto, Canada, University of Toronto Press, 1973
15. Masters WH, Johnson VE: Homosexuality in Perspective. Boston, MA, Little, Brown, and Company, 1979
16. Money J, Zubin J: Contemporary Sexual Behaviors: Critical Issues in the 1970s. Baltimore, MD, Johns Hopkins University Press, 1972
17. Rivers C, Barnett R, Baruch G: Beyond Sugar and Spice. New York, G. P. Putnam's Sons, 1979
18. Stevens-Long J: Adult Life Developmental Processes. Los Angeles, CA, Mayfield Publishing Co., 1979
19. Wolman BB: Handbook of General Psychology. Englewood Cliffs, NJ, Prentice-Hall, 1973

Section V

ADULT WOMAN:
MENOPAUSE AND BEYOND

11

Physical Changes Related to Aging

Susan Shreve McCarter

Part I—Menopause

The word menopause, from the Greek words meaning "month" and "cessation," means the permanent end of menstrual flow. The ceasing of menstruation, however, is only one of the events of the menopausal process. The entire period of transition is called the climacteric, from Greek words meaning "rung of the ladder." The climacteric is divided into the premenopausal, menopausal and postmenopausal periods. The term for the entire timespan is perimenopause.

In the latter half of the nineteenth century, gynecology textbooks described menopause as an illness, and menopausal and postmenopausal women were treated as invalids. Women in the nineteenth century were considered inherently frail. The "scientific" reasoning used to support this idea was the so-called "conservation of energy law." According to this "law" the human body contained a set quantity of energy which was used by each organ and body function [14].

Women supposedly expended a great deal of their total energy supply on menstruation and childbearing functions. They were thus advised not to squander any energy on mental, athletic, or sexual pursuits. When menopause arrived, they were thought to have used so much energy in reproduction that their doctors ordered them to bed. Invalidism in later life, so frequently seen in nineteenth century upperclass women, could be considered a result of improper budgeting of energy during childbearing years. This certainly kept women away from studying, participating in athletics, or even much interest in sex!

More recently, the climacteric was considered a deficiency disease. With the discovery in the 1920s of estrogen and its function in the female reproductive system, the idea of replacing the deficient hormone during menopause was born. Certain adherents to this theory advised beginning a woman on estrogen replacement in her premenopausal years and continuing the hormone throughout her entire life.

One proponent of the deficiency disease theory was Dr. Robert Wilson whose book *Feminine Forever* was read by millions of women. They were promised escape from "the horrors of this living decay" and came to look on estrogen as a means of preventing symptoms of aging [21]. By 1975, millions of women in the United States were being "treated" for menopause with estrogen therapy.

In 1975, research results were published which linked estrogen replacement therapy with endometrial cancer. This research, and more recent studies which seem to confirm it, has stimulated a reevaluation of estrogen therapy by both the medical profession and women. The theory of the climacteric as a deficiency disease is no longer accepted by most medical experts.

Few gynecologists today would suggest estrogen to an asymptomatic menopausal woman. Additionally, social scientists, perhaps encouraged by the women's movement, are reexamining the status of the older woman in today's society. It is now widely recognized that menopause is not only part of a biological process, but that sociocultural factors also influence this period in a woman's life.

Spontaneous, gradual, functional decline of the female reproductive system is normal. The majority of women (80–85 percent) have either no signs of menopause or have minor discomfort with which they can easily cope. About 15–20 percent require intervention for relief of severe symptoms [15]. For these reasons the term "symptoms" will be used only when referring to menopause-related problems which require medical intervention. Since menopause is not an illness, the terms "signs" or "indications" will refer more accurately to changing body processes and their manifestations. It is important to remember that although reproductive function ceases, sexual function does not.

In the United States, spontaneous menopause may occur from ages forty-one to fifty-nine years, with forty-seven to fifty-two being the most frequent age span, and fifty as the average age. In the 1920s, Dr. Alan Treolar began a linear study which conclusively shows that there is no correlation between age at menarche and age at menopause [19]. Therefore, a woman cannot predict an early menopause because she had an early puberty.

There are two approaches for determining the time span of the climacteric. Physiologically, it is measured from the first early signs of menstrual irregularities (usually during the forties) until a year after the last menstrual period. This timespan may cover ten to fifteen years. More commonly, menopause is considered to begin a year or two before cessation of menses when dramatic manifestations first appear, and to end shortly after menstrual periods cease. With this last definition, the span of menopause is four to five years.

Surgical menopause occurs at any age as a result of removal of both ovaries. This is often done in association with hysterectomy and removal of the tubes for treatment of pelvic infection, endometriosis or cancer. The problems these women face are physically more severe and socially different.

PHYSIOLOGY OF MENOPAUSE

As with the other reproductive processes throughout life, the physical events associated with menopause are directed by the endocrine system. In some ways, these endocrine events can be viewed as a reversal of those that occur during puberty. The physical changes, of course, are not as dramatic.

Changes related to menopause begin at the hypothalamic level. For some unknown reason, the sensitivity of the hypothalamus to estrogen begins to decline. This results in an interruption of its positive feedback system with estrogen. In turn, the anterior pituitary release of FSH and LH will reflect the altered hypothalamic release of LH-RH. Of course, this will affect the ovarian production of estrogen as well as ovulation. The less frequent ovulation results in changing estrogen levels, which further interferes with hypothalamic function.

The fluctuating hormone levels bring about the physical manifestations commonly associated with menopause. It is possible that if the hormonal decline is gradual and steady, the woman will notice fewer unpleasant symptoms. It is known that women with abrupt, surgical menopause following bilateral oophorectomy have more severe symptoms of hormone deficiency than women experiencing a more gradual, natural decline.

It has become clear that menopause is not caused by ovarian "shutdown." Instead, the ovarian and other physical manifestations are reflections of changes in the hypothalamus and pituitary. Production of estradiol by the ovary gradually declines and extragonadal sources of estrogen become increasingly available. These sources include the adrenal cortex, fatty tissue, and the brain.

A review of the previous ideas will show two main thoughts. The first is that there will be specific physical changes at the menopause in relation to changing hormone patterns. The second is that a woman's production of estrogen continues after menopause. The importance of this is that many changes once thought to be directly related to estrogen deficiency are now considered part of the normal aging process that occurs for everyone.

In keeping with these ideas, we will first discuss reproductive system changes specifically related to menopause. We will then briefly review more general changes associated with aging. Because of the time-overlap of these two processes, their associated signs are not always so clearly delineated.

Physical Changes of Menopause

Since menopause is not a specific event but an ongoing process, early changes that occur are referred to as premenopause signs. The completion of menopause is recognized in retrospect. If more than a year has elapsed since the last menstrual period, the woman is said to be postmenopausal.

Breast changes. With the hormonal fluctuations and high peaks of estrogen, the breasts at times become engorged and painful. Changes occur in the glandular network and there is an increase in subcutaneous fat.

Ovaries. Changes in structure and function of the ovaries occur with menopause. Ovulation becomes more sporadic as the ovary becomes less sensitive to gonadotropins. For this same reason, when ovulation does occur there is often incomplete development or early failure of the corpus luteum with a resultant decline in progesterone. The ovary decreases in size and is rarely palpable in a postmenopausal woman.

Uterus. The changing estrogen and progesterone levels are reflected in the endometrium. The result is that premenopausal menstrual periods often cannot be definitely predicted. They may be scanty and infrequent, heavy and frequent, and some women maintain their same menstrual pattern throughout this time. Clearly, menstrual patterns will vary from one woman to another during the premenopausal years.

As described in chapter 18, irregular bleeding may also be due to underlying pathology. Since many pathological conditions may occur during this same time period, it is important to note bleeding patterns and report them to a physician.

Vasomotor. The most common vasomotor response is the hot flash or flush. The typical hot flash is a feeling of great warmth from the chest to the scalp, which may be accompanied by a flushing of the skin and perspiration. The flash may be followed by a chilling sensation, and cold clammy skin. It has been estimated that about two-thirds of premenopausal women experience hot flashes, with about 10 percent severe enough to prompt the woman to seek relief.

The perception of hot flashes is very individual. Some women are acutely embarrassed and are sure that it is readily apparent to everyone that they are having a hot flash. Others are able to take them in stride. From this difference in perception and feeling it should not be construed that the hot flashes are psychosomatic in origin. The causal factor is the disturbed equilibrium of the hypothalamic-pituitary-ovarian axis and its resultant effect on the autonomic nervous system is dilation of the cutaneous blood vessels, especially those above the waist.

The hot flashes may begin a short while before menopause and continue for one to five years after cessation of menses, although there are women who report experiencing them into their seventies and eighties. They are occasionally seen at other ages and with other physical conditions, but generally hot flashes appear only during the climacteric. The average hot flash lasts only seconds, with one minute usually being the upper limit. A woman may experience them a few times a day, or several times an hour. They do seem to increase in frequency and strength with emotional distress, hot weather, too much clothing, increased physical activity, and during illness.

Hot flashes seem to be more uncomfortable when they occur at night. They cause the woman to awaken, hot and sweaty, and throw off her covers. Sometimes she sweats so profusely that it is necessary for her to change her bed linen. The insomnia that menopausal women frequently complain of is most likely attributable to hot flashes rather than to an estrogen deficiency.

Other vasomotor disturbances seen with the hot flashes or in place of them are palpitations, numbness and tingling of the extremities, cold hands and feet, and a peculiar sensation on the skin. This skin sensation is often described as the feeling of crawling ants and is known as formication. Many women do not know that these all may be part of menopause vasomotor response. Instead, they may imagine that they have heart trouble or a serious disease instead of menopausal signs that will eventually cease spontaneously.

Both vascular (migraine) and tension headaches occur during the premenopausal years just as they do before this time. Vascular headaches seem to be related to estrogen in that they usually disappear after menopause. They will reoccur or continue if estrogen replacement therapy is given. The exact relationship between estrogens and migraines is not clear. Tension headaches may be relieved by analgesics and alleviation of the tension.

ESTROGEN REPLACEMENT THERAPY AND ALTERNATIVES

Until late 1975, estrogen replacement therapy (ERT) was employed by many physicians to relieve most of the physical and psychological symptoms of menopause. Some physicians even advised ERT as preventive therapy for all pre- and postmenopausal women. Those subscribing to the theory that menopause was a deficiency disease felt that ERT was necessary from menopause to death. Drug companies advertised in medical journals that ERT was helpful not only for recognized estrogen deficiency symptoms but also for depression, anxiety and fatigue.

One advertisement showed a dull-looking, unhappy woman and her handsome, concerned husband with the caption reading, "For her symptoms that bother *him* the most." Not only did physicians and drug companies push estrogen, but women themselves asked for treatment as soon as they reached forty. Didn't the book say they could be "feminine forever?" Large numbers of middle and upperclass women in the United States, the group who could afford frequent visits to physicians, were taking estrogen prior to the cancer studies.

In 1975 the *New England Journal of Medicine* published two retrospective studies on the relationship between exogenous estrogen and endometrial cancer [15, 22]. The studies showed that women who took estrogen during their climacteric years had a five- to fifteen-fold increase in the incidence of cancer of the endometrium when compared to women who did not take estrogen.

Since these studies, and others published following them, the rationale for ERT has changed considerably in regard to symptoms relieved by estrogen, contraindications, dosages, and the length of time estrogen is to be used. The Food and Drug Administration has published special warnings with accompanying information for patients. The National Institutes of Health conducted a consensus meeting on estrogen replacement therapy in September, 1979.

Combining the recommendations by the Food and Drug Administration and the National Institutes of Health, the following regime for ERT is presently suggested:

• ERT should be used only to relieve hot flashes.

• After oophorectomy, ERT should be employed to make the transition from normal to low estrogen more gradual.

• Estrogen should be prescribed in the lowest dosages to relieve the symptoms, and for the shortest length of time necessary. Reevaluation of therapy should take place every six months.

• Women with contraindications for the use of oral contraceptives or who give a history of estrogen-related problems that worsened during pregnancy should not be given ERT.

• ERT should not be employed longer than three years, unless given for osteoporosis. In osteoporosis, an orthopedic assessment should be made before prescribing estrogen. The NIH physicians deliberated over the trade-off between the risk of endometrial cancer and the debilitating effects of osteoporosis. They advised that for women with preliminary signs of osteoporosis, estrogen therapy was the lesser risk.

• Any vaginal bleeding during ERT should be evaluated immediately. The NIH physicians discussed the prudence of taking a sample of the endometrium to evaluate it for hyperplasia and cancer. They reported that this should be done by endometrial biopsy or suction curettage on all women taking estrogen, bleeding or not, at least once a year.

• ERT should not be employed to relieve emotional symptoms. The NIH report agreed that improvement in emotional well-being does accompany ERT, but suggested that it was related to alleviation of the physical symptoms.

One of the more recent developments in ERT is the addition of progestins for several days of the estrogen cycle. This produces endometrial shedding and has been shown in at least one study to provide protection against endometrial cancer [5]. The FDA labeling advises against progestins. The NIH Consensus Report, although admitting such protection possibly does exist, urges caution. To date, no consensus agreement has been reached about the use of progestin/estrogen therapy. However, many physicians now add progestins to ERT feeling that this reduces the problems associated with unopposed estrogen on the endometrium.

There is no convincing evidence that estrogen alone increases the risk of thromboemboli, stroke, or heart disease in menopausal women. Recently one study seemed to indicate an increase in breast cancer in menopausal women taking estrogen, but other studies do not show this risk [13]. There is evidence that gallbladder disease does increase in women taking estrogen during the climacteric [3].

Both the FDA, in its physician and patient labeling, and the NIH Consensus Report agree that the decision to take estrogen for menopausal symptoms should be a joint one between the woman and her physician. A woman should know all the possible risks and be able to make her decision based on benefit versus risk. She should also be aware that not everything is known about the subject of ERT and that much additional information is still needed.

There are two types of estrogen preparations available for treatment of menopausal symptoms. There are the so-called natural compounds extracted from the urine of pregnant mares, and the synthetic preparations approximating natural estrogen. In the United States, the "natural" conjugated estrogen manufactured by the Ayerst Laboratories called Premarin (PREgnant MAre's uRINe) accounts for over 90 percent of the market. Estrogens are also available in combination with androgens or tranquilizers although the value of these preparations has not been determined.

The usual regime is 0.3mg or 0.625mg daily for three weeks, followed by one week's rest. If progestin is prescribed it is taken during the third week of estrogen, in which case menstrual shedding will occur during the week's rest. The most common side effects of estrogen are nausea, breast swelling and tenderness, endometrial hyperplasia, headaches, enlargement of uterine fibroids, liver disease and increased risk of liver adenomas, fluid retention, skin rash or chloasma, or both, hair loss, and inability to use contact lenses. Estrogen replacement therapy many aggravate asthma, epilepsy, migraine headaches, cardiac or liver disease [3].

Until recently, alternatives to the use of estrogen for relief of menopausal symptoms were rare. Even today when women ask for other, nonhormonal ways to relieve their symptoms, not much information is available. For women whose main complaint is nighttime hot flashes, Bellergal®, which is a combination of phenobarbital, ergotamine, and belladonna derivatives, may help.

Use of vitamins and minerals to relieve menopausal problems is increasing, although valid research findings that support their effectiveness are lacking. A great many books on women's health, often written by nonmedical people, discuss natural treatments of menopausal symptoms, especially hot flashes. With the understanding that many of these treatments are empirical, we shall discuss some of these alternative preparations.

Many women claim that Vitamin E has given some relief, especially for hot flashes. Seaman and Seaman in *Women and the Crisis in Sex Hormones* claim it works by preventing too much FSH and LH production [14]. The dosages they suggest are much higher than the recommended daily allowance. The Seamans suggest beginning with 100 IU's (30 IU's is the recommended daily allowance) and increasing up to 600 IU's a day for short periods as necessary to relieve the symptoms. The vitamin should be taken after a meal containing fat or with lecithin, which contains fatty acids to help ensure absorption from the GI tract. Women with heart problems, high blood pressure, or diabetes probably should not use this treatment.

B complex vitamins are thought by some to help relieve depression, stress symptoms, and headaches. There are on the market today several "stress formula" B complex preparations that contain high levels of vitamins B and C. Vitamin D and calcium may slow down postmenopausal bone loss. Calcium is available as calcium lactate, calcium carbonate or calcium gluconate. It may also be combined with magnesium as in dolomite, or with phosphorus and other minerals as in bone meal. Seaman also claims that calcium and Vitamin D taken at bedtime have a mild sedative effect [14].

Nurses have long been familiar with the effectiveness of education and therapeutic listening. These two techniques are just as useful as intervention with the woman experiencing menopausal difficulties as they are in other situations. Being able to talk about her problems as well as learning about this normal process may help decrease a woman's anxiety. In addition, women should be encouraged to share their experiences and feelings with each other and with family members.

CONTRACEPTION DURING PREMENOPAUSE

Contraception should be used until the woman has experienced one, and some suggest two, complete years without a menstrual period [4]. Ovulation in the years approaching menopause is frequently sporadic and the eggs produced may have chromosomal changes. If one of these eggs is fertilized, it may result in spontaneous abortion, stillbirth, or abnormalities such as Down's Syndrome. In addition, because of factors related to aging, pregnancy at this time is related to a higher incidence of maternal complications [5]. The sexually active woman should be aware of these menopausal risk factors. She can then take them into account during earlier years of family planning as well as with contraceptive planning during this time.

• Because of associated risk factors, the birth control pill is not acceptable as a contraceptive method for women over forty.

• The IUD is also not a recommended form of contraception for premenopausal women. Since IUD's often cause irregular bleeding, a woman of this age may mistakenly attribute intermenstrual bleeding to her IUD and thus dismiss a warning of a serious problem.

- Because of irregular ovulation at this time, rhythm may be an unreliable contraceptive.
- The barrier methods of diaphragm, spermicidal jelly or foam, and condoms are the safest methods of contraception for premenopausal women.
- Sterilization for both men and women is available and becoming increasingly popular. Currently in the United States, sterilization is the most common method of fertility control for couples over thirty [7]. A woman may wish to discuss with her partner whether tubal ligation or vasectomy best suits their needs. For a more detailed discussion of contraception see chapter 14.

Part II—Beyond Menopause

Growth and development bring changes to all people during a lifetime. An early obvious developmental change occurs at puberty with the onset of women's reproductive capability. Later, menopause is another signal of ongoing development. Advancing years bring gradual changes both to the reproductive system and to the rest of the body. These changes are influenced by hormonal, genetic, and environmental factors.

Breasts. Fat deposits in the breasts begin to diminish as do both the stroma and the gland field. These changes may result in the breasts assuming a pendulous shape. Pigmentation of the nipple and areola is lessened and erectile tissue becomes somewhat less responsive.

Vulva. The mons and labia become less prominent from loss of fatty deposits. Pubic hair thins and decreases and the skin becomes thinner. Eventually there may be lessened muscle tone in the perineal body, and urinary and anal sphincters. This will result in some degree of urinary or fecal incontinence. There does not seem to be a diminishing of clitoral sensitivity [10].

Vagina. The vaginal epithelium becomes thinner, the rugae disappear, and there is a loss of elasticity of the muscle and connective tissue. The vaginal canal is somewhat dryer because of decreased vascularity and a reduction in cervical secretions. The pH becomes neutral or alkaline, discouraging lactobacillus growth. The alkalinity and thinner vaginal walls make a woman more susceptible to vaginal infections and irritation.

Uterus. The uterine body diminishes in size at a greater rate than does the cervix, reverting the body/cervical ratio to about that at puberty, 1:3 (see Figure 3-14). This is caused by vascular and muscle fiber changes. Although the endometrium is normally nonfunctioning, it remains capable of responding to estrogen throughout life.

Ovaries and tubes. The Fallopian tubes exhibit a loss of tissue folds and villi. The muscle fibers in the walls become thin and constricted. The ovary diminishes in size and becomes nonpalpable. Follicular growth and atresia continue for an indefinite time beyond menopause, although ovulation is rare, since cyclic hormonal support has diminished. Thus estradiol levels decrease, although the ovary continues secreting estrone.

Sexual response. The sexual response cycle occurs in the same four phases as it has before. However, there are some changes related to aging that become apparent. Women experiencing these changes in themselves and their partner may become alarmed if they do not understand the underlying physical process. For a more detailed description of the following phases see chapter 22.

1. *Excitement phase.*

The excitement phase builds more slowly. Vaginal lubrication is lessened in amount and takes longer to achieve. Clitoral response remains much the same, but the labia show less swelling. Nipple erection remains one of the first signs of sexual excitement, but breast enlargement is less pronounced. Muscle tension may be lessened. All of these responses are mirrored in the male with the most obvious change being a longer time to achieve erection.

2. *Plateau phase.*

For women, events of this phase are similar to those of their younger years but the responses are less pronounced. In the male, full erection may not take place until this phase and may be somewhat reduced. There may be lessened or absent pre-ejaculatory fluid.

3. *Orgasmic phase.*

Orgasmic contractions may be fewer in number and less intense. Otherwise the orgasmic phase is similar to that experienced by younger women. For men the experience is also less intense but equally satisfying.

4. *Resolution phase.*

Both men and women rapidly return to the preexcitement phase.

Sexual activity is not age-dependent. It can continue as long as a woman wishes. Just as at other ages, the elderly woman must deal with problems associated with her sexuality. These problems can be primarily biological or psychological. Concern over slower sexual arousal may inhibit a woman and cause her to avoid sexual situations fearing she is abnormal. Education and talking through the problem may be all that is needed to resolve it.

Many times elderly women complain of dyspareunia. The use of a vaginal lubricant, such as K-Y jelly, may provide relief. Because estrogen creams are rapidly absorbed through the vaginal mucosa they are not recommended for relief of dyspareunia. Many women find that regular sexual activity keeps the vagina dilated and lubricated.

Vaginal infections may increase at this time because of the thin walls and altered pH and bacterial flora. Treatment is the same as in the other age groups. However, if the problem is persistently recurrent, an estrogen cream may be indicated to build up the vaginal epithelium.

The support structures of the pelvis lose tone and strength with aging. If these structures have been previously injured through childbirth, rape, gynecological surgery, or any other trauma they become less efficient. As a result the pelvic structures, including the uterus, bladder, and rectum, are displaced downward to varying degrees. The resultant conditions are known as: *cystocele*, the protrusion of the bladder against the weakened anterior vaginal wall causing a bulging into the vagina; *rectocele*, the pressure from the rectum causing a bulging in of the posterior vaginal wall; and *uterine prolapse*, a descending of the uterus into the vagina.

With a cystocele the woman may find that she loses urine when she laughs, coughs, sneezes, or does heavy lifting. She may dribble urine constantly and worry about both hygiene and odor. With a rectocele, the problem may become so severe that a bowel movement can be accomplished only by exerting manual pressure on the posterior vaginal wall. With uterine prolapse, the cervix may become ulcerated.

Kegel's exercise will often help all of these conditions. The woman is instructed to tighten her perineal muscles as if to stop urination or defecation. She repeats this exercise ten to fifteen times, several times a day. This exercise may be done almost any time, anywhere. If the muscle relaxation worsens with age, eventually the Kegel's may no longer help. In these instances surgery may provide the only relief. (See chapter 25.)

General effects of aging. There is much ongoing research concerning the process of aging. Although details are still obscure, it is becoming apparent that many problems previously attributed to aging are treatable disease processes. In other cases, genetic factors are responsible for age-related changes.

Examples of changes currently thought to be related to aging include reduced sensory perception, decreased strength and endurance of skeletal muscle, degenerative changes in elastic and connective tissue, reduced capacity of the cardiovascular and respiratory systems, and a reduction in the regenerative and protective capabilities of the body. As a result of these physiologic changes, aging women experience wrinkling skin, thinning hair (with changing distribution, such as appearance of facial hairs), digestive problems, and a general slowing down. Good health practices, such as proper diet, adequate rest, exercise, and good hygiene, will help prevent disease and minimize the effects of aging.

Osteoporosis is the loss of calcium from bones causing a reduction in bone mass. Both men and women exhibit this calcium loss. However, the process begins ten to fifteen years earlier in women about the time of or shortly before menopause. The first actual symptoms are not usually seen until the postmenopausal years and continue into old age.

Symptoms include back pain, loss of stature, the so-called "dowager's hump" from vertebral compression, and an increase in fractures, especially of the hip. In elderly women these problems can be life-threatening because of the long periods of immobilization necessary for healing with resultant complications such as pneumonia.

At present, it cannot be stated with certainty whether these changes are a result of the natural aging process or of estrogen deficiency. It is true that the process begins much earlier in women, but by age eighty the incidence of osteoporosis is equal in both men and women. In addition 75 percent of postmenopausal women do not ever develop severe symptoms.

Osteoporosis seems to be a result of a combination of factors. These include inadequate calcium and protein intake over many years, insufficient exercise, and the unknown effect of a reduction in steroid levels. Treatment then consists of improved nutrition and establishing an exercise regime. Some physicians prescribe Vitamin D.

As previously mentioned, many physicians feel that estrogen thereapy is a valuable aid in treating osteoporosis. It has been established that ERT will not result in improvement of the condition but may retard its progress. Therefore, the best results from using estrogen therapy are obtained when it is started early. An orthopedic consult should precede initiation of therapy. Contraindications to estrogen use should, of course, be considered.

What aging means to most people is a change, a slowing down, but not a falling apart. The same diseases can be found in the elderly as in the young. Unfortunately, it is easy to dismiss symptoms as being part of the aging process rather than conducting a thorough medical investigation.

Part of the solution to managing the health problems of the elderly person lies in choosing a physician who is interested and skilled in treating older patients. Alex Comfort tells old people to avoid physicians who begin consultations with "Well, of course you *are* . . ." and then mentions the patient's chronological age [2]. The other half of the solution is in the mind-set of the older person. A woman who understands the changes of age, reacts by compensating rather than giving up, and insists on treatment for problems, will continue to lead a rewarding, interesting life well into old age.

REFERENCES

 1. Burnside IM (ed): Nursing and the Aged. New York, McGraw-Hill, 1976
 2. Comfort A: A Good Age. New York, Crown, 1976
 3. Department of Health, Education, and Welfare, Food and Drug Administration: Estrogen Labeling. Federal Register, Vol. 41 No. 190, September 29, 1976
 4. Ehrenreich B, English D: Complaints and disorders. Glass Mountain pamphlet, No. 2, Old Westbury, NY, The Feminist Press, 1973
 5. Hafez ESE, Evans TN (eds): Human Reproduction: Conception and Contraception. Hagerstown, MD, Harper and Row, 1973
 6. Hammond CB et al: Effects of long-term estrogen therapy. American Journal of Obstetrics and Gynecology, Vol. 133 No. 5, March 1, 1979, pp. 525-547
 7. Hatcher RA et al: Contraceptive Technology 1980-1981, 10th ed. New York, Irvington Publishers, 1980
 8. Kart CS, Metress E, Metress J: Aging and Health: Biologic and Social Perspectives. Menlo Park, CA, Addison-Wesley, 1978
 9. Kinsey AC et al: Sexual Behavior in the Human Female. New York, Pocket Books, 1970
10. Masters W, Johnson V: Human Sexual Response. Boston, Little, Brown, and Company, 1966
11. National Institutes of Health Consensus Development Conference Summary; Estrogen Use and Postmenopausal Women. Vol. 2 No. 2, Bethesda, MD, National Institute of Aging, September 13-14, 1979
12. Penjelley ET: Sex and Human Life, 2nd ed. Reading, MA, Addison-Wesley, 1978
13. Ross RK et al: A case-control study of menopausal estrogen therapy and breast cancer. Journal of the American Medical Association, Vol. 243 No. 16, April 25, 1980
14. Seaman B, Seaman G: Women and the Crisis in Sex Hormones. New York, Rawson Associated Publishers, 1977
15. Smith D et al: Association of exogenous estrogen and endometrial carcinoma. New England Journal of Medicine, Vol. 293 No. 23, December 4, 1975, pp. 1164-1167
16. Sloane E: Biology of Women. New York, John Wiley and Sons, 1980
17. Speroff L, Glass RH, Kase NG: Clinical Gynecologic Endocrinology and Infertility, 2nd ed. Baltimore, Williams and Wilkins, 1978
18. Tietze C, Lewitz S: Mortality and fertility control. International Journal of Gynaecology and Obstetrics, Vol. 15 No. 2, 1977, pp. 100-103
19. Treolar AE: Menarche, menopause, and intervening fecundity. Human Biology, Vol. 46 No. 1, February 1974, pp. 89-107

20. U.S. Bureau of Census: Estimates of the population of the U.S. by age, sex, and race. Current Population Reports, Series P-25, No. 721, Washington, DC, 1978
21. Wilson RA: Feminine Forever. New York, M. Evans and Co., 1966
22. Ziel IIK, Finkel W: Increased risk of endometrial carcinoma among users of conjugal estrogens. New England Journal of Medicine, Vol. 293 No. 23, December 4, 1975, pp. 1167-1170

12

Psychosocial Growth in Later Years

Susan Shreve McCarter

Part I—Menopause

Menopause has always been a time of great mystery to women. Unlike other periods in their lives, menopause is not a time women have traditionally shared with one another. They go through this period alone, often denying to themselves and others that anything is wrong. Unlike puberty, marriage, and childbirth, menopause is not marked in any way; it becomes a nonevent. Despite attempts to ignore or deny it, the period of middle age is a period of momentous change, both bodily and socially.

After years of neglect, menopause is at last being recognized as an important event by medicine, sociology, and psychology. One reason is that more women, in fact the vast majority, are living through and beyond menopause. In 1970 there were 22 million women between the ages of forty five and sixty four. That total had increased by another million in just seven years. It is projected that by the year 2010 there will be 36 million women in this age group [2]. In addition, the women's movement of the 1970s has affected women in their middle years as well as younger women. These women have shown their younger sisters that the status of the middle-aged and older woman is in great need of improvement. The spotlight of attention on menopause has sparked discussion, questions, and a great determination to change things.

The unfortunate stereotype of the depressed, anxious, irritable menopausal woman persists in the minds of many—including, unhappily, women themselves as well as their physicians. Some women do notice a heightening of emotional distress during climacteric years. Many cope through an understanding of these symptoms and their causes and with help from supportive family and friends. Some turn to their physicians and are given estrogen, tranquilizers, mood elevators, or combinations of the three. Some seek therapy with psychiatrists, psychologists, and other mental health professionals.

ETIOLOGY OF EMOTIONAL SYMPTOMS

There are several theories about the etiology of emotional "symptoms" during menopause. One, a deficiency disease theory, suggests that the symptoms are caused by decreasing hormone levels. This theory is not currently accepted by most medical authorities. However, some still point to the feeling of "well-being" associated with estrogen as evidence that hormones and emotional symptoms at menopause are somehow related. More research is needed in this area.

Another theory states that emotional symptoms of menopause are psychological in origin. Largely based on Freudian theories of female psychology, this theory states that at menopause the ability to mask or compensate for latent psychologic disturbances is lost. A simplistic explanation of this idea is that the female is a victim of penis envy, which is finally compensated for by motherhood, although she continues to have some latent sense of deficiency and inferiority. When faced with the end of fertility, the woman loses that compensation, and feelings of loss and resentment cause depression and anxiety.

More recently, social scientists have been examining cultural factors and the social roles assigned to women in the United States. The women's movement and many women entering the social sciences have sparked an interest in the sociocultural aspects of menopause. Recent studies on menopause focus on the conditioning of women by our western culture. Women in our culture seem to be programmed to have emotional and psychological problems at menopause.

A most telling indication that culture plays a large part in the emotional problems of middle-aged women is to study them in various other cultures. Dr. Pauline Bart studied the changing status of midlife women in thirty societies around the world. She considered the indications of high status to be increased respect, special privileges, freedom (especially from taboos), and power and influence. In seventeen of these cultures, she found that the status of women went up in middle age, went down in two cultures, and stayed the same in eleven. Whatever the role of women during their fertile years, Dr. Bart found that role was apt to be reversed at menopause [1].

In her study of Rajput women, Marsha Flint found that their status was increased at menopause. These women had little difficulty with, nor did they pay much attention to menopause [14]. Margaret Mead cites Balinese postmenopausal women as being allowed more freedom of speech and activities. They are allowed to attend ceremonies from which they had been barred during their childbearing years. They also are freed from the modesties of speech and action that were required of them in younger years [17]. In China an older woman is called a *lao-nien*, indicating a stage of life where she is at last freed from the control of men; first of her father, then her husband and finally her son. In fact, she often achieves domination over men.

In the U.S., pioneer women were traditionally thought of as being strong, valued and independent. Women of the 1920s and 1930s were also independent compared with later generations. They had lived through World War I and a depression, during which many of them worked to help support their families. Through the years of the Second World War, women again had an important role. Rosie the Riveter was a working woman who had a valued job at good pay. It was she who kept her family together, living in a world in which men, as heads of families, were often absent.

After the war, returning men felt it necessary to reestablish their dominance and they did so by sending the women back to the home. During the late 1940s and 1950s, when most of today's menopausal and postmenopausal women were first entering adulthood, they limited their careers to childrearing and "homemaking.'' The feminine mystique was born.

The birth rate was higher then than in any generation since 1890. Families moved to the suburbs and women became immersed in family life to the exclusion of nearly everything else. The working mother was thought to be depriving her family of proper care and attention. The career woman was considered a neurotic competitor with men, who really just needed a man to dominate her and give her lots of children. During this period of time, marriage and motherhood were considered women's careers.

Once this pattern is accepted, a woman is caught up in a process that will dead end—or so we have traditionally believed. Her reproductive capacity ceases about the time that her children leave home. Essentially, she is forced into an ''early retirement.'' If women experienced depression at this particular time it was assumed to be brought on by regret over the children leaving and so was referred to as the ''empty nest'' syndrome [18].

In fact, studies show that women accept the ''launching'' of their children and menopause with much more equanimity than the ''empty nest'' theory would suggest [18]. Neugarten and Kraines questioned women of all ages about physical and emotional symptoms and found that women in the empty nest period reported high levels of life satisfaction. Neugarten's studies show that women do not report any major disruptions in their lives from menopause [19].

A recent longitudinal study by Baruch and Barnett adds support to Neugarten's conclusions. Their research reports that many women feel their mid years are their best years. At mid life they feel more self-assured and more positive about decision making and their future. Many women seem to feel that after spending their younger years caring for children and a husband, they can fulfill their own dreams [20].

Bart did a study on middle-aged women which gives a more detailed picture of the ''empty nest'' syndrome [2]. It shows that women who are overprotective and overinvolved with their children are more likely to experience menopausal depression. It also shows that society shares the responsibility for creating this depression.

The society which places high priority on the exclusive careers of marriage and motherhood for women, builds a trap for them at middle age. Over and over in Bart's interviews, these women declared their belief that motherhood was a woman's *only* role and that they would be rewarded for being a good mother. They believed in a pay-off and instead they were deserted. Their lives did not turn out the way they expected, and now it was too late. They felt cheated and angry. However, since expressed anger is not considered acceptable behavior for women, these mothers turned the hostility and anger that should have been directed outward, in upon themselves. Depression, rather than aggression, became the response to disappointment and anger [2].

Unlike women in some cultures, ''secure'' and ''coveted'' does not describe the role of the older woman in the United States. Ours is a culture that has valued women for reproduction and nurturing. Applying Bart's theory of reversal, it is not surprising that women past childbearing, no longer nurturing a family, are greatly reduced in status. At no time in recent history has the tendency to limit a woman's role to motherhood been stronger than in the generation of women now in their forties and fifties.

Another value our culture holds for women is that of youth and beauty. Everywhere an American middle-aged woman looks, she is reminded of the importance of being young, or at least looking young. Television commercials talk about moisturizing creams to keep away the wrinkles, hair coloring that cannot be detected, and diets and exercises to keep slim. The models who sell products are young and pretty. Middle-aged women are shown as the nagging mother-in-law or the nosy neighbor or the user of false teeth cleaner.

Furthermore, a double standard exists. Men are seen to improve with age. The forties and fifties in a man's life are seen as his peak years. Gray hair is distinguished in a man; in a woman it is unattractive and a sign of old age. Older men can date younger women and be rewarded with envy and admiration. Women who date or marry younger men are often objects of scorn and ridicule. Obviously, for women youth and beauty are highly valued; the loss of these is a dreaded event. For many women this dreaded event is emotionally related to menopause.

A woman who has spent a great deal of her time and effort staying attractive and who believes that "looks are everything," will likely have a difficult time during menopause. She will be fighting a battle she knows she will eventually lose. This woman, so often scorned for her vanity and self-absorption, in reality deserves compassion and understanding. She bought the idea that her face was her fortune and she built her life around it. Now as she loses the firm body, the high breasts, the smooth skin and the glossy dark hair of youth, she finds herself laughed at and ridiculed as she struggles to maintain some of her youthful features. If she gives up and allows her aging to show, she feels that she will lose everything she once considered important to her.

For the most part, the previous ideas describe middle and upper class women in the United States. There are other groups of women in this country for whom menopause is not a traumatic event and perhaps not even noticed. Women involved in satisfying careers do not report significant problems with menopause [20]. Although studies are limited, certain subgroups within the American culture report little or no difficulty with menopause.

The author once spent several months visiting a total of twenty black senior citizen groups in Washington, D.C. Although the women in the groups were considerably past menopause, it was thought that it would be interesting to talk with them about their experience. Most did not remember having any special menopausal symptoms. Some admitted having an occasional hot flash, but their attitude was that these had been petty annoyances which were easily forgotten or ignored. One women in all of those who were interviewed had gone to her doctor about her hot flashes. When he suggested estrogen she scornfully turned it down. She just wanted to know if the flashes were normal. She certainly didn't think she needed treatment.

Bart suggested several reasons for the black woman's nontraumatic menopause. She notes that black families are often multigenerational, extended families. The mother and grandmother have a very important matriarchal role throughout their lives. Black women go outside the home to work in large numbers and are important contributors to the family income. They do not have time to become involved with their children to the exclusion of all other interests [2]. This picture of the asymptomatic black menopausal woman may change as she is studied more closely, and also, if black families emulate white culture patterns. To date, no studies of menopausal patterns of black women exists.

MID-LIFE PROBLEMS

Besides the concerns associated with change of role and loss of youth, other problems begin to appear at the time of menopause. Difficulties associated with changes in marital status or career may happen coincidentally with menopause. The focus of concern may be directed at menopausal signs rather than the difficulty itself. This leads to the belief that there is a cause and effect relationship between menopause and these psychosocial problems rather than seeing them as unrelated events occurring simultaneously.

In the U.S., many women will experience a change in marital status during the menopausal years. Our society is currently reflecting a rise in midlife divorce. In addition, over 3 million women between the ages of forty and sixty-four become widows [1]. This is due partly to the fact that women have a longer average life-span than men. In addition, they often marry men older than themselves.

The increase in divorced and widowed women has produced a newly-recognized group called displaced homemakers. These are women older than forty and younger than sixty-five whose role had always been homemaking until divorce or widowhood caused them to lose their job. Too young for programs for the elderly or social security, often ineligible for benefits for minor children, ineligible for unemployment insurance because homemaking is not considered employment, these women fall between the cracks of programs to help women. Although a National Displaced Homemaker Bill providing benefits and training has been before Congress for several years, the bill has yet to pass.

For many women, divorce or widowhood represents a change in their economic situation. In order to survive, they must work. Some have skills that have grown rusty after years of disuse, while others have never worked and have no marketable skills. This situation demands all of the adjustments of any career change plus an adjustment in the woman's self-image.

Another problem experienced by divorced and widowed mid-life women relates to the need for intimacy. Intimacy involves both psychological and intellectual sharing as well as a sexual relationship. Establishing a new social network may be difficult. Dating mores will have changed and there is only former experience to rely upon. If that was long ago or very limited, the transition will be even more difficult.

Much to many women's surprise, sexual needs do not diminish with the loss of a partner. Sexual drives opposing her own and others' stereotyped ideas and expectations for her behavior may create tremendous conflicts. Until she can in some way come to terms with her sexuality, these conflicts will remain.

COPING

Many communities today have a woman's center and mid-life women have been included in their programs with special events directed towards them. Mutual help networks are springing up. Many colleges, especially community colleges, have an increased enrollment of older women students and are trying to respond to their special needs. In the past, the few books available about menopause were by and for physicians. Today scores of popular books are available.

These books deal with subjects such as physical and mental health, finances and jobs, political action, and sexuality and self-esteem. (See chapter 26.)

All of these activities represent ways women are coping with problems that occur at mid-life. Education serves several purposes. It teaches a woman what to expect during menopause and how to deal with problems which may occur. It provides a means of increasing skills to ease financial problems. For single women it may also provide a means of building a new social network.

Self-help and discussion groups are ways that some women use to reestablish control over their lives and find better ways to relate to family members. These social networks help them redefine themselves. In a more general way, proper diet and exercise are being recognized as vital factors in maintaining good health at any age. They are especially important in stressful situations. Women who establish good health practices will be better able to manage problems that arise at any time.

Part II - Beyond Menopause

The last of Erikson's eight stages is Integrity vs. Despair. He describes it as the time when the individual can "ripen the fruit" of the previous seven stages. A review of one's life culminates in an "acceptance of one's one and only life cycle as something that had to be and that, by necessity, permitted of no substituting" [12]. This results in a sense of ego integrity. If previous development was not satisfactory, the individual feels despair or disgust. There is not enough time to start over or to try an alternate road to integrity. It is too late to develop all of the previous seven ego qualities needed. The psychological tasks of this stage are accompanied by the physical changes of aging and the sociological changes brought about by retirement, changes in economic matters, and deaths of family and friends. The result is a review of one's life to determine "Who am I?" [13]

It is important to bridge the gap between theory and reality. It may seem that an individual with a sense of ego integrity will adjust to old age with a minimum of difficulty. However, the reality is that our society poses some very real problems for the elderly. A sense of ego integrity only provides a firmer basis for approaching these problems.

An individual may experience psychological difficulties when trying to cope with both the physical changes of aging and the sociological problems for the elderly imposed by our society. If there are unresolved emotional conflicts from earlier years their problems will be compounded. For many the stereotype of a blissful old age may be more myth than reality.

Dr. Robert Butler said, "The problems of old age in America are largely the problems of women" [8]. Since women have a longer age span than men, women over sixty-five greatly outnumber men in the same age range. In addition, women are at a distinct disadvantage under the United States legal, social security, and pension systems.

DILEMMAS FOR AGED WOMEN

There is a great amount of interplay in the biopsychosocial changes of aging.

Not all of these changes create problems and some have both positive and negative aspects. Changes which have a major impact on many women include retirement, finances, housing, physical appearance, sexuality, and companionship.

Retirement may bring freedom from the demands of a daily work schedule and allow time for pursuing other interests. For those who were totally involved in their work, retirement may be seen as loss of an important part of their identity. For most people there is some ambivalence in feelings surrounding retirement.

These retirement issues and adjustments will be present whether it is the woman herself who is retiring or her spouse. One's whole life must be reorganized. The external structure provided by a work schedule is gone as well as the meaning that it gave to one's life. Now new meaningful activities must be developed as well as the time frame in which they can be accomplished.

If it is the woman's spouse who retires, his changes will be imposed on her established routines. Retirement will have an impact on both partners calling for compromise and consideration from each. Both the stability of the relationship and the stability of the individuals are important factors in the ease with which they adjust.

Financial concerns are major issues for the elderly in our society. As at other ages, financial needs center around such things as food, clothing, shelter, entertainment, and leisure activities. Chronic and debilitating diseases may occur with aging causing increased expenditures for health care. Retirement brings a fixed and probably reduced income even though cost of living remains stable or increases.

Sources of income for the elderly may include Social Security benefits, private pension plans, and personal savings and investments. Federal and state aid programs including Medicare, Medicaid, food stamps, and veterans benefits may also help. Local programs established to help the elderly may vary but include things such as Meals-on-Wheels, reduced transportation costs, counseling, legal services, and low-income housing.

Despite the fact that these financial difficulties exist for all aged people, women are at an even greater disadvantage than men. Many of the programs mentioned still provide unequal benefits and women receive lesser incomes. In many cases inheritance laws and pension plans may be written so that upon her husband's death, the woman receives little or nothing.

These sources of income and financial aid programs vary and laws governing them keep changing. For younger people, especially women, developing a financial plan for old age is a necessity. Women need to become familiar with the details of their or their husband's pension plans, insurance benefits, Social Security regulations, and inheritance laws. It is more difficult for those who reach old age without benefit of such planning. They, in particular, need to be put in touch with locally available resources.

Living arrangements become one of the areas of greatest change in the social patterns of elderly women. Whereas in the past aging women used to live with their children or in old age homes, today they are often found living alone. Some reasons for this change are a more mobile society, and increasing costs of institutional care. In addition, many people have found the available types of institutional care to be unacceptable. Finally, many younger women must work and so are not available to care for aging parents.

Alternatives were clearly needed and are being developed. These include public housing for old people, private retirement communities, and apartment complexes. For the elderly who live alone or with families who are working, community day care programs provide activity, companionship, and supervision. Nursing homes are still available for those who need more comprehensive health care.

Even though these alternatives are an improvement, they do require adjustments by the older person. If the move is of great distance, they must leave family and friends behind and disrupt long-established living patterns. Even a move of a few miles will be into a new community with new routines. If the move is to a community or home for the elderly, it may have both positive and negative aspects. While they may gain more peer companionship, the loss of stimulation from a mixture of ages may be deeply felt.

Many residences for the elderly are being built convenient to shopping, churches, health care, and recreational facilities. In some, these services are contained within the residence. The pros and cons are represented by the convenience versus the segregation from the surrounding community. In addition, these living arrangements are expensive and often require that a lifetime of savings and other resources be turned over to the residence.

In any case, a move to a nursing home or retirement community will be a big and often agonizing decision for all involved. Part of the difficulty is due to the constraints placed by financial costs and medical needs. For those who are healthy, day care programs provide the minimal supervision and socialization which they need. For those with medical problems, some insurance programs provide for skilled home-nursing care. It is hoped that in the future existing home-care benefits will be expanded and funded to provide the supervision and assistance required to maintain independence.

Body changes brought by aging are interpreted and handled by women in different ways. Their perception of aging is influenced by their own sense of self as well as our society's emphasis on youth and appearance. Thus, some women spend large amounts of money, time, and energy to retain their youthful appearance by use of hair dyes, cosmetics, and surgical procedures. Other women remain comfortable with the changes that aging brings to their appearance.

Sexuality continues throughout life. However, there are barriers which interfere with elderly women being able to meet their sexual needs. These include lack of a partner, the belief that old age sex is wrong, the disapproval of one's children, and lack of privacy in living quarters. In addition, the elderly woman may be surprised and embarrassed to find that her sexual needs continue. Education of the elderly and those who are involved in their care should include ways to fulfill this normal need such as masturbation and provision for privacy.

Loneliness is one of the major problems which older women face. Because women have a longer lifespan, they may outlive their spouse and/or male friends. A woman's children are often busy with their own lives and families. Increasingly restricted financial situations make it more difficult to afford normal social outlets. The socialization of women in our society encourages them to be passive and assume that someone will take care of them. When this does not happen, they often become angry and depressed, further alienating those around them. All of these are contributing factors in making loneliness the monumental problem it is for elderly women.

COPING

Dr. Alex Comfort lists four needs for elderly people, including dignity, money, proper medical services and useful work [9]. In order to meet these needs elderly people must rely on friends, family, and community in addition to their own resources. The more restricted the input from any one of these sources, the more difficult it will be to meet the needs that Dr. Comfort outlines.

Studies show that people who remain active and involved in life make the most successful adjustment to aging. Ways in which elderly people maintain involvement are through social, community, and political activities. Examples of these include senior citizens groups, volunteerism, and political organizations such as the Gray Panthers.

It must be recognized that all older people do not have the mobility, finances, or health to participate in these types of activities. Currently, there are very few resources available to give meaning to such peoples' lives. Our society is just beginning to recognize and become responsive to this need.

Community resources vary from one locale to another. Many churches, schools, and libraries provide services and programs for the elderly. Volunteer organizations such as women's groups and Boy and Girl Scout troops often develop activities involving older people. YMCA and YWCA programs can be found specifically directed toward involvement of senior citizens. Many communities have organized legal aid and transportation services for the elderly.

Local social service agencies coordinate services such as transportation, housing, food stamps, and financial assistance. In addition, they can also make referrals to other community agencies. Many large communities have a separate Department of Aging Services and Programs. For additional information on resources for aging see chapter 26.

REFERENCES
1. Bart PB: Why women's status changes in middle age. Sociological Symposium, Vol. 3, Fall 1969
2. Bart PB: Depression in middle aged women. *In* Gornic V, Moran BK (eds): Women in Sexist Society. New York, New American Library, 1972
3. Block MR, Davidson JL, Grambs JD, Serock KE: Unchartered Territory: Issues and Concerns of Women Over 40. College Park, MD, University of Maryland, 1978
4. Boston Women's Health Collective: Our Bodies, Ourselves. New York, Simon and Schuster, 1976
5. Bumagin VE, Hirn, KF: Aging is a Family Affair. New York, Thomas Y. Crowell, 1979
6. Burnside IM (ed): Nursing and the Aged. New York, McGraw-Hill, 1976
7. Busse EW, Pfeiffer E (eds): Behavior and Adaptation in Late Life. Boston, Little, Brown, 1977
8. Butler RN: *preface in:* The Older Woman: Continuities and Discontinuities: Report of the National Institute on Aging and the National Institute of Mental Health Workshop. Bethesda, MD, National Institutes of Health, September 14-16, 1978
9. Comfort A: A Good Age. New York, Crown, 1976
10. Duetsch H: The Psychology of Women. New York, Grune and Stratton, 1944
11. Elderly Widows. Statistical memo No. 33, Washington, DC, DHEW, 1976
12. Erikson E: Childhood and Society. New York, W. W. Norton, 1963

13. Erikson E: Identity in the Life Cycle. New York, W. W. Norton, 1980
14. Flint M: Menarche and Menopause of Rajput Women. Ph.D. Dissertation. New York, City University of New York, 1974
15. Gruis ML, Wagner NN: Sexuality during the climacteric. Post Graduate Medicine, Vol. 65 No. 5, May 1979
16. Kinsey AC, Pomeroy WB, Martin CE, Gebhard PH: Sexual Behavior of the Human Female. Philadelphia, W. B. Saunders, 1948
17. Mead M: Male and Female. New York, Dell, 1970
18. Neugarten BL, Datan N: The middle years. *In* Ariti S (ed): American Handbook of Psychiatry, Vol. I, 2nd ed. New York, Basic Books, 1974
19. Neugarten B, Kraines RJ: Menopausal symptoms in women of various ages. Psychosomatic Medicine, Vol. 27 No. 3, March 1965
20. Rivers C, Barnett R, Baruch B: Beyond Sugar and Spice. New York, G. P. Putnam's Sons, 1979
21. Toth SB, Toth A: Empathetic intervention with the widow. American Journal of Nursing, Vol. 80 No. 9, September 1980

Section VI

ADOLESCENT AND ADULT HEALTH ISSUES

13

Breast Problems

Janet Stearns Wyatt, Sandra L. Tyler, Gail M. Woodall

The breasts are specialized epithelial glands and as such are subject to many of the same problems as other epithelial tissue. They are also an integral part of the reproductive system and again can share its problems. In many cultures, they become symbols of sexuality and motherhood and thus are bestowed with tremendous psychological significance. Because the breast serves a variety of physical and psychological functions, the range of possibilities for breast-related problems is great.

For the most part, much of the information about breast problems has centered on a discussion of cancer. As a result of the fear generated by this word, many women panic when a breast symptom appears. In order to maintain perspective, this chapter discusses a wide range of breast problems including cancer.

Presently, at least 25 percent of the women in the United States who see a physician do so because they are concerned about an abnormal breast finding. Most often the breast complaint concerns the presence of a lump, but other complaints have ranged, in order of frequency, from breast pain to nipple changes, skin changes and axillary masses. Generally any one or a combination of these symptoms can be associated with a number of different breast problems. Although the topic of breast cancer has often eclipsed other problems, it is important to point out that more than 70 percent of all breast problems are benign or not cancerous [7].

Generally, breast problems may be categorized according to their benign or malignant nature. The accompanying outline offers a classification of breast problems. Methods of diagnosis and treatment will be included as each problem is discussed.

    I. BENIGN BREAST PROBLEMS
        A. Genetic and developmental
            1. Accessory nipples
            2. Breast hypertrophy
            3. Small breasts
        B. Benign mastopathies
            1. Fibrocystic disease
            2. Infections
            3. Tumors and lumps
                a. Fibroadenoma
                b. Trauma or fat necrosis
                c. Galactocele

BENIGN BREAST PROBLEMS

Genetic and Developmental Breast Problems

The genetic breast disorders include such problems as accessory or rudimentary breasts, abnormal breast and nipple forms, and absence or non-development of one or both breasts. Developmental breast problems usually occur at or after puberty or with pregnancy. They include breast underdevelopment, asymmetry, and breast hypertrophy. Although the actual physiological significance of any of these problems may vary, the psychological impact may be the element that actually prompts treatment.

Treatment of either genetic or developmental breast problems may involve surgery or hormonal therapy. Hormonal therapy with estrogens is most often prescribed for those women with underdeveloped breasts. The remaining forms of treatment generally involve a variety of surgical methods.

Accessory nipples: Accessory nipples or extra breast tissue is most frequently found along the mammary line. (See chapter 3.) Usually, the presence of extra-mammary tissue is physiologically insignificant. If glandular tissue is present, it may be subject to the same disease as other breast tissue. In any case extra breast tissue may cause emotional discomfort or embarrassment so that many women elect to have it removed. Simple surgical excision generally leaves minimal scarring.

Breast hypertrophy: Breast enlargement or hypertrophy may occur in relation to breast growth at adolescence, or secondary to obesity or pregnancy. Normally, breast development ceases when regular ovulation is established and progesterone is available to inhibit prolactin [1]. However, for some women, the breasts may continue to grow for one to two years after puberty, resulting in an unusual increase in breast size. For all women with breast hypertrophy, the physical and psychological problems may be great.

Physical problems include shoulder, back, neck and breast pain as well as poor posture. In addition, "grooving" of the shoulders from bra straps may occur. Often the discomfort of oversized breasts can be relieved only by lying down.

The psychological problems of the adolescent with breast hypertrophy are often complicated. Breast hypertrophy may seriously interfere with the psychosocial tasks of adolescence and compromise the growth of positive personality traits and self-esteem. In addition, obesity is often perpetuated in many women as they attempt to balance breast and body size. Although breast size may diminish somewhat after pregnancy and weight loss, the primary mode of treatment is surgical breast reduction.

Requests for breast reduction have come from women ranging in age from twelve to seventy-six years. Reduction surgery offers an approximately normal breast shape and contour for these women. Surgical scarring is minimized by placing incisions under the breast or around the nipple. In the absence of infection and hemorrhage, healing will be rapid and complete [12].

There are, however, a number of considerations that should concern women who are contemplating breast reduction. Often, breast sensation is reduced and may only minimally return over a two year postoperative period. In addition, breast feeding is often discouraged, since this may again cause an increase in breast size. For some women, breast feeding may be impossible because much of the gland field has been removed. Preoperative counseling should include a thorough explanation of the physical changes which surgery will bring. Counseling should also explore the woman's existing self-concept and expectations she may have about the surgical outcome and its implications.

Small breasts: Because we live in a society that is preoccupied with perfection, many women perceive their breast size or shape to be inadequate. For some, particularly those with a poor self-concept, this "physical defect" is seen as a limiting factor in the quality of their lives. This concern may be real enough to prompt them to request breast augmentation.

Augmentation is a procedure involving placement of a prosthesis against the pectoralis major muscle and behind the breast glandular tissue. These implants are specialized rubber pouches filled with silicone gel or saline. They are made in different sizes and shapes allowing a woman to attain a breast contour which is consistent with her desired body image. (Figure 13-1.)

Breast augmentation may be done as an outpatient procedure. However, it does require close postoperative monitoring for acute pain, infection, hematoma, or unusual swelling. An additional complication may result from the natural healing process. During the first month after surgery, a fibrous capsule of scar tissue forms around the implant.

Although this capsule has the beneficial effect of securing the implant, and preventing slippage, in some women it becomes excessively thick resulting in a spherical shape, unnatural firmness, and pain. When this occurs, it can be corrected by closed compression as an office procedure or by surgical incision under anesthesia. Often there is an associated loss of nipple and breast sensitivity following surgery. However, full return of sensation may occur during the next six months to two years.

Normally, breast implants last a lifetime. Because the implants are placed behind the normal breast tissue they do not limit a woman's ability to do self-breast exam. It is important to note that implants have not been associated with an increased risk of breast cancer although frequent medical follow-up is advised.

Although breast augmentation does not physiologically interfere with breast feeding there is controversy as to its advisability. Any abscess formation that might occur during lactation would necessitate removal of the implant and may limit chances for further implant placement.

Often following breast augmentation, many women do not experience the hoped-for resolution of their problems. An adjustment in body shape may do nothing to alter a negative self-concept. Preoperative counseling should allow

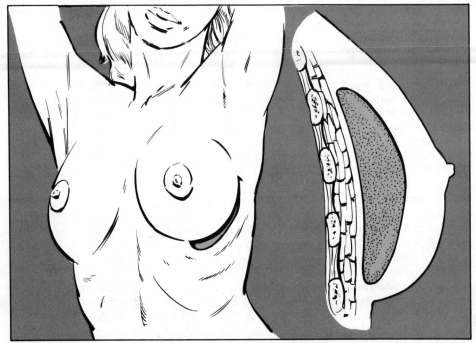

Figure 13-1. Placement of implant for breast augmentation.

exploration of each woman's motives for surgery so that every aspect of her breast problem may be discussed.

Benign Mastopathies

Most of the breast diseases that concern women are benign and may be treated without major complications. While some benign breast disorders cause a variety of signs and symptoms, others present with only one or two characteristics. Three categories of benign breast disease include fibrocystic disease, infections, and tumors and lumps.

Fibrocystic Disease. Fibrocystic breast disease (cystic disease) is the most common breast disease for American women. For many years the terminology for, and the description of, fibrocystic breast disease has been very confusing. Some examples of names for this disease are chronic cystic mastitis, fibroadenomatosis, mastodynia, and sclerosing adenosis. Haagensen and others use the inclusive term "cystic disease." All of the stages from microscopic to gross disease then fall into this category [5].

Because cystic disease seems to be estrogen dependent, gross cystic disease generally becomes evident only after ovulation is well established. At this time visible or palpable lesions may occur in one or both breasts. These lesions are usually apparent in the upper outer breast quadrant, and are often accompanied by symptoms of cyclic premenstrual pain, tenderness and breast firmness.

Generally, the lesions of cystic disease are round, freely movable and well delineated. They may feel hard and firm if filled with fluid or if a fibrous capsule has developed around them. They may also feel soft and fluctuant if the fluid level is low.

These changes in consistency along with changes in lesion size are frequently related to the menstrual cycle. For the most part cystic disease seems to improve during pregnancy and lactation. Although some women experience symptoms of cystic disease from age forty to fifty, menopause often resolves the problem.

Treatment of cystic disease usually involves palliative measures to reduce discomfort. A mild analgesic such as aspirin is often recommended along with warm compresses. A well fitted, supportive bra may also help alleviate discomfort. To reduce breast swelling and fluid retention at menses many clinicians also recommend a reduction in dietary sodium or prescribe short-term use of a mild diuretic.

Studies by Minton show a connection between cystic breast disease and the use of methylxanthines which are present in caffeine, theophylline, and theobromine. When use of products with these substances was reduced, the symptoms of cystic disease were reduced [10].

In another study results were more dramatic when women discontinued smoking as well as methylxanthines. Adjunctive therapy with Vitamin E has also produced both subjective and objective improvement of fibrocystic breast disease in limited studies [9]. It would seem to follow that some women may benefit by giving up coffee, tea, cola drinks, chocolate, unprescribed use of respiratory medications and smoking. Further research should reveal more information to help women participate in their own treatment plans.

Often the palliative measures for cystic disease are insufficient. If the cyst is extremely uncomfortable or persistent the surgeon may elect to aspirate the fluid. In addition to differentiating it from a solid tumor, this will serve to resolve the cyst. If the aspirant is hemorrhagic, if the cyst refills, if a mammogram done two weeks later is abnormal, or if cytology studies of the fluid are abnormal, an excisional biopsy is indicated [7]. There is a difference of opinion as to the value of cytology, and some physicians elect not to have it done.

Infection. Because the breast is a specialized epithelial tissue it is subject to any of the systemic or local diseases which affect the skin anywhere. Some of the common infectious breast problems that may occur include folliculitis, herpes simplex virus, Montgomery gland infections, sebaceous cysts, and lactational mastitis and abscess.

The most common of these problems is lactational mastitis. When nipples become cracked and irritated as a result of nursing, bacteria may enter and cause an acute inflammatory reaction. Usually this inflammation will subside with the use of aspirin, warm compresses and bra support. However, chronic inflammation may create a deep subareolar abscess. Incision and drainage of the abscess is then required with follow-up antibiotic therapy to prevent reinfection.

Often infectious problems of the breast are accompanied by a discharge that results when the nipples are squeezed. Herpes simplex and Montgomery gland infections commonly create a "pseudo" nipple discharge that responds well to local antibiotic or steroid therapy along with good hygiene.

Tumors and lumps. A breast lump or tumor creates a great deal of fear for many women since this symptom is often the first noted sign of breast cancer. However, benign neoplasms occur more frequently and create few, if any, treatment complications.

FIBROADENOMA. A fibroadenoma is a mixed tumor containing both fibrous and glandular elements. It is a disease of young women, occurs more often in black women, and usually does not develop past menopause. Estrogen stimulates its growth so these tumors are commonly seen during adolescence, pregnancy, and with exogenous estrogen use.

The size of the fibroadenoma varies but the average range is 1 to 5 cm [7]. These solid tumors are usually round, rubbery, and well delineated, although they may be lobulated and if calcified will feel hard. They are freely movable, do not cause skin retraction, and are typically painless. Evidence does not support the fact that fibroadenomas become malignant or predispose a woman to breast cancer [5].

If the woman is under twenty-five and the tumor shows little or no growth, reexamination in two to three months is recommended. If the tumor persists or grows, excision is advised. Surgery may be scheduled at her convenience if a woman is under twenty-five or more immediately if she is at high risk.

TRAUMA OR FAT NECROSIS: Trauma to the breast is manifested by the usual signs of injury including bruising, redness, swelling, and tenderness. Because the breast is composed of both glandular and fatty tissue, a common complication is fat necrosis. This necrosis occurs either directly from the injury or indirectly from tissue compression resulting from hemorrhage.

In the healing process the necrotic tissue becomes fibrosed and clinically may resemble a malignant mass. It may take only a day or up to several weeks after injury for the mass to occur. The mass is firm, usually fixed, and slowly increases in size over a period of time. It often causes skin or nipple retraction and dimpling of the overlying skin. It is important to note that the mass is usually rounded and well delineated. This helps to distinguish it from the more common characteristics of carcinoma.

There is no evidence to support the idea that trauma causes breast cancer. However, a malignancy may have been present prior to the trauma. Since there is no way to prove that a mass was caused by trauma or is not malignant, excision and biopsy are recommended.

GALACTOCELE. A galactocele has all the characteristics of a benign neoplasm in that it is rounded, well delineated and movable. It is a cyst containing thickened milk and is usually located in the central breast area. Such cysts result from abrupt termination of lactation. If there is a history of termination of breast feeding within the past year a galactocele may be suspected. Diagnosis and treatment consist of aspiration of the thick milky fluid from the cyst cavity.

DUCT ECTASIA. Mammary duct ectasia may be described as an inflammatory process of the terminal lactational ducts of the breast. Symptoms of this process include periareolar pain, itching, areolar swelling, and a nipple discharge that may range in color from clear serous fluid to yellow, green, bluish, or black. This benign condition is uncommon and usually does not occur before menopause. Often the swelling that occurs with this problem resembles a tumor or mass so that biopsy is recommended. Treatment of duct ectasia usually involves surgical excision of the affected mammary ducts.

INTRADUCTAL PAPILLOMA. Although multiple papilloma may develop through-out a duct system, solitary papillomas are more common and will be discussed here. They may appear in any age group following duct development at puberty. This lesion neither becomes malignant nor is it associated with an increased evidence of malignancy.

The presence of a papilloma in a breast duct causes a serous, serosanguinous, or clear discharge. This discharge is the most common presenting symptom. The tumor may or may not be palpable. Very rarely there may be skin dimpling or nipple retraction.

Since the symptoms of benign papilloma may mimic those of carcinoma, clinical differentiation is important. If the tumor is palpable it will be excised and biopsied. A nipple discharge without a palpable tumor is rarely associated with malignancy[5]. Therefore, if nipple discharge is the only symptom, treatment will be delayed and careful follow-up is necessary. Occasionally, the tumor will regress spontaneously.

GALACTORRHEA. Galactorrhea is the secretion of a milky fluid from the nipples at any time not directly related to pregnancy or lactation. It is seldom seen before puberty. It is not related to any specific breast disease, but rather to more generalized causative factors. It occurs as a result of increased prolactin release. See chapter 3 for review of prolactin control and release.

Some of the most common galactorrheic syndromes are:

1. Excessive estrogen intake such as with the use of oral contraceptives or synthetic estrogen drugs.

2. Special drugs which may disrupt prolactin levels including amphetamines, tricyclic anti-depressants, phenothiazines, reserpine derivatives, and methyldopa.

3. Hypothyroidism.

4. Benign pituitary adenomas.

5. Stress, trauma, and surgical anesthesia.

6. Prolonged intensive stimulation such as might occur during sexual manipulation.

Medical evaluation is necessary to rule out organic cause. Once this has been done treatment, education, and reassurance may be initiated as indicated. If at all possible, the determined causative factor should be avoided or corrected.

MALIGNANT BREAST PROBLEMS

Although there are over one hundred different varieties of breast cancer, a diagnosis of breast cancer will usually involve one of two major diagnostic groups. *Lobular carcinoma* accounts for approximately 25 percent of all breast cancers and affects the glandular tissue of the mammary lobules, that is, adenocarcinomas. *Ductal carcinoma* accounts for 65 percent to 70 percent of all breast cancers and describes those carcinomas originating within the ductal system [7].

Once a malignancy is classified the extent of growth of the neoplasm is measured and labeled. A localized malignancy is described as non-invasive or as carcinoma "in-situ." When surrounding tissue is affected, it is called invasive or infiltrative. Generally prognosis is better if the malignancy is found while it is still noninvasive.

While research into the cause of breast cancer continues, epidemiological studies have revealed a number of special characteristics which put women at a greater risk for developing cancer of the breast. (See Table 13-1.) At present researchers do not know if a special combination of these risk factors has to occur or if one particular factor might be the clue to predicting breast cancer. Often women will have many of these factors as part of their medical history and yet never experience a breast malignancy. The study of all aspects of breast malignancy will certainly continue since the female breast remains the leading site for cancer in American women and the major cause of death of women between forty to forty-four years of age [3].

---

*TABLE 13-1.*_____

Factors thought to put women at an increased risk for developing breast cancer.

Age forty or over
Obesity
High socioeconomic status
Caucasian
Jewish
Residence in North America and Europe
First pregnancy after the age of thirty (two times the risk)
No pregnancies (two to three times the risk)
Early menarche
Late natural menopause
Hypothyroid conditions
High dietary intake of fats
Estrogen ingestion
Previous history of breast cancer
Previous history of cancer of the reproductive organs
Family history of breast cancer—especially if along maternal lines (fifty times increase in risk if both mother and sister have breast cancer).
History of chronic fibrocystic breast disease
Chronic exposure to ionizing radiation
Chronic psychological stress
Triad of obesity, hypertension and diabetes

Factors have also been identified which seem to offer some form of "protection" against breast cancer. At one time a history of breastfeeding was thought to lower a woman's risk, although studies now show that this is not true. It has also been proposed that women who have experienced a full-term delivery before the age of twenty have two-thirds less chance of developing breast cancer. Until the cause(s) of breast cancer are determined, women and physicians must continue careful monitoring for breast disease.

The major signs and symptoms of breast cancer include many characteristics of benign breast diseases. Breast lumps which are cancerous are usually firm and may be fixed and poorly delineated. Pain seldom accompanies a malignant lump but may occur as part of an inflammatory reaction to a tumor growth. Nipple discharge as a sign of cancer is uncommon but if it does occur is frequently spontaneous and hemorraghic in quality. Dimpling of the skin, retraction of the nipple or other changes in the breast contour may also occur if the tumor is growing near the skin surface or chest ligaments. Nipple crusting, itching, and areolar erosion are uncommon but may occur with a form of malignancy known as *Paget's disease* of the breast. The axillary masses are most often due to lymphatic metastasis or to a tumor in the tail of breast tissue which extends into the axilla.

Special diagnostic tests are used to confirm diagnosis of breast cancer. The three main tests are mammography, thermography and biopsy. A discussion of the technical aspects of these procedures can be found in chapter 24.

Because mammography has been a controversial testing method for use in breast cancer screening and diagnosis, special guidelines for the use of this test have been published by the American Cancer Society. They recommend a baseline mammogram for women between the ages of thirty-five to forty and a yearly mammogram after age fifty. In the years between forty and fifty, the frequency of mammography may be determined by the consideration of risk factors. To date, biopsy remains the only method that provides definitive diagnosis.

Following confirmation of malignancy by biopsy, treatment will consist of one or a combination of surgery, radiation or chemotherapy. The form of treatment that will be used should be decided by both the woman and her physician. A delay of up to two weeks between biopsy and initiation of treatment does not involve increased risk. This allows the woman time to begin adjusting to the implications of her disease as well as actively participating in choosing the treatment best for her.

Recently much controversy has been generated concerning the various plans for treatment of breast cancer. Although some form of breast surgery is still generally recommended when a malignancy is found, the Halsted radical mastectomy is now thought by many to be unnecessary for women with non-invasive carcinomas.

In recent years, total mastectomy, lumpectomy, radiation, oncologic agents, castration, and adrenalectomy have offered additional or alternative methods of treatment. A Consensus Development Conference was held at the National Institutes of Health on June 5, 1979, to discuss the viability of these alternatives to radical mastectomy [3].

Three categories of acceptable surgical procedures were defined. They included radical mastectomy, total mastectomy with removal of axillary lymph nodes and preservation of the pectoralis muscle, and lesser surgical procedures with or without radiotherapy. The consensus of the panel was that total mastectomy is recommended treatment for women who have Stage I and selected Stage II breast cancer. (See Table 13-2 for staging.) The Halsted procedure is still recommended for Stage III. Stage IV breast cancer is considered inoperable and suggested treatment consists of chemotherapy and/or radiotherapy.

It cannot be stressed enough that survival depends upon early detection. Since lumps are the most frequent initial sign of cancer, breast self-exam is a woman's best defense against this disease. Once a lump has been discovered, a woman must promptly seek medical care. Certainly, the diagnosis itself and the treatment for breast cancer are frightening and awesome. However, the possibility of less radical surgery as well as involvement in the choice of treatment allows a woman to maintain some control over the sequence of events happening to her.

Breast reconstruction is an option for some women following mastectomy but cannot be done for at least six months after the initial surgery. It usually follows the same procedure used for breast augmentation. However, if there has been extensive removal of skin and tissue another approach may be needed. The flap method of reconstruction involves the transfer of skin and tissue from other body sites to form a breast mound. In addition, a nipple and areola may be grafted.

The use of implants following mastectomy for cancer is controversial. Arguments for implantation include a more natural post-operative recovery. For example, not having to cope with an external prosthesis allows more freedom in choice of clothes and results in a more normal body image. Arguments against implants center around the fact that recurrent cancer growing beneath the implant may be undetectable. Physical and mammographic examination is compromised. Saline implants may improve visualization but details still remain limited.

Discussion of Breast Issues

Breast diseases whether benign or malignant cause similar symptoms because of disruption of normal physiological processes. Because of the similarity of the symptoms, it is easy to jump to conclusions and assume a malignancy. Even though chances are high that the problem will be benign, a malignancy is always a possibility. For this reason as well as to reduce a woman's anxiety, a prompt definitive diagnosis is imperative.

Eliciting detailed information about the presenting symptom as well as associated symptoms such as pain and swelling is necessary. For example, it is important to know whether a woman's nipple discharge is accompanied by a lump. In addition, portions of an overall history assume special significance. The day of the last menstrual period and date of termination of last pregnancy as well as lactation are important to know. A careful contraceptive and sexual history as well as a family history of breast diseases is needed. Additional helpful information includes any history of trauma and use of drugs such as caffeine, tranquilizers, estrogen, or anti-hypertensives.

One of the most effective ways to reduce a woman's anxiety, fear, and feelings of helplessness is to make her an active participant in her own care. Basic to accomplishing this is giving the woman information about breast anatomy and physiology. This gives her a way to understand whatever pathological process is occurring or treatment which has been prescribed. She is then more likely to follow recommendations as well as to perform regular breast self examination as outlined in chapter 23.

The woman who has had a malignancy diagnosed, as well as her family, will need additional resources. They will need emotional support, sometimes financial support, help with decision making and help with any individual concerns. The American Cancer Society is an excellent resource for education as well as referral. It sponsors a program called "Reach to Recovery" which is designed to help both the woman and her family following mastectomy. Additional education and resources can be found in The Breast Cancer Digest which can be obtained by writing to the Office of Cancer Communications, National Cancer Institute, Building 31, Room 4-B, 39 Bethesda, MD 20205. See chapter 26 for additional resources.

TABLE 13-2.

Breast cancer staging as prepared by the American Joint Committee for Cancer Staging (Adapted from **Breast Cancer Digest**).
Classification System of Breast Carcinoma

Stage I. A tumor less than 5 cm with minor skin involvement, either affixed or not affixed to the chest wall, muscle, or fascia; nodes not considered to contain growth; no evidence of metastasis.

Stage II. A tumor less than 5 cm with possible muscle or chest wall fixation; nodes are movable, but may not contain growth; no evidence of metastasis.

Stage III. A tumor larger than 5 cm with or without fixation or extension to fascia and chest wall; any amount of nodal involvement; no evidence of metastasis.

Stage IV. A tumor of any size with extension to chest wall and skin; any amount of nodal involvement; evidence of metastasis.

REFERENCES

1. Bidlingmaier F, Knorr D: Oestrogens: Physiological and Chemical Aspects. Basel, Switzerland, S. Karger, 1978
2. Bethume GW: Office evaluation of breast problems. Primary Care, Vol. 3 No. 2, June 1976
3. Breast Cancer Digest, Vol. 79, 1691, Bethesda, MD, United States Department of Health Education and Welfare, March 1979
4. Gallagher SH et al: The Breast. St. Louis, C. V. Mosby, 1978
5. Haagensen CD: Diseases of the Breast, 2nd ed. Philadelphia, W. B. Saunders, 1971
6. Koch SJ: Augmentation mammoplasty. American Journal of Nursing, Vol. 80 No. 8, August 1980
7. Leis HP: Diagnosis and Treatment of Breast Lesions. New York, Medical Examination Publishing Company, 1970
8. Leis HP, Kwon SC: Fibrocystic disease of the breast. Journal of Reproductive Medicine, Vol. 22 No. 6, June 1979
9. Medical News. Journal of the American Medical Association, Vol. 244 No. 10, September 5, 1980
10. Minton JP et al: Caffeine, cyclic nucleotides, and breast disease. Surgery, Vol. 86, No. 7, July 1979
11. Wilcox PM, Ettinger DE: Benign breast disease: Diagnosis and treatment. Primary Care, Vol. 4 No. 4, December 1977
12. Woods J et al: Experience with and comparison of methods of reduction mammoplasty. Mayo Clinic Proceedings, Vol. 53, August 1978

14

Contraception

From puberty until menopause, women who are heterosexually active will risk pregnancy. There will be occasions during this time span when some women will choose to become pregnant, but for the majority of these fertile years, women will need contraception to prevent pregnancy.

It is important to remember that not all sexually active women are heterosexual. Lesbian women may give a positive response when asked if they are sexually active since there are some gynecological concerns related to sexual activity. To insist on the need for contraception merely creates embarrassment and ill will. A suggested approach would be to inquire whether the woman is heterosexually, homosexually or bisexually active and proceed from there.

Perhaps the most important thing to be considered in any discussion of contraception is that it must be regarded within the context of a woman's sexuality. To approach the issue of contraception only from the point of view of failure rates, medical contraindications and instructions for use may doom a woman to failure. A truly effective birth control counselor needs to be comfortable talking about sex.

Nurses may be confronted with two types of situations in which birth control counseling is needed. The first is a straightforward request from an individual who has acknowledged the need for contraception. The second situation is that of a woman who is heterosexually active yet has not acknowledged a need for birth control. All too often, women who do not acknowledge contraceptive needs receive their first counseling at a prenatal or an abortion clinic.

Some women, particularly those in the teen years, are not able to acknowledge their sexual activity with men and deny it by not planning for it. There may be other reasons for this so-called "lack of responsibility." These include embarrassment, peer or partner pressure, cost, fear, and ignorance. In addition, it is conceivable that, for some women, sexual pleasure is heightened by risk-taking.

It is said that the "perfect" contraceptive should meet the following criteria:
100 percent effectiveness
Simple to use
Removed in time from act of intercourse
Safe
Cheap
Reversible
A comparison of the available methods of contraception with these criteria, shows the lack of perfection of all of them.

When reference is made to method effectiveness, it is important to understand the difference between theoretical and use effectiveness. *Theoretical effectiveness* refers to the number of pregnancies that would be expected in 100 women over a period of one year if the method was used consistently and instructions were explicitly followed. *Use effectiveness* reflects human error. This may be a result of inconsistent or incorrect use. It may also be a reflection of error by the health provider, such as an incorrectly sized diaphragm, an improperly inserted IUD, or inaccurate or inadequate instruction for use.

When women ask for information regarding effectiveness this difference should be explained. Nurses who do not understand this may inadvertently direct a woman away from a perfectly good method by quoting theoretical effectiveness rates of one method and use effectiveness rates of another.

THE MYTHICAL METHODS

The following methods are not mythical in terms of their existence, but only in terms of their effectiveness.

Douching

Solutions vary according to local custom, but may include vinegar or baking soda in water, commercial douche preparations, soapy water or Coca Cola. Since there are millions of highly motile sperm in a single ejaculation, it is not surprising that douching has a failure rate of approximately 40 percent [14]. In addition, the action of the douching solution may actually speed the sperm on their way.

Holding Back

It is thought by some women that they cannot get pregnant without an orgasm. The idea of "holding back" and not allowing an orgasm to occur is, of course, ineffective.

Sponges and Tampons

Sponges, tampons, and pieces of cloth placed in the vagina do not prevent the sperm from entering the cervical os.

Scrotal Hyperthermia

The scrotum is conveniently placed outside the male pelvis as spermatogenesis does not take place at temperatures above 36°C. Men in hot climates whose religion or custom requires wearing constrictive clothing on the genitals have a lower fertility rate than men whose custom does not require them to wear such clothing [11]. However, for practical purposes, hot baths and the use of jock straps are not recommended as birth control methods.

First Intercourse

Unfortunately, the idea that a woman cannot become pregnant the first time she has intercourse is still a fairly common misconception. First intercourse can, and frequently does, result in pregnancy.

THE NATURAL METHODS

The following methods do not require any chemical, hormone, device or equipment. They vary greatly in effectiveness and acceptability.

Abstinence

This method is the only one of all the methods that meets the criteria of being 100 percent effective. Religion, age, illness or environment may demand periods of abstinence for some people. However, for all but a small percentage of people, total abstinence is neither practical nor acceptable.

Breast Feeding or Prolonged Lactation

Although breast feeding may prolong post partum amenorrhea and may interfere with implantation, it is not considered to be a highly effective method. In women who supplement breast feedings with bottle feedings its effectiveness drops even more since resumption of menses and ovulation will occur even sooner. A couple truly wanting to postpone or prevent another pregnancy would be well advised to use another method (See Figure 14-1).

Withdrawal

Withdrawal is not a highly effective method of contraception. However, some people do use it as a primary method while others may use it as a back-up method. Therefore it is important to examine its advantages and disadvantages.

The effectiveness of withdrawal depends upon avoidance of ejaculation inside the vagina. The male must withdraw the penis from the vagina just at the time of ejaculatory inevitability and deposit the semen outside the vagina. Care must be taken not to ejaculate on or near the female genitals since sperm can swim up the vaginal canal if they are deposited on moist surfaces close to the vaginal opening. This may be the way the rare phenomenon of a "splash pregnancy" occurs in a woman who has never had intercourse.

Alternatives to Vaginal Intercourse

Years ago, many of the following methods were probably included in the broad but vague term "heavy petting." They all provide effective contraception since there is no intra-vaginal ejaculation.

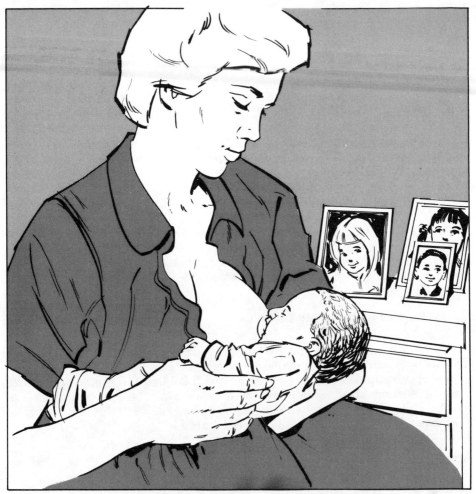

Figure 14-1. *Breast feeding is not an effective contraceptive method.*

In addition, many heterosexual couples regularly include these forms of sexual expression as a pleasurable part of their sexual relationship. Lesbian women also incorporate these forms of sexual stimulation into their lovemaking.

As with any type of sexual stimulation, these alternatives may have some side effects if practiced without caution. Acceptance by both partners is, of course, of primary importance.

Oral-genital stimulation. This type of stimulation seems to have increased in recent years, probably coincidental with the liberalizing of attitudes towards sex and the encouragement of freer expression of sexuality. It has two main disadvantages. Injury can be caused to the clitoris, labia, or penis with vigorous practice. Also, bacteria or viruses may be transferred from one site to another. The most common conditions spread in this manner are herpes, gonorrhea, and yeast.

Anal stimulation. A generally unaccepting attitude towards this type of stimulation prevents many couples from obtaining accurate information about it and thus unknowingly harm each other. Improperly practiced, it can result in problems such as chronic recurrent vaginitis, urethritis in the male, and rectal fissures or relaxation of the rectal sphincter. Often people feel uncomfortable asking advice about anal stimulation. Few nurses feel comfortable initiating questions regarding this practice due to their own uneasiness or to the threatening effect such questions often have on others.

When it is suspected that a problem may be related to anal stimulation, after discussing other possible causes, the nurse might add, "If anal stimulation is a part of your sexual practice, it is wise to take the following precautions:

1. Use adequate lubrication.
2. Entry should be made very slowly allowing for gradual stretching of the tight rectal sphincter.
3. If intercourse is practiced, then anal stimulation should be last in the sequence. This prevents spread of bacteria to the vaginal area.
4. A male who is susceptible to urethritis might consider the use of a condom.
5. A condom could also be used and then removed or changed before vaginal entry."

This approach avoids putting a person on the defensive, while still providing important information.

Mutual masturbation, vibrators, stimulators, and artifacts. The main precaution with any of these or other types of stimulation is an awareness of the chance of injury related to excessive pressure or duration of use. Early warning signs of tissue damage are a painful tingling or burning sensation. These sensations should be regarded as a signal to stop.

The Calendar Rhythm Method

This and the three methods that follow are based on three assumptions:
- Ovulation takes place fourteen days plus or minus two days before the onset of the next menstrual period.
- The egg is viable for approximately twenty-four hours.
- Sperm are viable for two to three days [8].

Abstinence is recommended around the time of ovulation with a margin of safety ranging from three to four days before and after the presumed date of ovulation.

The calendar method is based on predicting the probability of the time of ovulation by keeping records of past menstrual cycles. It is generally recommended that a woman keep a careful record of her menstrual cycle for six to twelve months before relying on this method. A menstrual cycle is always counted from the day of the onset of bleeding of one period to the onset of the next period. The woman subtracts eighteen from the number of days in her shortest cycle and eleven from the number in her longest cycle. This calculation determines the period of abstinence. For example, a woman having cycles that range from twenty-six to thirty days would need to abstain from day eight to day nineteen of each cycle. That is, twenty-six minus eighteen equals eight, and thirty minus eleven equals nineteen.

The long periods of abstinence or reliance on other types of sexual stimulation make this method unacceptable to many couples. Additionally, many things can cause a change in what is usually considered by a woman to be a very predictable pattern. These include illness, emotional or physical trauma, weight loss or gain, and travel. These are all fairly common occurrences in a woman's life. An additional problem is that sperm have been known to remain viable for longer than two to three days. Pregnancies have been known to occur with a single exposure seven days before documented ovulation [10].

The calendar method and its imperfections make it apparent that a more accurate method of determining ovulation is desirable. The two methods that follow are an attempt to give these calculations a more scientific base.

Basal Body Temperature or Thermal Method

The BBT is the lowest body temperature reached during waking hours and usually occurs immediately after awakening. Progesterone, which is present from the time of ovulation until just prior to the next menses, causes a rise of 0.4–0.5°F in the BBT. (See chapter 3.) By carefully taking and recording her first waking temperature, a woman can determine when ovulation occurred.

Careful instructions to a woman interested in using this method should include the following points. The temperature can be taken either rectally or orally, but once a site is chosen it should be maintained. A special thermometer calibrated in 0.1 degree increments makes reading easier and more accurate but is not a necessity. The woman should take her temperature each day immediately upon awakening before eating, drinking, smoking or going to the bathroom.

Special emphasis needs to be placed on helping her to interpret the data which she collects. A rise in temperature may be related to illness, exhaustion, or excitement. If such a relationship is suspected, it should be noted on the chart. A rise in temperature related to ovulation will be sustained and will last until the onset of the next menstrual period.

Assuming a twenty-four to forty-eight hour period of viability for the egg, a woman can be told that the "safe" period for intercourse usually begins on the third consecutive day of temperature elevation. The preovulatory "safe" period is far more difficult to determine. The preovulatory phase differs vastly from one woman to another and somewhat from one cycle to another in a given individual. See Figure 14-2.

Since the BBT cannot predict ovulation, for highest effectiveness a woman would need to restrict intercourse to the postovulatory phase. In actual practice, most women probably begin a period of abstinence anywhere from day three to seven of a cycle. The poor predictive nature of the BBT method and the need for long periods of abstinence have generated interest in a method that could help a woman determine imminent ovulation.

The Ovulation or Billings Method

Drs. John and Evelyn Billings of Australia have described a method of determining fertile and infertile phases of the menstrual cycle by observing changes in the cervix and cervical mucus. By becoming aware of these symptoms and learn-

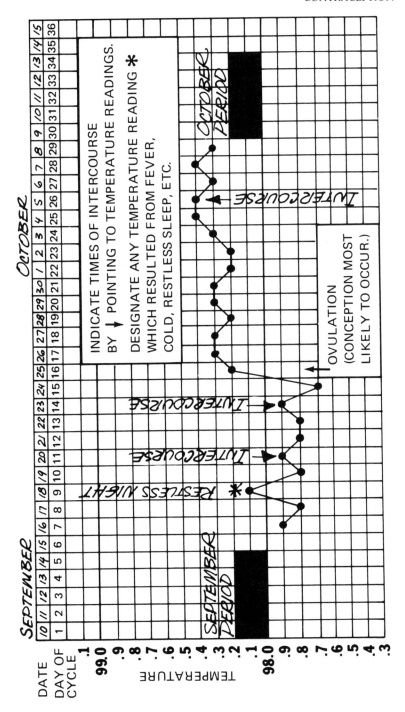

Figure 14-2.   *Example of a properly completed basal body temperature chart.*

ing the significance of them, it is hoped that a woman can not only tell when ovulation has occured, but also can know days in advance that it is going to occur.

The cervical mucus at the time of ovulation has certain recognizable characteristics. It becomes profuse, clear, and stretchy with an egg white consistency. The spinnbarkeit test, one parameter which is used to determine imminent ovulation, measures the number of centimeters which the mucus can be stretched before breaking. This can be done between two cover slips or, more simply, by the woman stretching the mucus between two fingers.

Ovulatory mucus can also be determined microscopically. Cervical mucus which has been put on a slide, dried, and examined under a microscope, will show a typical fern pattern. This is caused by the crystallization of the sodium chloride in the mucus. The ferning will rapidly decrease and disappear in the days following ovulation when estrogen decreases and progesterone becomes the dominant hormone. See Figure 14-3.

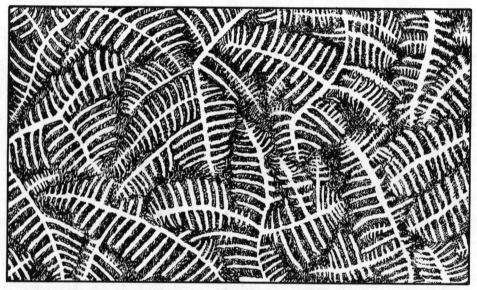

Figure 14-3.   Ferning of cervical mucous.

The arrangement of mucin fibers in cervical mucus during the fertile stage permits easy passage of sperm. They lie parallel to each other and to the cervical canal. Mucin fibers during the infertile phases form a crisscross pattern and prevent sperm entry. These characteristics of fertile-phase mucus are caused by the effect of estrogen on the mucous-producing glands in the cervix. See Figure 14-4.

Women may also be taught to become aware of other changes. These are the softening of the cervix as ovulation approaches, the crampy one-sided adnexal pain that many women experience and ovulatory spotting or bleeding. The pain that is experienced is referred to as "mittleschmertz" (mid-cycle pain).

A couple using the Billing's method is advised to abstain during the menstrual period. Menstrual blood would mask the presence of fertile-phase mucus if the woman were ovulating extremely early in that cycle. Any dry days following the

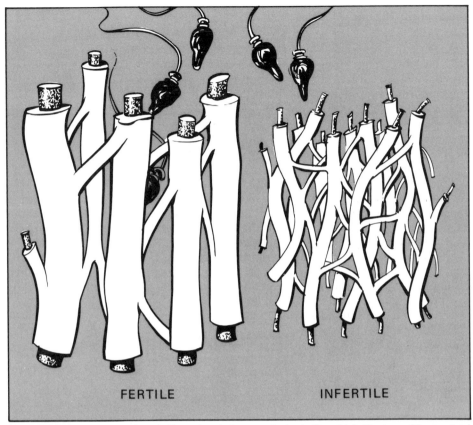

Figure 14-4.   Arrangement of mucin fibers of cervical mucous during fertile and infertile stages of the menstrual cycle.

menses are considered infertile. As soon as she becomes aware of any genital wetness she enters the fertile phase of her cycle and must abstain. This fertile phase lasts until the evening of the fourth day past the peak mucus production. The dry days that follow are considered infertile. The postovulatory infertile phase ends with the onset of the next menstrual period.

Strict adherents to this method allow intercourse only every other day during the "dry days." This is because the semen in the vagina may mask fertile-phase mucus. For the same reason, the combination of this method with use of contraceptive foams or jellies is unacceptable.

The Billings authored a workbook for women interested in this method called *Natural Family Planning: The Ovulation Method*. It is available from the publisher [1]. Initially, instruction should be given by specially trained counselors. Additional information regarding this method as well as assistance in finding local resources can be obtained by writing to the following organization:

The Human Life Foundation of America and The Natural Family Planning
  Federation of America
1511 K Street, N.W.
Washington, D.C. 20005

The Sympto-Thermal Method

As the name suggests, this method is a combination of the cervical mucus and BBT methods. In an attempt to increase the effectiveness of any one method, it asks the woman to observe symptoms as well as the temperature shift. In addition she observes the guidelines given for the calendar rhythm method.

Successful use would require adhering to the instructions already mentioned, but allowance is made for overlap. For example, instructions for the postovulatory infertile phase would be to abstain until the evening of the fourth day after peak mucus OR until the evening of the third day of temperature rise after the thermal shift, *whichever comes later*.

Proponents of this method claim higher effectiveness rates than for any of the methods used alone. This seems to have been confirmed by a study comparing the use-effectiveness of the sympto-thermal with the ovulation method. A failure rate of 9.4 percent was reported during the year of study [17]. This compares to 24.8 percent with the ovulation method.

Other than the apparent difference in effectiveness, the advantages and disadvantages are similar in both methods. Careful instruction by trained counselors is of utmost importance. An additional resource for people interested in the sympto-thermal method is:

The Couple to Couple League
P.O. Box 11084
Cincinnati, Ohio 42511

BARRIERS AND CHEMICALS

Foams, Jellies, Creams and Suppositories

Chemical preparations contain a spermicide chemical in an inert base. Although the base differs from one preparation to another, they all are designed to form a thick occlusive barrier to the sperm. In addition, the sperm is immobilized and killed.

There has been relatively little research done on side effects caused by spermicidal preparations. For the most part they have been presumed harmless with the exception of an occasional allergic reaction by the man or woman. However studies that have been done suggest the possibility of an increased incidence of birth defects should conception occur during or shortly after spermicide use. Because data is tentative at this time, women should be aware of further information as research makes it available [9].

Used alone the theoretical effectiveness rate is 95–97 percent. However the use effectiveness rate of these preparations may be as low as 78–80 percent [14].

Instructions for use:

Shake foam container vigorously.

Place high in the vagina to ensure covering of cervix.

Insert no more than twenty to thirty minutes before intercourse. (Body heat causes these preparations to liquify and run out of the vagina.)

Once the preparation has been inserted the woman should remain lying down.

Follow instructions on individual packages to ensure insertion of the proper amount.

Insert additional applications before each act of intercourse.

If douching is desired it must be delayed for eight hours after the last time intercourse occurs.

Condoms

The condom is a thin sheath that fits over the erect penis for the purpose of containing the ejaculate. Condoms are made of thin latex rubber or the cecum of young lamb intestines. Occasionally an allergy to rubber is reported by either partner; otherwise, the major complaint seems to be the decrease in sensitivity of the glans. This sometimes results in an inability to enjoy intercourse and occasionally the inability to maintain an erection. Theoretical effectiveness of this method is 97–98 percent. However, in actual use the effectiveness rate is 85–90 percent. [14]

Instructions for use:

Do not use condoms that are older than two years.

Do not expose condoms to heat. This would preclude carrying them in glove compartments of cars or in wallets or back pockets for long periods of time.

A condom should be rolled down over an *erect* penis. This can be done by either partner.

About one-half inch of space should be left at the tip of the condom to catch the ejaculate. Some condoms come with a nipple tip for this purpose. If condoms without nipple tips are used, care should be taken to allow for this space. This can be done by pinching the tip of the condom until it is in place.

If lubrication is used, avoid vaseline since it deteriorates rubber. Contraceptive foams or jellies or K-Y jelly may be used.

The condom should be held in place at the base of the penis while withdrawing to prevent slippage. Withdrawal should be made before loss of the erection for the same reason.

If the condom breaks or slips off, immediate insertion of contraceptive foam may be helpful.

Foam and Condom Combination

When discussing either of the above methods it is wise to remind a person that the combination of foam and condom used consistently approaches 98–99 per-

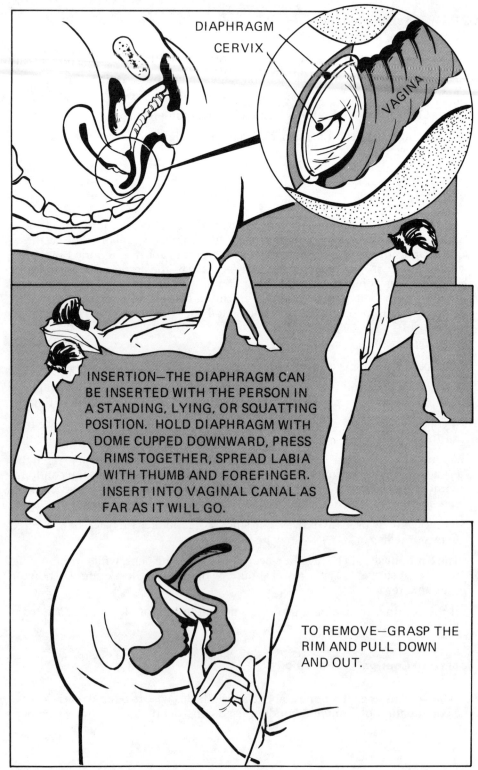

DIAPHRAGM

CERVIX

VAGINA

INSERTION—THE DIAPHRAGM CAN BE INSERTED WITH THE PERSON IN A STANDING, LYING, OR SQUATTING POSITION. HOLD DIAPHRAGM WITH DOME CUPPED DOWNWARD, PRESS RIMS TOGETHER, SPREAD LABIA WITH THUMB AND FOREFINGER. INSERT INTO VAGINAL CANAL AS FAR AS IT WILL GO.

TO REMOVE—GRASP THE RIM AND PULL DOWN AND OUT.

Figure 14-5.   Suggested technique for inserting and removing a diaphragm.

cent effectiveness. The advantages and disadvantages remain the same as with either method used alone. Although the effectiveness of this method is well proven, the most consistent complaint from users remains the necessity to have to bother with something "at the last minute."

Diaphragm

The diaphragm combined with contraceptive cream or jelly acts as both a mechanical and a chemical barrier to sperm. The device itself is a dome-shaped latex rubber cup with a flexible rim. This is designed to fit snugly behind the pubic bone anteriorly. Posteriorly, the rim extends beyond the cervix and rests in the vaginal cul-de-sac. The lateral walls of the vagina expand to accommodate the diameter of the diaphragm. When placed in this manner, the cervix is covered with the rubber cup. (See Figure 14-5.)

Since the sperm are microscopic, a diaphragm cannot provide a tight enough barrier to prevent all of them from reaching the cervix. Therefore it must be used with a contraceptive cream or jelly. Any sperm that manage to get around the rim are then immobilized and killed by the spermicide.

Side effects with this method are few and some are similar to those with foam and condoms. There have been reports of allergies to the jelly, or perhaps to the rubber itself.

Occasionally the rim of the diaphragm will cause discomfort or trauma to the vaginal walls. This may be caused by a diaphragm that is too large. It may also be due to a poor choice of rim style. The pressure of a rim on the anterior vaginal wall can sometimes cause enough trauma to "set the stage" for a urethritis in a woman prone to urinary tract infections. Frequently a change in size or in rim style will correct such a problem.

The size of a diaphragm refers to its diameter. They are available in 5mm increments ranging from 50–100 mm. Rim styles include arcing, coil spring and flat rim.

The main difference between the coil spring and the flat is the narrower rim of the latter. The arcing is often preferred because of the ease with which it can be accurately placed, but its more rigid rim is more likely to cause discomfort. (See Figure 14-6.)

There are very few absolute contraindications to diaphragm use. Allergy to rubber or spermicide would be one. An inability to attain a proper fit would be another. Conditions such as uterine prolapse, cystocele, rectocele and other pelvic abnormalities may make it impossible to attain a good fit. However, with some patience on the part of both the clinician and the woman, and a trial of different styles and sizes, a proper fit can usually be made. Frequently recurring urinary tract infections which seem to be related to the use of the diaphragm may necessitate discontinuing the method.

Complete inability to properly insert and remove the diaphragm is seldom a problem with adequate instructions. Lack of motivation, aversion to touching the genital area, and sexual inexperience are factors which may interfere with proper use of a diaphragm. However, these need not be automatically considered contraindications. It is only rarely that use of a diaphragm would be discouraged.

A woman who has never had intercourse can almost always be fitted for a diaphragm. A possible exception to this may be a woman with a tight hymen. However, if she can use tampons it is likely that she can insert a diaphragm. The inner dimensions that determine fit do not change after having intercourse. Therefore, the diaphragm can be accurately sized regardless of whether or not a woman is a "virgin."

As with all the methods, the effectiveness of the diaphragm depends largely on proper use. The diaphragm's theoretical effectiveness is 97–98 percent. Actual use-effectiveness figures are often stated as 80–90 percent [2]. The reasons for diaphragm failure are usually inconsistent use, improper placement, or failure to use adequate amounts of spermicides. The true "diaphragm baby" is probably a rarity.

Instructions for use: It is essential that a woman be given thorough instruction if the diaphragm is to be used effectively. Ideally, at the time of her diaphragm fit, she will be taught the following skills: To locate and be able to identify her cervix; to insert and remove the diaphragm; and to check for proper placement.

Adequate time must be allowed so that she can practice these skills a sufficient

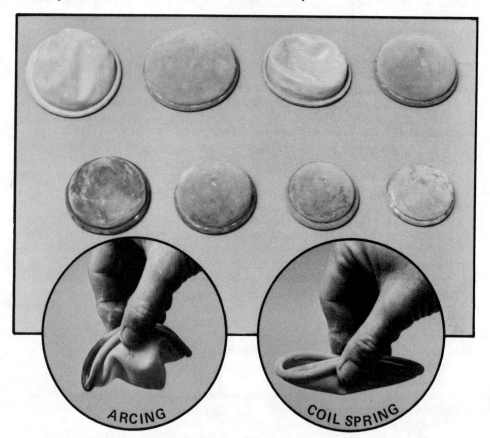

Figure 14-6.   Various rim styles and sizes of diaphragms are available.

number of times. If she can gain confidence in her ability to master these techniques her compliance will be greater and discontinuance rates lessened. A supportive and encouraging clinician is crucial.

An alert and observant clinician can identify problems in technique before they become intolerably frustrating. She can listen for comments that might indicate embarrassment, uncertainty or fear of the method. Nonverbal cues such as facial expressions and general comfort with one's body can also be indicators of successful diaphragm use.

At the end of a practice session the following instructions should be given in writing and reviewed verbally:

Use the diaphragm each time you have intercourse.

Always check to make certain that the rubber is covering the cervix and the front rim is securely tucked behind the pubic bone.

Apply an adequate amount of jelly or cream. Beginning inside the rim, place a ring of jelly around the diaphragm and about a teaspoonful in the center. A thin coating on the outside of the diaphragm provides extra protection.

Insert the diaphragm no more than two to three hours before intercourse. It can also be inserted at the time of intercourse but before penetration. This can be incorporated into foreplay if the couple desires.

Leave it in place for at least eight hours after the last episode of intercourse.

An applicator of additional spermicide needs to be inserted each time intercourse is repeated. Additional cream or jelly must also be applied if the diaphragm has been in place more than two to three hours before use.

Do not douche until the diaphragm has been removed.

The diaphragm should not be left in place more than about twenty-four hours since, as with any foreign body left in the vagina for long periods of time, an infection may result.

After removal clean the diaphragm with mild soap and water. Dry thoroughly with a towel and lightly dust it with cornstarch. This avoids the likelihood of putting it away wet which would hasten the deterioration of the rubber. Do not use perfumed soaps or talcs.

Store the diaphragm in its case away from direct sunlight and extreme heat.

Check frequently for holes or weak areas. This can be done by holding it up to a light and firmly stretching the rubber.

Do not use vaseline or cold cream on a diaphragm.

With proper care a diaphragm can last for two to three years or more.

A return appointment in one to two weeks is important. This provides an opportunity for the woman to identify any problems that may have occurred during practice and for the clinician to check for proper placement and size. Occasionally a diaphragm that seems to fit well at the end of a diaphragm fitting will actually be too small when the woman is fully relaxed. This is often discovered on the follow-up visit.

During the interval between fitting and follow-up, it is wise to use the diaphragm with a condom. It might also be suggested that the diaphragm be inserted and worn for eight to ten hours as a trial to check for comfort.

Frequent questions about the diaphragm:
Will it be felt by my partner?

No. A properly fit and correctly placed diaphragm should not be felt by either person.

Must I limit my physical activity during the hours that I need to wait before removing the diaphragm?

No. You may jog, participate in any sports, shower, bathe or swim.

Can any position for intercourse be used? I have heard that the diaphragm may slip out of place if the woman is on top.

In general, a diaphragm that fits snugly and is neither too large nor too small is unlikely to slip. However, it may be more possible to have this happen in the woman-superior position. Slipping may also be more likely if an excessive amount of jelly or cream has been used.

Are the spermicidal creams and jellies harmful if ingested?

No. However most of them have an unpleasant taste.

Am I likely to ever need a change in size of diaphragm, and if so, when?

It is advisable to have the size checked following a ten to twenty pound weight change, full term delivery or pelvic surgery.

Is it necessary to use my diaphragm during my period?

Consider it always necessary. It is rare, but not unheard of for a woman to ovulate during a menstrual period. The diaphragm holds back the menstrual flow and makes intercourse at that time more asthetic for many couples.

HORMONAL METHODS

Oral Contraceptives

The combination oral contraceptives contain both estrogen and a progestin. Together, these exogenous synthetic hormones act in four ways to prevent conception.

Inhibition of ovulation at the hypothalamic level. This in turn suppresses release of pituitary FSH and LH.

Interference with the tubal transport of the ovum if ovulation does occur.

Creation of an inadequate endometrium for implantation if fertilization does occur.

Changes in cervical mucus making it scanty, thick and relatively impenetrable to sperm.

The various brands of contraceptive pills contain synthetic estrogens and progestins in different combinations and in different doses. The number of possible combinations is great. For more detailed information regarding the estrogenic and progestational potencies of the various preparations refer to *Managing Contraceptive Pill Patients* by Richard P. Dickey [4].

While using oral contraceptives, the menstrual period is almost always lighter, shorter, and occurs with predictable regularity. The reason for menstrual regularity is that the period is actually a withdrawal bleeding. It occurs during the seven days when no pills are taken. This follows twenty-one days during which hormone-containing pills are taken. It is lighter and shorter because of the smaller buildup of endometrium under the influence of the synthetic hormones.

Complications and side effects. It appears that the major, potentially life-threatening complications as well as most of the lesser side effects of the Pill are primarily related to its estrogen component. Once this was suspected, pills containing less estrogen were developed, researched and marketed. The lower doses are thought to have fewer risks of the major Pill-related complications. These risks include the following:

Thromboembolic disease and myocardial infarction
Gallbladder disease
Benign liver tumors
Post-pill amenorrhea
Cancer

Certain conditions place women at a higher risk for developing these complications. These conditions include obesity, smoking, diabetes, and age greater than thirty-five. In addition there is a synergistic effect created by these conditions. That is, the more of them present, the higher the risk.

In view of these potential complications, careful evaluation of a women's gynecological history as well as a thorough physical examination must precede the use of oral contraceptives. Contraindications are often divided into the following categories.

Contraindications:
Absolute Contraindications.

Presence or history of deep thrombophlebitis, thromboembolic disorders, or myocardial infarction.

Cerebral vascular or coronary artery disease.

Known, suspected, or previous history of carcinoma of the breast.

Known or suspected estrogen dependent carcinoma.

Abnormal genital bleeding.

Known or suspected pregnancy.

Impaired liver function.

Strong Relative Contraindications.

Severe vascular headaches.

Hypertension with diastolic pressure greater than 100.

Diabetes.

Gallbladder disease.

Long leg casts, serious leg injury, or conditions that impair good venous return.

Sickle cell disease.

Planned elective surgery.

Age greater than thirty-five.

Possible Contraindications.

Irregular menstrual cycles or profile suggestive of anovulation.

Heavy smoking.

Problems such as mental retardation, alcoholism or previous history of unreliable Pill taking [4].

In addition to the serious or potentially life-threatening problems previously mentioned, the Pill has medically minor side effects. These can be so uncomfortable or annoying to a woman that she will discontinue use of the Pill. Forewarning and reassurance may avoid unnecessary alarm.

The following side effects can usually be attributed to either the estrogen or progestin component of oral contraceptives:

Nausea
Fluid Retention
Increased appetite and weight gain
Chloasma (mask of pregnancy)
Acne
Excessive facial or body hair
Headaches
Intermenstrual spotting or bleeding
Missed periods
Depression
Change in libido

Often a change in pill type will alter the hormone balance enough to correct the problem. In addition, many of these problems will correct themselves when the body has had time to adjust to the Pill, but this may take as long as two to three months.

Effectiveness. The Pill can be considered virtually 100 percent effective in theory. A theoretical effectiveness rate of 0.1–0.3 pregnancies per 100 women years is usually mentioned. The reasons for failure are not entirely clear. They may be due to gastrointestinal disturbances that affect absorption of the Pill or interaction with some drugs that may decrease its effectiveness. (See questions and answers about the Pill.)

Use effectiveness of the Pill ranges around 95–96 percent. The most common reasons in this category of failure are missed pills or pills taken at irregular intervals. A thorough education given at the time a woman begins oral contraception has a positive effect on successful pregnancy prevention.

Instructions for use and follow-up. Manufacturers of oral contraceptives package their product in two ways. Each pill type comes in both a twenty-one-day and a twenty-eight day version. In either case, there are twenty-one pills which are "active" and contain estrogen and progestins. In the twenty-eight-day package the last seven pills are "inert." Some manufacturers put iron in the inert pills but most do not.

The purpose of the inert pills is to help a woman keep track of the days on the "off week." Many women who choose the twenty-eight-day package do not actually swallow the inert pills but instead punch one out and throw it away each day. This seems to help reinforce the habit of taking pills regularly.

The first package can be started on the fifth day of a menstrual cycle or during the first Sunday following the onset of the menstrual period. If using the "Sunday start" and the period begins on a Sunday, the first pill should be taken that same day. The main advantage of the "Sunday start" to many women is that menstrual periods will not occur on weekends.

Theoretically, contraceptive protection is provided starting from when a woman takes her first pill. However, should a woman ovulate during that first week, pill "protection" would come too late. Therefore, a back-up method such as abstinence, foam, condoms, or a diaphragm is often recommended during the first pill cycle.

Pills should be taken at the same time each day. The effectiveness of the Pill depends on maintaining an adequate blood level of the synthetic hormones. It is designed to be taken every twenty-four hours to maintain this level. If a pill is missed for ten to twelve hours, that level may dip down enough for ovulation to occur during that cycle.

If a pill is not taken at the usual time, it should be taken as soon as remembered. This may mean taking two pills on the same day. In addition, a back-up method should be used for the remainder of that cycle.

It is common for bleeding to occur as a result of missing or taking pills late. This bleeding may sometimes continue until the end of the package. If three or more pills are forgotten, they should be stopped and re-started on the following Sunday or on the fifth day of the resultant menstrual bleeding. After restarting, a back-up method should be used during the entire package.

Theoretically, bleeding does not occur during the first twenty-one pills of each package. If there is spotting or bleeding which is NOT due to a missed pill it is insignificant and can be ignored. It does not mean lowered effectiveness but it can be annoying. If it persists for two or more cycles the clinician will probably prescribe a different pill with a different hormone balance.

If withdrawal bleeding does not occur during the last seven days of the cycle it does not necessarily mean that the woman is pregnant. If there were no missed or late pills, the chance of pregnancy is minimal and the next package can be started. If a second period is missed a clinician should be contacted. A pelvic examination and pregnancy test should be done. If no problems are found, a different pill type will be prescribed. If there were missed or late pills, pregnancy is a possibility.

Pills should be discontinued and an alternate method used until pregnancy is confirmed or menstrual bleeding begins.

Each woman who is taking oral contraceptives should become thoroughly familiar with symptoms associated with serious problems. Examples of these are severe leg pain, visual changes, severe headaches, chest pain or shortness of breath. Detailed information is contained in the FDA circular given with each package.

A commonly suggested follow-up schedule for a woman taking oral contraceptives is to have an initial three month assessment of blood pressure, weight and well-being. If this proves to be normal, similar follow-up is often done every six months. A yearly GYN examination is essential.

Frequent questions about the oral contraceptives:

Is it normal to have a breast discharge while I am on the Pill?

> A discharge from the breast which is not associated with pregnancy or lactation cannot ever be assumed to be normal. Such discharge is sometimes associated with oral contraceptive use in the absence of pathology. However, anyone with this problem needs to have a thorough investigation.

Am I protected from pregnancy during the seven days of each cycle when no hormones are taken?

> Yes.

Is it necessary to take a break from the Pill every two years or so?

> Opinion on this varies. The "Pill break" was recommended to reassure both the woman and her clinician that her cycles would re-establish themselves. This is no longer widely recommended for two reasons. Spontaneous resumption of menses during one break does not accurately predict what will happen on the next. The pregnancy rate is fairly high when women are forced into discontinuing their method of choice. Many physicians feel the risk/benefit ratio does not justify an enforced interruption of pill use.

My friend was put on the Pill to regulate her periods. My periods come every three to four months. Why won't my doctor put me on the Pill?

> The Pill suppresses normal endocrine and ovarian function. When a cycle is very irregular, clinicians are reluctant to further suppress it. To do so may compromise your future fertility. However, each woman should be allowed to establish her own priorities after being informed of the risks.

I have heard that some medications decrease the effectiveness of the Pill. What are they?

> There have been some reports that antibiotics and some of the anti-epileptic and anti-tubercular drugs may interfere with action of the oral contraceptives. This is probably more a theoretical risk than an actual one. It would be wise for an individual on long term therapy with these drugs to discuss this with her clinician.

I have heard that I should take a vitamin supplement while on the Pill. Is this true?

Although there is some evidence to support lower blood levels of Vitamin B_6 and B_{12} in women on the Pill, these levels do not represent a deficiency of these vitamins for most women. Therefore, vitamin supplementation is generally unnecessary.

I am planning to have plastic surgery done on my face. Must I stop the birth control pill before the operation?

There are not any firm guidelines for making a decision regarding the use of oral contraceptives when surgery is planned. Consequently you may find that your answer will vary from one physician to another. Since it is known that oral contraceptives are associated with an increased risk of circulatory clotting disorders, it seems prudent to be cautious. Many physicians feel that surgery which will not involve postoperative bed rest and limitation of movement can safely be done without discontinuing use of the method. However, it is probably advisable to discontinue use of oral contraception prior to orthopedic, abdominal, pelvic, or circulatory system surgery. The physician should be consulted regarding specific time recommendations for stopping and re-starting oral contraceptives. Of course it is important to use an effective interim method.

The Mini Pill

Mini Pills are oral contraceptives containing only progestin. They have been marketed in the United States since 1973, and were developed to be used by women who had contraindications to the use of estrogen. Their theoretical effectiveness is 98–99 percent, making them less attractive than the combined pill, but putting them into the same range as the IUD. There are very few published use-effectiveness rates for these preparations.

The Mini Pill is taken daily and the bleeding that occurs is a type of breakthrough bleeding. It appears at irregular intervals between twenty-five to forty-five days. The irregular bleeding, higher incidence of spotting and lower effectiveness rate cause many women to discontinue this method.

Morning-After Contraception

For most women unprotected intercourse usually causes great concern. They may seek information regarding risks and options. The risk of pregnancy from a single exposure may be as little as 2 percent and would not exceed 30 percent [8].

A woman who can accept abortion or a pregnancy may choose to take a "wait and see" approach. Morning-after contraception may be an acceptable alternative for a woman who would find abortion or pregnancy difficult to handle. For this reason, counseling at this time is extremely important.

A woman must be given as much information as possible about the risks associated with each option. She needs to be made aware of the fact that "morning-after" is only effective if given within seventy-two hours of the probable time of conception. The closer it is given to the time of unprotected intercourse, the more effective it will be. She also needs to be made aware of any risks to the fetus associated with the method should it fail.

There are three approaches to morning-after contraception.

Hormonal. It has been demonstrated that conception can be prevented by giving high doses of estrogen over a period of five to six days. The estrogens that have been shown to be most effective are diethylstilbesterol (DES), ethinyl estradiol, and Premarin®. The high doses of estrogen build up a thick but non-nourishing endometrial lining. When the fertilized ovum reaches the uterus, implantation cannot take place. There may also be interference with tubal transport.

Complications and contraindications are similar to those of oral contraceptives. Any woman who cannot take oral contraceptives for medical reasons should not be given the morning-after pill. The doses of estrogen given are equivalent to that found in forty to fifty tablets of birth control pills each containing 50 mg of estrogen. This level often results in nausea or vomiting, which may become severe. To counteract this problem, an anti-nausea preparation may be prescribed to be taken along with the estrogen.

Effectiveness is over 99 percent when treatment is started as close to exposure as possible (within 72 hours) and continued for the full five to six days. Failures are usually a result of severe nausea which results in incomplete treatment or to an undetected, preexisting pregnancy. True method failures are rare.

High doses of estrogen taken during the first few months of pregnancy can be damaging to the fetus. This has been documented with in utero exposure to DES. Therefore a woman must realize that if this method fails, abortion would be recommended. The woman should also be told that the use of estrogen for morning-after contraception is not FDA approved except in cases of rape or incest.

Mechanical. Studies using copper IUD's as morning-after contraception are currently underway. The FDA has not yet approved this use of the IUD. An IUD inserted within 5 days following conception would probably interfere with implantation of the ovum. This would seem to be a useful approach for someone needing an ongoing contraceptive method who does not have contraindications to use of an IUD.

Menstrual Extraction. Suction is used to extract the endometrium around the time of the expected menstrual period instead of waiting for confirmation of pregnancy. Since this is the same procedure used for performing a first trimester abortion, the risks are, for the most part, the same as those described in chapter 24. Additional risks of abortions performed very early in pregnancy include a higher incidence of incomplete abortion and uterine perforation. Another factor to be considered is that a woman may be subjecting herself to an unnecessary procedure. Because of these reasons many physicians prefer not to perform menstrual extractions.

This method seems to have particular appeal for a woman who does not want to know that she is pregnant and thus be forced to make a decision about abortion. In such situations sensitive counseling and exploration of basic attitudes towards sex are very important. Many of these women have not yet come to terms with their sexuality and the consequences of sexual activity. These women might benefit more from help with values clarification than with standard contraceptive education.

INTRAUTERINE DEVICES

The contraceptive effectiveness of objects or devices placed inside a human or animal uterus has been recognized for thousands of years. However, it was not until the 20th century that the use of IUD's became widespread. The development of suitable materials, the improvement of insertion techniques, and the appearance of antibiotics to combat infection were all responsible. See Figure 14-7.

The present day IUD is a small plastic device infused with barium to make it radio-opaque. There are five FDA approved IUD's of various shapes currently on the market. The Lippes Loop and Saf-T-Coil are plain plastic devices. To increase their effectiveness, the Copper 7 and Copper T are wound with a thin copper wire and the progestesert contains progesterone. Since both the copper and progesterone are released slowly from the IUD, these devices lose effectiveness over a period of time. The copper-bearing devices are effective for three years and the Progestesert for eighteen months.

The Loop and Coil are available in different sizes to fit uterine cavities of different depths. All IUD's have one or two strings that protrude through the cervical os. The strings serve to confirm the presence of the IUD as well as to facilitate removal. See Figure 14-7.

The presence of an IUD within the uterus is thought to prevent implantation of a fertilized ovum or to disturb a newly implanted blastocyst. There are numerous

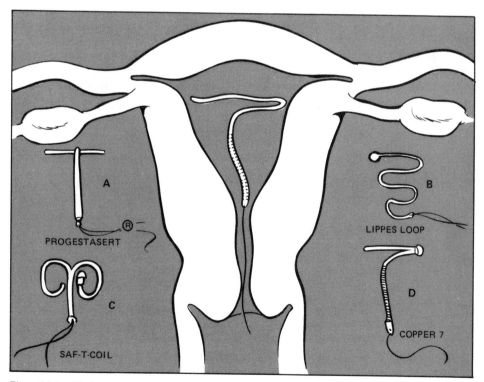

Figure 14-7.   Various types of IUDs. Inset shows IUD placement in the uterus with strings in vaginal canal.

theories as to just how this is accomplished.

There may be some alteration in the motility of the Fallopian tube. A local inflammatory response of the endometrial lining may cause phagocytosis of sperm cells or lysis of the blastocyst. This same inflammatory response may so alter the uterine lining as to make it an unlikely place for implantation.

It is also thought that the presence of a foreign body in the uterus stimulates production of prostaglandins. The increased uterine contractions caused by the prostaglandins may interfere with implantation or disrupt an already implanted ovum.

The copper is thought to interfere with implantation by disrupting enzymes in the uterine lining or by interfering with the uptake of estrogen by the uterine mucosa. In addition, copper is toxic to sperm. The effect of progesterone in the Progestesert is much the same as progestin taken orally.

Since the IUD probably does not prevent fertilization, but only implantation of an already fertilized egg, it may be unacceptable to some women who view it as an abortifacient. This needs to be taken into consideration during counseling. Each woman's views on this sensitive subject deserve careful exploration.

General recommendations regarding IUD insertion are:

• An IUD should be inserted during a menstrual period to minimize chances that the woman is pregnant. (This is not an absolute requirement, but many clinicians prefer it.)

• Eight to ten weeks should be allowed following a full term delivery or two to three months following Cesarian section.

• Three to four weeks should be allowed following therapeutic abortion.

• At least three months should pass after an episode of PID.

Complications and side effects:

• PELVIC INFECTION
     Symptoms: lower abdominal pain or tenderness; painful intercourse; fever
                       or chills; unusual vaginal discharge or bleeding.

The presence of an IUD significantly increases a woman's risk of infection of the uterus, ovaries or tubes. This may be due to infection introduced at the time of insertion by improper technique, inadequate sterilization of equipment or presence of pathological organisms in the vagina or cervix.

Most IUD related infections are not life-threatening if diagnosed and treated early. Future fertility may be impaired by the scarring that follows a severe infection. Therefore, knowledge of early warning signals of infection are important.

Treatment consists of antibiotic therapy, bed rest if severe, and, generally, removal of the IUD. The presence of the IUD may aggravate the infection and retard recovery. This could lead to an increased risk of sterility. However, if an infection seems mild, some clinicians will leave an IUD in place if response to therapy seems adequate and rapid. Careful observation is very important.

• PREGNANCY
     Symptoms: delayed or abnormal period; associated signs of pregnancy in-
                       cluding nausea, vomiting or breast tenderness.

If a woman becomes pregnant with an IUD in place, the risk of miscarriage is possibly as high as 50 percent. Some women spontaneously abort during the early months of a pregnancy without knowing that they are pregnant.

It is highly recommended that an IUD be removed from a pregnant uterus because of the increased risk of infection. The combination of pregnancy and infection can be fatal for mother and fetus. Although a pregnancy sometimes remains undisturbed during IUD removal, the procedure frequently results in spontaneous abortion. A woman considering this method of contraception needs to be aware of this when she is deciding about using this method.

- ECTOPIC PREGNANCY
  Symptoms: sudden one-sided lower abdominal pain; late or unusually light
            period; dizziness; faintness.

An ectopic pregnancy is one that develops outside the uterus. The most common site where this occurs is in one of the Fallopian tubes. This is a dangerous and potentially life-threatening situation. As the pregnancy develops the tube may burst resulting in massive hemorrhage and sometimes death.

IUD users are ten times more likely to develop an ectopic pregnancy than are women using other methods of contraception [13]. This may be due to impaired tubal transport. There may also be unknown factors related to the higher rate of ectopic pregnancies in IUD users.

- PERFORATION
  Symptoms: absent strings; abdominal pain; fever.

Perforation of the uterine wall by an IUD is more likely to occur at the time of insertion than at any other time. The risk of perforation with insertion is increased when the clinician is inexperienced, when the uterus is soft (such as immediately after delivery or abortion) or with extremes of anteversion or retroversion of the uterus.

Occasionally an IUD will migrate through the uterine wall after a period of time. This does not always cause symptoms. Sometimes it is first detected when a routine check reveals that the strings are not visible or palpable. The copper IUD's will often cause local irritation and inflammatory response in the abdominal cavity.

- EXPULSION
  Symptoms: cramping; absence of strings.

The uterus has a tendency to contract and attempt to expel a foreign body placed inside it. Expulsion of an IUD is most common within the first few weeks or months after insertion. After the third month the incidence of expulsion decreases as the uterus adjusts to the presence of the foreign body.

Some of the small IUD's can be expelled without symptoms. Therefore a string check is the only reliable way to determine whether an IUD is present. A woman can feel the string or strings by inserting a finger into her vagina and reaching back towards the cervix. The material feels somewhat like fishing line. If firm plastic is felt at the os or a significant change in length of strings is noted, it may indicate partial or complete expulsion.

- INCREASED BLEEDING AND CRAMPING

Many women experience more cramps with their menstrual periods during the first few months of IUD use. The cramping usually diminishes over a period of time. However, for some women the discomfort remains great enough to necessitate removal.

Increased amount and duration of menstrual flow is often a side effect. Intermenstrual spotting also is seen with greater frequency in IUD users. These abnormal bleeding patterns usually diminish over a period of a few months. However, it is frequently severe enough to require removal of the device.

Contraindications:

Absolute contraindications

    Acute or subacute PID.

    Known positive gonorrhea culture.

    Pregnancy.

Relative contraindications

    Rheumatic or valvular heart disease.

    History of ectopic pregnancy.

    Wilson's disease or copper allergy (would contraindicate a copper device).

    History of PID.

    Nulliparity if a woman desires future pregnancies (conservative approach).

    History of dysmenorrhea or heavy periods.

    Anemia.

    Inaccessability to health care facilities for routine follow-up or emergency treatment.

Effectiveness. The theoretical effectiveness of IUD's ranges from 95–99 percent. The different effectiveness rates from one IUD type to another can be attributed to characteristics such as size, shape, and presence of copper or progesterone. The use effectiveness of the IUD is 90–94 percent. The similarity in effectiveness rates is because the woman using an IUD can make relatively few errors in use.

Instructions for use and follow-up. The most important responsibility for the woman with an IUD is to periodically check the strings. In the first few months this should be done frequently. Thereafter it is advisable to check after each menstrual period. A change in length or absence of strings should be reported to a clinician.

   ● For increased effectiveness use a second method of birth control around the time of ovulation and during the two to three months following insertion.

   ● Pay attention to the early warning signs of IUD problems.

   ● Missed periods should be reported to a clinician.

   ● The woman should not attempt to remove an IUD herself. The best time to make an appointment for IUD removal is during a period.

   ● Appointments for annual pelvic, Pap smear, and breast examination are essential.

Frequent questions about the IUD:

If I have never been pregnant can I use an IUD?

Women who have had a full or late term pregnancy have a lower IUD complication rate and higher effectiveness. However, many women who have not been pregnant use IUD's successfully.

Why do I have to check my strings? Wouldn't I feel it if my IUD was being expelled?

Not necessarily. Most women do have increased cramping at the time of expulsion. However, some women apparently expel their IUD's during a period. The cramps may be indistinguishable from normal menstrual cramps. The IUD may be flushed down the toilet unnoticed.

Will my partner feel the strings?

Occasionally a man will complain about discomfort from an IUD string. This is most common if the string is cut very short and protrudes straight from the os. A longer string usually bends out of the way during intercourse.

STERILIZATION

Sterilization is becoming an increasingly popular form of fertility control. In the United States it is now the most common form of birth control used by married couples over the age of thirty [8]. There are many reasons for the increase in numbers of sterilization procedures being done.

Sexually active women have many years of fertility during which they may prefer not to become pregnant. Many of the available contraceptive methods bring with them a high risk of pregnancy. During most of a woman's later reproductive years the Pill, which is the most effective reversible method, carries the highest health risk.

Many younger women have made a decision to remain childless. This may be due to concern over world population problems or to the greater acceptance of women pursuing ambitious academic and professional goals. For some women, motherhood does not promise the same satisfaction as pursuit of their career goals.

A woman desiring sterilization can now legally have this procedure regardless of her age, marital status, number of children or consent of spouse. A woman using federal funds must be twenty-one years of age and mentally competent. If she is married or in an otherwise stable relationship, consent of both partners is preferred, but not required by law in most states.

Counseling for sterilization should include three issues.

1. Sterilization must be considered a permanent, irreversible method. Although there have been limited successful surgical procedures to regain fertility, these are expensive, not widely available, and very disappointing when unsuccessful. A person considering sterilization should be helped to explore unpleasant but realistic possibilities that are often ignored. These include divorce or death of a spouse with remarriage to someone desiring children, or the loss through illness or injury of one or more children.

2. When a counselor becomes aware of ambivalence on the part of an individual, care should be taken in recommending this method. Questions relating to sperm banks or operations to restore fertility should be carefully explored for underlying uncertainty. However, when an individual is able to accept the permanence of his or her decision, is aware of the risks involved and can fully accept the responsibility of the decision, there should be no reason to deny it.

3. When a couple reaches a mutual decision for a permanent contraceptive

method, they must then decide which partner will have the procedure. There are pros and cons for either male or female sterilization. Many of them involve psychological concerns rather than procedural risk.

Vasectomy for the male is a safer, simpler and less expensive procedure than are any of the female sterilization methods. Success can be determined by doing a sperm count. However, some men have concerns about impotence or a decreased sexual drive following vasectomy. If education about anatomy and physiology does not dispel these fears, vasectomy might not be the preferred method. Since a woman must go through the pregnancy and childbirth experience, she may be more willing to go through the necessary procedure.

Effectiveness. Male and female sterilization cannot be considered 100 percent effective. Occasionally the ends of a severed tube rejoin and pregnancy occurs. This can happen following vasectomy or tubal ligation. However, the failure rates of permanent sterilization are generally considered to be 0.04 to 0.2 percent [8].

Description of Sterilization Procedures

Tubal ligation or occlusion. Sterilization is accomplished by disrupting the Fallopian tubes in order to prevent passage of the ovum. This can be done by cutting and then tying or cauterizing the ends of the tubes, by damaging sections of the tubes with cautery, or by placing a clip on a folded loop of the tube in order to occlude the lumen. This can be done by one of three approaches. Either laparoscopy, abdominal, or vaginal incision may be used. (See chapter 25 and Figure 14-8.)

The main risks involved in these procedures are related to anesthesia, blood loss, and burning or injury to adjacent organs such as the bowel. Laparoscopic sterilization by cautery, when done by an experienced surgeon, results in fewer than 0.5 burn injuries per 1,000 cases [6]. Contraindications to the above procedures would include active pelvic infection, scarring of tubes from previous surgery or infection, serious medical problems that would increase risk of surgery, and obesity.

Hysterectomy. Although hysterectomy results in sterility, it is not generally accepted as a method of sterilization unless removal of the uterus is desired or necessary for other reasons. If a woman has large uterine fibroids, a history of abnormal Pap smears or endometrial biopsies, or severe episodes of dysfunctional uterine bleeding *and* desires sterilization, this approach is valid. However, the surgical risk associated with hysterectomy is so much greater than with the other sterilization methods that it is not recommended for that reason alone. (See chapter 25.)

Vasectomy. Vasectomy interrupts the two vas deferens. These are the tubes which ascend from the testes and are the transport system for sperm. The procedure is relatively easy to perform.

Complications from vasectomy are rare and when they do occur are usually short term and minor. Occasionally the ends of the vas will meet and rejoin and thus restore fertility, although this is rare. Other complications include hematoma, infection, and formation of a sperm granuloma.

There has been concern over the fact that as many as one-half to two-thirds of

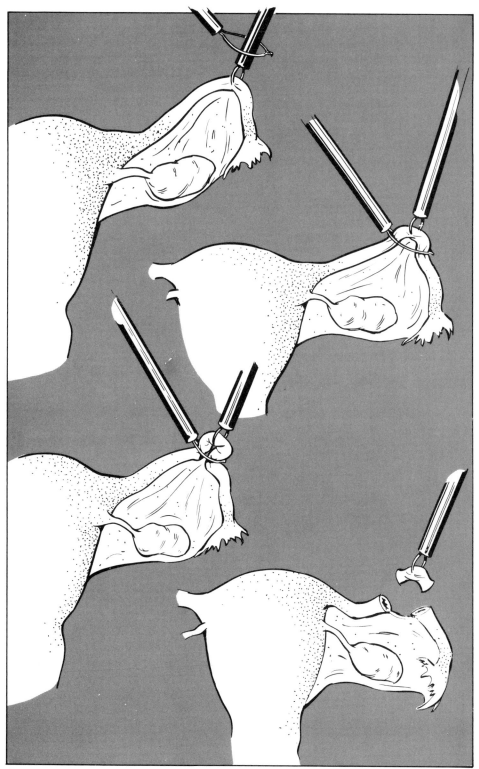

Figure 14-8.   Procedure used in laparoscopic tubal sterilization.

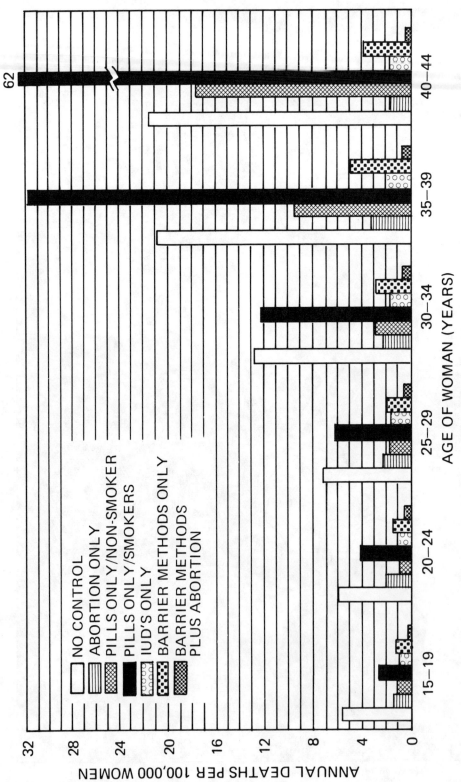

Figure 14-9.   *Annual number of deaths associated with births and birth control per 100,000 women in developed countries, by regimen of control and age of woman. Used with permission of Christopher Tietze from Induced Abortion 1979, a Population Council Fact Book.*

those with vasectomies will develop sperm antibodies. It has been feared that this may be associated with future systemic pathological conditions. To date there has been no statistically signficant data to support this concern [8].

It is important for men undergoing vasectomies to understand that sterility is not achieved immediately. Another birth control method must be used until he has had two consecutive negative sperm counts. The first sperm count should not be done until there have been at least ten ejaculations. The second count can be done about four weeks later.

CONCLUSION

Both pregnancy and the use of contraceptives involve risk for the heterosexually active woman during her reproductive years. Complications may range from mere annoyances to death. Although it is not often thought of in these terms, pregnancy carries a far greater risk for some women than do any of the contraceptive methods. Figure 14-9 summarizes the mortality associated with various types of contraception and pregnancy.

REFERENCES

1. Billings JJ: Natural Family Planning: The Ovulation Method, 3rd ed. Collegeville, MN, The Liturgical Press, 1975
2. Bradbury B: Preventing the "diaphragm baby syndrome:" A matter of technique, teaching, and time. Journal of Obstetric, Gynecologic, and Neonatal Nursing, March/April 1975
3. Britt S: Fertility awareness: four methods of natural family planning. Journal of Obstetric, Gynecologic, and Neonatal Nursing, Vol. 6 No. 2, March/April 1977
4. Dickey RP: Managing Contraceptive Pill Patients. Aspen, CO, Creative Infomatics, Inc., 1977
5. Diller L, Hembree W: Male contraception and family planning: A social and historical review. Fertility and Sterility, Vol. 28 No. 12, December 1977.
6. Engel T: Laparoscopic sterilization: Electrosurgery or clip application? Journal of Reproductive Medicine, Vol. 21 No. 2, August 1978
7. Flesh G: The intrauterine contraceptive device and acute salpingitis. American Journal of Obstetrics and Gynecology, Vol. 135 No. 3, 1979
8. Hatcher R et al: Contraceptive Technology, 10th ed. New York, Irvington Publishers, 1980
9. Jick H et al: Vaginal spermicides and congenital disorders. Journal of American Medical Association, Vol. 245 No. 13, April 3, 1981
10. Kistner RW: Gynecology Principles and Practice, 3rd ed. Chicago, Yearbook Medical Publishers, 1979
11. Peel J, Potts M: Textbook of Contraceptive Practice. New York, Cambridge University Press, 1969
12. Roitman M: Laparoscopic sterilization: Falope ring technique. Journal of American Osteopathic Association, Vol. 76 No. 107, 1977
13. Rosenfield A: Oral and intrauterine contraception: A 1978 risk assessment. American Journal of Obstetrics and Gynecology, Vol. 132 No. 1, September 1978
14. Ryder N: Contraceptive failure in the United States. Family Planning Perspectives, Vol. 5, 1973
15. Tietze C, Lewit S: Life risks associated with reversible methods of fertility regulation. International Journal of Gynaecology and Obstetrics, Vol. 16, 1979

16. Timby B: Ovulation method of birth control. American Journal of Nursing, Vol. 76 No. 6, June 1976

17. Wade M: A randomized prospective study of the use-effectiveness of two methods of natural family planning: An interim report. American Journal of Obstetrics and Gynecology, Vol. 134, July 1979

15

Upper Reproductive Tract Disorders

The function and structure of the organs in the female pelvis can be impaired by trauma, infection, benign cysts and tumors, or malignancy. The damage to the uterus, tubes or ovaries can range from problems that are minor and need no treatment to those that require major surgery. The problem may be one the woman is unaware of until it is found during a routine pelvic examination or one that causes severe symptoms such as pain or bleeding.

An assault on these organs either by disease or by trauma may threaten a woman's gender identity. Loss of pelvic organs before or during reproductive years means forfeiting future pregnancy. Women of any age may feel a threat of disfigurement or a loss of femininity.

This chapter will discuss infection, benign cysts and tumors, and malignancies of the upper reproductive tract. Trauma to the reproductive organs will not be discussed in detail, but one should be aware of damage caused by childbirth, accidents, or sport-related injuries. The implications for nursing interventions remain the same for all upper reproductive tract disorders.

The conditions discussed in this chapter may occur in any woman regardless of whether she is homosexual, heterosexual, or bisexual. Lesbian women probably

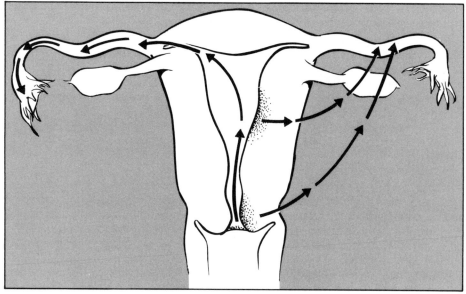

Figure 15-1.   *Two different routes of spread of pelvic infection.*

have a lower incidence of pelvic inflammatory disease although this has not been documented. This idea may be helpful to keep in mind when trying to determine the cause of a pelvic problem

INFECTION

Pelvic Inflammatory Disease (PID) is a generalized term describing an infection of the pelvic organs. The sites involved may be the endometrium (endometritis), the Fallopian tubes (salpingitis) or the ovaries (oophoritis). Frequently there is also involvement of adjacent organs or supporting structures resulting in abdominal or pelvic peritonitis. See Figure 15-1.
Tuberculous PID is extremely rare in the United States but is still found in under-developed countries. Sexually transmitted PID is responsible for 65 to 75 percent of all cases. There is increasing evidence to support the fact that organisms other than *N. gonorrhea* are responsible for acute pelvic inflammation. Although the gonococcus may be the most frequent causative organism, other causes may include *E. coli, Streptococcus* and *Chlamydia*.

Acute Phase

The initial phase of this disease is an infection of the cervix (see chapter 16). The upper tract infection is a result of delayed or inadequate treatment of the lower tract infection. The organisms ascend and spread by surface invasion along the endometrium to the Fallopian tubes and then to the ovaries. The spread is trans-mucosal and often occurs at the end of or just after a menstrual period. At that time there is a loss of the normal cervical mucous barrier. Also, menstrual blood provides an excellent growth medium for bacteria.

The bacteria tend to remain localized to mucosa and serous surfaces and do not spread via the bloodstream and lymphatics. Most of the damage occurs in the tubes, ovaries, and surrounding pelvic and abdominal peritoneum. The tubes and ovaries become inflamed and edematous and there is generally an abundance of purulent exudate. The endometrium is rarely involved because of the cyclic sloughing.

Chronic Phase

If treatment of the acute phase is inadequate, absent, or delayed the purulent exudate pours from the tubes into the peritoneal cavity. The body defense mechanisms, with or without the aid of antibiotics, are mobilized in order to local-ize and control the acute infection. It is this walling-off process and eventual fibro-sis of areas where exudate has developed that results in the problems encoun-tered in chronic PID.

If gonorrhea or secondary bacteria once again gain access to the cervix and ascend, the already trapped exudate provides an ideal environment for growth. Even in the absence of exudate, the process flares up once again.

Signs and Symptoms. Pelvic pain is the most common symptom in the acute phase. The pain is occasionally mild to moderate, but often it is severe. Although there can be generalized abdominal tenderness, more often the pain is in the lower abdomen and is usually bilateral.

Frequently a woman will also have noticed a heavy, purulent discharge from the vagina. This occurs as a result of cervicitis which is the initial stage of the disease. Fever may be present and occasionally is accompanied by chills, nausea and vomiting. Lab tests may show a leukocytosis and elevated sedimentation rate.

When a pelvic exam is done, the woman usually complains of severe discomfort. Any manipulation of the cervix will cause considerable pain, the so-called "chandelier sign." Pain and involuntary guarding may make the pelvic examination difficult and inadequate. When this occurs, adnexal masses may be best evaluated by ultrasound (see chapter 24).

When PID becomes subacute or chronic, pain is usually milder and may be felt as persistent cramps, lower abdominal tenderness, back pain, dyspareunia or dysmenorrhea. Intermenstrual spotting or bleeding may result from impaired ovarian function.

Diagnosis. Skillful counseling and a nonjudgmental attitude are very important in eliciting a history of sexual activity. If the woman has had intercourse with a male who has a known or suspected venereal disease, PID may be a likely diagnosis. Other problems should be considered and ruled out before making a definite diagnosis. Conditions that have symptoms similar to PID include appendicitis, ruptured ectopic pregnancy, twisted ovarian cyst, acute pyelitis, and diverticulitis. The diagnosis can be aided by culdocentesis and ultrasound. Occasionally laparoscopy or laparotomy may be necessary.

Treatment. The acute phase of an initial attack is usually treated with antibiotics, limited activity, increased fluids, and analgesics. Severe cases will require hospitalization with complete bedrest and I.V. fluids. Once a diagnosis is made, frequent pelvic exams should be avoided since they tend to "stir up" the infection.

If a large pelvic abscess is present it may be drained through the cul-de-sac, although laparotomy is usually required. When a tubo-ovarian abscess is thought to have ruptured, emergency surgery is necessary. This complication carries a high mortality rate, and often necessitates total hysterectomy and oophorectomy.

Surgery plays a much smaller role in treatment of acute PID than it did twenty to thirty years ago. This is primarily due to two factors. The first is improved treatment with the advent of antibiotics. The second is the increased routine screening done for gonorrhea at the time of pelvic examination. Early treatment affords the best means of preventing serious complications.

Surgery does play a larger role in the treatment of the chronic phase. Some women will have recurrent episodes of acute infection due to the impaired defense mechanism of the damaged tubes and ovaries. Other women will have persistent chronic pain, dysfunctional uterine bleeding, dyspareunia, and secondary dysmenorrhea. When these symptoms cannot be relieved and cause severe disability, hysterectomy with bilateral salpingo-oophorectomy must be performed.

Risk factors and sequelae. Approximately 10–17 percent of women with cervical gonorrhea will develop PID. Of these, almost 25 percent will experience recurrent disease. Recurrences may be gonococcal or nongonococcal. Of those women with a previous history of PID who develop gonorrhea, more than one-third will develop PID in contrast to the 10–17 percent mentioned earlier [1].

Intercourse with an infected partner at the time of menstruation will increase a woman's risk of PID. Also, a history of previous infection or use of an IUD increase her risk. Thus, the three major risk factors are menstruation, IUD use, and a previous episode of PID. The long-term sequelae of PID include: recurrent episodes of PID, pelvic pain such as dysmenorrhea and dyspareunia, and infertility.

Pyogenic PID

Pyogenic or septic PID is caused by organisms that gain access to the pelvic organs following abortion, childbirth, gynecological surgery, or instrumentation. The incidence of pyogenic PID has significantly decreased since the legalization of abortion. This type of infection travels via the lymphatics and bloodstream (see Figure 15-1). It primarily involves the interstitial layer of the tube with little involvement of the mucosa.

The gravid, postpartum or postabortal uterus is extremely vulnerable to infection. The edematous, highly vascular uterine wall provides little resistance to invading bacteria. In addition, retained products of conception provide a medium for growth.

The bacteria commonly involved are extremely virulent and include *Peptostreptococcus*, *Bacteroides*, *E. coli*, *Staphylococcus*, and occasionally *Clostridium*. If treatment is not started early and pursued vigorously, pyogenic pelvic inflammatory disease can lead to septicemia and an overwhelming and possibly fatal outcome.

Symptoms and examination findings. A woman with pyogenic PID will usually have a high fever, rapid pulse, shaking chills, and extreme pelvic pain. In addition she will often have vaginal bleeding and a purulent, foul smelling discharge. Pelvic examination will usually reveal extreme pelvic pain and tenderness. The cervical os may be dilated and occasionally placental fragments can be seen.

Diagnosis. Once again, the history is very helpful in diagnosing the problem. A recent pregnancy, abortion, or gynecological procedure will help establish the diagnosis of pyogenic PID. Cultures of the discharge as well as blood cultures can be helpful in identifying the specific type of bacteria involved.

Treatment. Early treatment consists of the use of broad spectrum antibiotics, I.V. fluids, and bed rest. Rapid resolution of fever and pain in twenty-four hours is anticipated with appropriate antibiotic therapy. When applicable, D & C for removal of retained products of conception may be required.

Risk factors and sequelae. In the past, criminal or self-induced abortion was the biggest risk factor in pyogenic PID. Puerperal infection followed delivery under unclean conditions and with the use of unsterile instruments. Both of these causes of PID are on the decline. Puerperal infection has decreased because of the use of sterile technique with hospital births or professionally attended home-births. Postabortal infections have decreased as a result of legalization of abortion.

Once a woman recovers from pyogenic PID, there are very few sequelae. Because of the lack of involvement of the tubal mucosa, sterility is rarely a problem. However, this disease carries a much higher mortality rate than does PID due to gonorrhea or other sexually transmitted organisms.

BENIGN TUMORS

Leiomyomas

Uterine leiomyomas are benign tumors which arise from muscle cells. They are commonly referred to as fibroids. They may occur singly but are more often found to be multiple. There are three types which are classified according to their location within the uterus including submucous, interstitial or intramural, and subserous. See Figure 15-2.

These tumors are almost always benign. They seem to be hormone-dependent and therefore grow with varying degrees of rapidity during the menstrual years. Because of their response to estrogen, oral contraceptives and pregnancy will

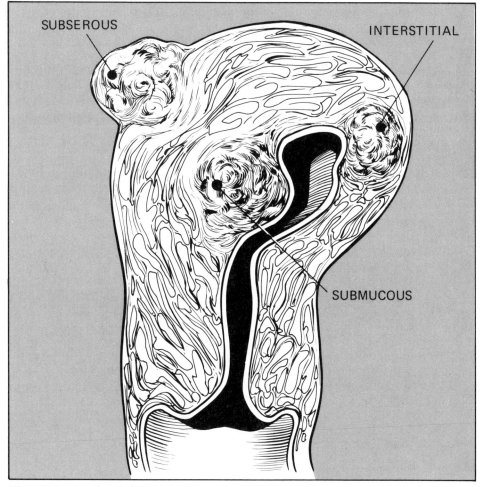

Figure 15-2. Location of leiomyomas.

stimulate growth. They often regress spontaneously in the postmenopausal years.

Symptoms: Very small leiomyomas may be asymptomatic. They may be incidentally discovered during a routine pelvic examination or during surgery. Symptoms which occur with large leiomyomas vary according to their location and size.

The growth of *submucous* leiomyomas will expand the uterine wall. This increases the surface area of the myometrium. The most common symptoms are heavy bleeding and cramps. Occasionally a submucous leiomyoma will protrude through the cervical os and cause postcoital bleeding.

Interstitial or intramural tumors may also cause some increased bleeding and dysmenorrhea. However, they usually remain asymptomatic until they become fairly large.

Since *subserous* leiomyomas are on the surface of the uterus, they often attain rather large sizes before causing symptoms. When symptoms do occur, they are related to the location of the tumor and may include bladder or bowel pressure and backache.

Diagnosis: Diagnosis of fibroids is usually made by history and the finding of a large, irregular uterus. Pregnancy must also be ruled out by menstrual history and appropriate testing. Ultrasound examination can further support the diagnosis and usually can distinguish a uterine mass from an ovarian mass. If the woman is asymptomatic, treatment is usually unnecessary. Yearly pelvic exams can monitor the rate of growth of the tumor. Since they usually grow slowly, a woman can often reach menopause without problems. Use of oral contraceptives and postmenopausal estrogen replacement are contraindicated.

If fibroid growth becomes rapid or symptoms become severe, surgery may be needed. Myomectomy is done if further pregnancies are desired and hysterectomy if a woman's family is complete. Recurrence following myomectomy is common and many women eventually need hysterectomy.

Endometrial Polyps

Polyps occurring in the endometrium are associated with endometrial hyperplasia. This is most often a result of excess estrogen which is unopposed by progesterone.

Endometrial polyps occur most frequently in premenopausal women when anovulatory cycles become more frequent. They also may result from the use of exogenous estrogen therapy for menopausal symptoms. Women with anovulatory cycles throughout their menstrual life are also susceptible.

Symptoms: Endometrial polyps are frequently asymptomatic. If present, symptoms include intermenstrual or postmenopausal spotting or bleeding.

Diagnosis and treatment: A woman with persistent, irregular bleeding should always have a D & C. If polyps are found, they can usually be removed by the use of a polyp forceps.

Cystic Ovarian Tumors

Nonneoplastic or functional cysts are so-called because they result from normal ovary function. (See chapter 3.) There are four types of functional cysts.

Follicle cysts may result when a ripe follicle fails to burst and thus remains active. They may also result when any of the less stimulated follicles fail to undergo normal atresia. These cysts are usually small but occasionally attain sizes up to six to eight centimeters.

Corpus luteum cysts arise as a result of hemorrhage into a persistent, mature corpus luteum. They generally tend to be larger than follicle cysts and range from 5–10 centimeters.

Bilateral polycystic ovaries are characteristic findings in Stein-Levinthal Syndrome and are discussed more fully in chapter 18. The ovaries contain numerous follicle cysts and have a thickened capsule. They are actually surrounded by a dense layer of collagenous tissue. Since ovulation rarely occurs, there is an absence of corpus lutea.

Endometriomas arise from ovarian endometriosis. They are commonly referred to as "chocolate cysts" since they are filled with a dark brown, bloody fluid. Their size and occurrence are variable.

There are three types of neoplastic ovarian cysts:

Mucinous cysts contain a sticky, gelatinous substance secreted by the tumor cells. They tend to become quite large and some attain enormous proportions. They are usually unilateral.

Serous cysts are more likely to be bilateral and do not attain the large sizes found in mucinous cysts. They contain a clear, straw-colored liquid.

Dermoid cyst is actually a misnomer and probably originated because of the frequency with which dermal elements (such as hair and teeth) are found within the cyst. The correct name, *benign teratoma,* refers to a tumor arising from all three germ cell layers. This tumor has the potential for developing any type of tissue found in the body. The bulk of the cyst is made up of fatty, semi-solid sebaceous material. These cysts usually occur during active reproductive years and occasionally during childhood.

Solid Ovarian Tumors

Fibromas are tumors of fibrous connective tissue. They are usually unilateral and vary in size from small nodules to large melon-sized masses. They are found most often in women during active reproductive years.

Brenner tumors are relatively uncommon and grossly are identical to fibromas. However, microscopically they are found to have small cystic spaces within them. They generally appear after menopause or during late reproductive life.

Symptoms: Many of the benign ovarian tumors are completely asymptomatic and are incidentally discovered during a routine pelvic examination. The following symptoms occasionally occur.

• *Menstrual irregularities* such as oligomenorrhea which is frequently encountered with polycystic ovaries. Both follicle and corpus luteum cysts may be accompanied by a delayed menstrual period with subsequent prolonged flow.

• *Lower abdominal discomfort* of a vague nature is sometimes noticed.

• *Abdominal swelling* may be noted with some of the tumors that attain large sizes.

• *Bladder and bowel irregularities* may result when the tumor reaches a size large enough to exert pressure on those structures.

• *Pain* is not usually a symptom of benign ovarian tumors except in cases of torsion of the ovarian pedicle or rupture of the cyst.

Diagnosis: When an adnexal mass is found during a pelvic examination, three questions must be answered. Is the mass ovarian in origin? Is it a functional or neoplastic mass? Is it benign or malignant?

A thorough pelvic examination and history can often help to clarify the first two questions. Pelvic x-ray and/or pelvic ultrasound are often used. Laparoscopy can be used to differentiate ovarian from uterine masses as well as physiological from neoplastic tumors. A benign or malignant diagnosis can be determined only by surgery.

Treatment: When a physiologic, nonneoplastic cyst is strongly suspected, treatment usually involves waiting four to six weeks and then reexamining the woman. Most of these cysts will spontaneously regress after one or two menstrual cycles. Since these cysts are dependent on pituitary gonadotropins, oral contraceptives often help to resolve them. Therefore, an enlarged ovary in a woman who uses oral contraceptives would lead one to suspect a neoplastic tumor.

Surgery is indicated for neoplastic tumors or for physiological cysts which persist or become larger. In most cases benign cysts and solid tumors can be removed while leaving the ovary intact. However, in the event of a very large size, rupture, or torsion, removal of the entire ovary and tube may be necessary. If there is malignancy or malignant potential, a salpingo-oophorectomy must be performed.

MALIGNANCIES

Endometrial Carcinoma

Endometrial carcinoma is the second most common gynecological malignancy [2]. Both its absolute and relative frequency has increased over the past years. This is due in part to the increasing longevity of the female population. It is also related to the decreasing incidence of cervical cancer secondary to mass screening for cervical disease.

Certain risk factors have become associated with this disease and a stereotype of the susceptible woman has emerged. Obesity, hypertension, metabolic disturbances such as diabetes, poor fertility, dysfunctional uterine bleeding during reproductive years, and a delayed onset of menopause are all frequently found.

The association of endometrial carcinoma with poor fertility, late menopause and extended episodes of dysfunctional uterine bleeding have long led many investigators to suspect that estrogen may play a role in this disease. This is because of the increased amount of endogenous estrogen present in these conditions.

Exogenous estrogen in the form of sequential oral contraceptives or replacement therapy for menopausal symptoms may also be a factor. The sequential birth control pills were taken off the market because of a possible link to endometrial cancer. It seems that unopposed estrogen is what creates this problem.

Until more definitive evidence is obtained these drugs need to be used with caution. The low dose oral contraceptives seem a wise choice when the Pill is desired. Menopausal estrogen replacement should probably be as brief as possible and in the lowest possible dosage. (See chapter 11.)

Symptoms: The main and often only symptom of this disease is abnormal bleeding. Because the incidence of this disease is higher in older women, the bleeding will usually be postmenopausal. In premenopausal women, intermenstrual bleeding may occur. Pain is almost never associated with early, endometrial carcinoma.

Diagnosis: Office procedures such as endometrial biopsies and aspirations can often diagnose endometrial carcinoma. Occasionally a Pap smear of the cervix will reveal malignant endometrial cells. The most accurate and only definitive diagnosis is by D&C. If the previously mentioned tests are negative in a woman with postmenopausal bleeding, a fractional curettage must be done. This procedure involves curetting both the endocervix and the endometrium to help determine the extent of the disease.

If spread of the disease is suspected, additional diagnostic tests might include barium enema, intravenous pyelogram, cystoscopy and proctoscopy. Occasionally the extent of disease cannot be determined until surgery.

Accurate staging of the disease is important in determining a treatment plan as well as in establishing a prognosis. The following classification devised by the International Federation of Gynecologists and Obstetricians (FIGO) is generally used.

Stage O = Carcinoma in situ (preinvasive or intraepithelial carcinoma).

Stage I = Carcinoma confined to corpus and has not penetrated the basement membrane.

Stage II = Carcinoma involves corpus and cervix.

Stage III = Carcinoma extends outside uterus but not outside true pelvis.

Stage IV = Carcinoma extends outside pelvis.

Treatment: Treatment of endometrial carcinoma depends upon the stage of disease and may involve radiation, surgery, or a combination of the two. Surgical removal of the uterus and adnexa is considered to be the keystone of therapy. Although radiation may precede or follow surgery, it is rarely used as the only therapy. An exception to this would be in the case of a woman who by reason of age or concurrent medical problems is considered to be a poor operative risk.

The five-year survival rate ranges from 55–80 percent [9]. This depends upon the stage of disease, the medical condition of the woman and the treatment given. The highest cure rate is found with the combination of surgery and radiation.

Cancer of the Ovary

As in the case of benign ovarian tumors, ovarian carcinomas may be cystic or solid. They may arise as a primary carcinoma, result from metastases from another primary site, or very rarely, be a result of malignant change in a previously benign tumor. Although the ovary is the third most common site of malignancy in the female reproductive tract, ovarian cancer is the leading cause of death from genital cancer [1].

Ovarian cancer is primarily a disease of older women. It usually occurs at or shortly after the menopause with the peak incidence from forty to sixty years. Risk factors for this disease include nulliparity and infertility. Recent studies indicate that multiple pregnancies as well as the use of oral contraceptives may be protective against ovarian cancer. This is presumably because they interrupt the repeated ovulation that increases risk [10].

Symptoms: Unfortunately, ovarian cancer is a silent disease. It rarely causes any symptoms until other organs are involved. When early symptoms do occur they usually consist of vague lower abdominal feelings of discomfort or pressure. Abdominal swelling may occur as a result of an enlarging tumor or with ascites. Bowel and bladder irritability might also be noted. Pain, when present, is associated with torsion of the pedicle, rupture of the tumor, or invasion of surrounding organs.

Diagnosis: Regular, periodic pelvic examinations remain the best means of early diagnosis of ovarian cancer. A palpable ovary in a postmenopausal woman is suspicious and should always be investigated. An adnexal mass in a younger woman also needs to be carefully followed.

Occasionally a routine cervical and vaginal Pap smear will show findings of ovarian carcinoma. However, this is uncommon and indicates that the tumor has broken through its capsule. This situation has a poorer prognosis.

Treatment: When diagnosed most ovarian carcinoma is advanced. Surgery may be done for the following reasons:

- To exclude the possibility of a benign, readily curable ovarian fibroma.
- To give symptomatic relief from an enlarging pelvic mass.
- To stage the malignancy in order to plan treatment.

Surgical treatment consists of total hysterectomy and bilateral salpingo-oophorectomy. If gross disease was left behind or if there is a high possibility of microscopic residual disease, radiotherapy and/or chemotherapy are given. Both provide a woman with metastases a longer symptom-free time following surgery. The five-year survival rates for cancer of the ovary are extremely poor since most cases are discovered only when they have already extended beyond the ovary.

REFERENCES

1. Barber HRK et al: Current concepts in the management of ovarian cancer. Journal of Reproductive Medicine, Vol. 20 No. 1, January 1978
2. Boutselis J: Endometrial carcinoma, prognostic factors and treatment. Surgical Clinics of North America, Vol. 58 No. 1, February 1978
3. Dimitriades M et al: Chemotherapy of ovarian cancer. International Surgery, Vol. 63 No. 2, February 1978
4. Eschenbach D: Acute pelvic inflammatory disease: Etiology, risk factors and pathogenesis. Clinical Obstetrics and Gynecology, Vol. 19 No. 1, March 1976
5. Eschenbach D: Pathogenesis of acute pelvic inflammatory disease: Role of contraception and other risk factors. American Journal of OB-GYN, Vol. 128 No. 8, August 1977
6. Green T: Gynecology: Essentials of Clinical Practice. Boston, Little, Brown, 1977
7. Greenhalf JO: The problem of pelvic infection. The Practitioner, Vol. 216 No. 1295, May 1976
8. Lees D: Surgery of endometrial cancer. Clinical Obstetrics and Gynecology, Vol. 5 No. 3, March 1978
9. Novak E: Gynecology. Baltimore, Williams and Wilkins, 1971
10. Suppression of ovulation by pregnancy and pill use—sharply decreases ovarian cancer risk. Family Planning Perspectives, Vol. 11 No. 6, November/December 1979

16

Lower Reproductive Tract Disorders

As with the upper reproductive tract organs, the cervix and vagina are also subject to problems caused by infection, benign or malignant growths, and trauma. Because of their proximity to the external genital area, symptoms of cervical and vaginal problems are often more readily noticed by a woman or her sexual partner than are problems in the upper reproductive tract. Vaginal discharges can be seen or sometimes smelled. Cysts and tumors can often be felt by the woman or her partner. They are sometimes first noticed when inserting a diaphragm or tampon. An abrasion or laceration of the vagina is often accompanied by pain or bleeding—either with intercourse or with tampon use.

Although many of the symptoms of these problems are visible, the areas themselves are not. The inside of the vagina is a poorly understood and somewhat mysterious place to most women. The function of the cervix and vagina in a woman's sexual life imparts significant meaning to problems when they occur. Consequently, questions regarding the vaginal area are among those most frequently asked.

Although the frequency of sexually transmitted infections is apparently less in the lesbian population, all of the problems discussed in this chapter may occur in both homosexual and heterosexual women. No matter how or from whom the disease was contracted, symptoms and treatment will be the same. Any sexually active woman is at increased risk for contracting a sexually transmitted disease; therefore she must assume the responsibility for receiving regular health care screening. Whether sexually active or not, all adult women (being subject to the development of any of the other problems discussed in this chapter) also must take responsibility for routine health examinations.

INFECTION

Before discussing the various types of vaginal and cervical infections a comparison of normal to abnormal discharges may be helpful. This review is summarized in Table 16-1.

The use of products to eliminate normal vaginal discharge should be discouraged. Douching often alters the normal flora which is the vagina's defense against infection. Improper douching or the use of chemicals may cause trauma or irritation to the vaginal mucosa. Vaginal sprays, powders, deodorant tampons and harsh soaps sometimes cause allergic reactions resulting in severe discomfort. These products are unnecessary, expensive, and potentially harmful.

A common but sometimes overlooked cause of abnormal vaginal discharge is the presence of a foreign body left in the vagina. The most common objects found

TABLE 16-1   Comparison of normal and abnormal vaginal discharges.

	Normal	*Abnormal*
Composition	Cervical mucus, vaginal epithelial cells, normal vaginal bacteria	Pus, pathogenic bacteria and viruses, possibly blood cells and epithelial cells, fungi or parasites.
Color	Clear or creamy white	Wide variation: grey-white, yellow or green, brown or rusty
Consistency	Mucoid (pre and postmenstrual) thin and stringy (mid-cycle)	May be clumpy and thick or thin and liquid
Amount	Changes cyclically with hormonal fluctuations; least amount following menses; heaviest near and at ovulation and before menses	Varies from almost none to profuse amounts requiring frequent change of clothing
Odor	None	May have yeast-like, mushroom, fishy or other strong odor
pH	Acid	Varies

in adult women are forgotten tampons and diaphragms. A variety of objects are sometimes inserted by children in the course of exploring their own bodies. A foreign body in the vagina usually results in a profuse discharge with an unpleasant odor.

Some of the infections that will be discussed in this chapter are sexually transmitted and others are not. Some have serious implications while others are merely annoying or uncomfortable. Most are preventable. Prevention techniques which are applicable to all vaginal infections are as follows:

- Condoms prevent the spread of sexually transmitted diseases.
- Daily cleansing of the genital area decreases the amount of bacteria.
- Wearing cotton instead of nylon underpants, wearing pantyhose infrequently and then only those with cotton crotch inserts, avoiding tight pants, wearing skirts and loose shorts during hot weather, and changing out of wet swimming suits promptly all help to minimize the warm, moist environment which aids bacterial growth.
- Wiping from front to back after a bowel movement prevents the spread of bacteria from the rectal area to the vagina and urethra.

● Avoiding the use of bubble baths, perfumed powders, and vaginal hygiene products reduces the chance of chemical irritation of the vaginal mucosa.
● Douche only with medical direction.
● Maintenance of good health through diet, proper rest and stress reduction, increases resistance to infection.

Yeast (Monilia) Vaginitis

Cause:	Most common organism is Monilia (Candida albicans). (See Figure 16-1.)
Influencing factors:	Use of antibiotics (disturbs balance of normal vaginal flora). Diabetes. Pregnancy. Premenstrual changes in vaginal environment. Oral-genital contact (may result in oropharyngeal infections).
Symptoms and signs:	Itching. Vaginal and vulvar irritation (may result in dyspareunia or pain with tampon use). Redness and swelling of vulva. Small hairline fissures or cracks in the skin of introitus or labia. Thick white ("cottage-cheese") type of discharge. Oropharyngeal infections: (sore mouth, tongue, and throat with patchy, white exudate).
Diagnosis:	Microscopic identification of spores, hyphae, and buds. Culture of causative organism.
Treatment:	Vaginal creams or suppositories. Gentian violet swabbing of the vagina. Nonmedical suggestions: yogurt, vinegar douche. Oropharyngeal infections treated by using mouthwash of nystatin oral suspension.
Prognosis:	Usually responds well to treatment. Recurrences may result even with adherence to treatment regimes and preventive measures since it is a normal vaginal inhabitant. No evidence to date that any serious consequences result.

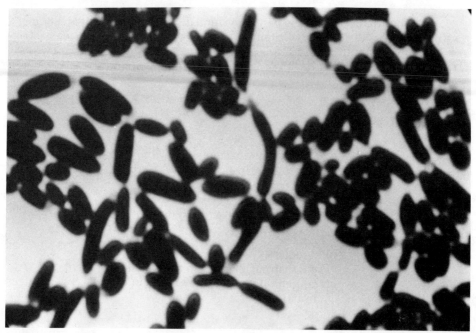

Figure 16-1.   Yeast hyphae and buds.

A yeast infection can be one of the most miserable feelings a woman experiences. Whether it is her first infection or one of many, she will need reassurance and education. Although yeast is not considered to be primarily sexually transmitted, the use of a condom or abstinence during the treatment period is sometimes advised. Some clinicians feel that yeast organisms harbored by a male may be responsible for recurrent infection in the female. In addition, some men react to contact with yeast by developing an itchy, irritating penile rash.

When recurrences seem to occur in conjunction with a menstrual period, treatment as described for three to four days before a period is often effective. This is usually done for two to three consecutive cycles. The possibility of diabetes must also be eliminated when there are recurrent yeast infections.

The most common reason for "recurrences" is failure to use all of the medication as prescribed. Symptoms usually are alleviated in two to three days. Since most preparations are messy to use, many women discontinue use as soon as the discomfort disappears. Women need to be encouraged to use all of the medication that has been prescribed.

Finally, it is somewhat comforting for a woman to know that she is not alone with her problem. Yeast infections are common. Although they are uncomfortable and treatment is expensive and messy, they do not seem to be a serious health threat.

Trichomonas (Trich) Vaginitis

Cause: Trichomonad, a microscopic, one-celled, flagellated organism. (See Figure 16-2.)

Influencing factors: Primarily sexually transmitted.
Potentially transmitted by wet towels, shared swimming suits, or improperly cleaned bathing facilities.

Signs and symptoms: Itching.
Profuse, runny, frothy, yellow-green discharge.
Discharge usually has odor.
Pelvic examination sometimes reveals petechiae on the cervix and upper vaginal walls (strawberry spots).

Diagnosis: Microscopic identification of Trichomonad.

Treatment: Oral metronidazole (Flagyl).
Flagyl is contraindicated during pregnancy; Betadine douches or gel may offer temporary relief.

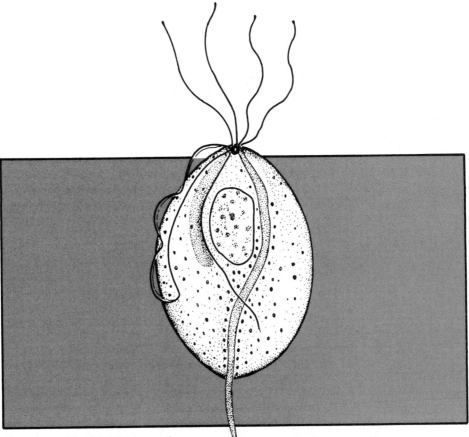

Figure 16-2.   Flagellated Trichomonad.

Prognosis: One course of Flagyl usually results in cure, particularly if partner has been treated at the same time.
May cause inflammatory changes which may result in abnormal Pap smears.
Considered by some to be a risk factor for cervical cancer. (See Figure 16-2.)

Since Trichomonas is primarily a sexually transmitted disease, treatment of partners is recommended. Where multiple partners are involved this may be unrealistic and ineffective. In such cases educating the woman regarding transmission and encouraging the use of condoms may be the best way of avoiding re-infection.

Unpleasant side effects from metronidazole (Flagyl) are extreme nausea and vomiting. This occurs if alcohol is used while taking the medication. Anyone being treated with Flagyl should be warned about this. It may also cause a disturbance in the vaginal flora with a resulting yeast infection. Repeated use of Flagyl has been found to depress white cell production in some people. Therefore, a repeat treatment soon after the initial treatment should be preceded by a complete blood count. It has also been found to be carcinogenic in mice.

For these reasons it is prudent to prescribe Flagyl only when Trichomonas has been confirmed by microscopic evidence of the Trichomonad. There is some concern that prolonged, untreated Trichomonas infections may increase a woman's risk of cervical cancer. Therefore, the possible risks of using Flagyl must be weighed against the risk of less effective treatments.

Other Types of Vaginitis ("Non-Specific")

Cause: Most common bacteria appear to be Hemophilus vaginales (Cornybacterium vaginale) and Chlamydia trachomatis. (See Figure 16-3.)

Influencing factors: Primarily sexually transmitted; male counterpart is non-gonococcal or nonspecific urethritis.
Poor hygiene may be a factor.

Signs and
symptoms: Very heavy discharge with strong odor; odor often described as "fishy."
Discharge is grey-white with creamy consistency.
Usually no itching or irritation.

Diagnosis: Hemophilus—Microscopic examination of saline preparation shows "clue cells" (epithelial cells covered with many short Gram negative rods).
Chlamydia—Organisms detected only by culture (procedure is time-consuming and expensive.)

Treatment: Hemophilus—Oral Ampicillin or Flagyl [9].
                        Chlamydia—Oral tetracycline.
                        Vaginal creams, suppositories, or douches for either of
                        these infections are of questionable value.

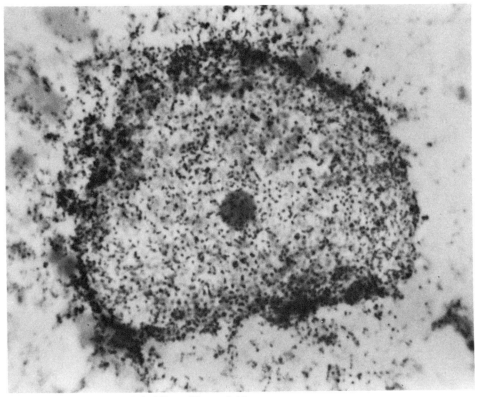

Figure 16-3.   Clue cells typical of Hemophilus vaginitis.

Prognosis: Both infections respond well when all partners are treat-
                        ed.
                        These organisms may cause non-gonococcal PID.
                        Infants delivered by women with Chlamydial infection
                        may contract trachoma inclusion conjunctivitis or
                        pneumonia [8].

There is an increasing awareness that these infections are sexually transmitted.
Treatment with vaginal preparations is often ineffective since it does not treat the
partner. Systemic treatment of the partner is often recommended.

When considering use of tetracycline, care must be taken to determine that a
woman is not pregnant. Tetracycline taken during pregnancy may result in a
discoloration of the permanent teeth of the child. Erythromycin or Ampicillin can
be used safely.

Gonorrhea

Cause:
Gonococcus or Neisseria gonorrhea; this is a Gram negative, intracellular diplococcus. (See Figure 16-4.)

Influencing factors:
Sexually transmitted; any other means of transmission is unlikely (due to fragility of organism); it dies rapidly on exposure to cold, oxygen, or drying.
Transmission is from one mucous membrane to another; this can be vaginal, anal, or oral-genital contact.

Signs and symptoms:
Very often asymptomatic; 50–80 percent of females and 40–50 percent of males may go many weeks or months without symptoms [1].
There may be a purulent vaginal discharge which originates at the cervix.
Stinging or discomfort with urination (particularly with involvement of Skene's glands).
Symptoms often go unnoticed until infection ascends the reproductive tract resulting in PID.
Gonococcal pharyngitis and tonsillitis may cause sore throat.
Rectal gonorrhea is asymptomatic.
Generalized rash and arthritis may result from untreated gonorrhea; this is rare but occurs with greater frequency during pregnancy.

Diagnosis:
Culture of organism.
Gram stain is unreliable in women since it is hard to differentiate the gonococcus from normal vaginal flora.

Treatment:
Follows Center for Disease Control (CDC) recommended schedule [13]:
A. *Uncomplicated gonorrhea* (cervical, rectal, urethral)
Aqueous penicillin G: 4.8 million units IM at two sites with 1 gm probenecid, orally,
OR
Tetracycline: 0.5 gm orally, qid for 5 days,
OR
Ampicillin: 3.5 gm orally, with 1 gm probenecid, (single dose).
OR
Spectinomycin: 2 gm, IM.

Note: It is recommended that probenecid be given ½ hour prior to the administration of the antibiotic to enhance absorption.

B. *Pharyngeal infections*
Aqueous procaine penicillin or tetracycline as outlined above.

C. *Penicillinase–producing Neisseria gonorrhea* (PPNG)
Spectinomycin: 2 gm, IM.

Prognosis: If treated early and correctly, gonorrhea is completely curable.

Severe problems result if infection spreads from the cervix to the endometrium, tubes, and/or ovaries.

Follow up cultures from cervix, throat and rectum must be done to document cure or discover treatment failure; these are usually done one week after completion of treatment.

True treatment failures of uncomplicated gonorrhea infections are rare. Most often a positive culture following adequate treatment is a result of reinfection. However, treatment with Spectinomycin is usually given for positive "test of cure" cultures. Although true PPNG strains are rare, such treatment would be effective therapy.

When reinfection occurs, careful and sensitive questioning is needed to determine the reasons. At times preventive measures such as abstinence and use of a condom may have been misunderstood. Many women do not realize that the contagious period lasts for approximately seventy-two hours following treatment.

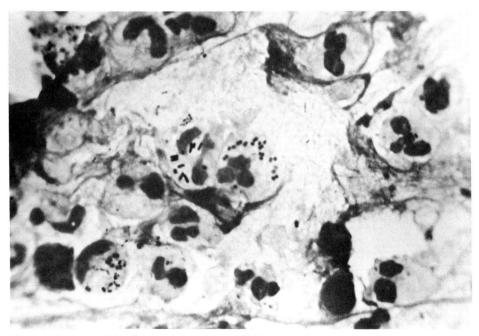

Figure 16-4.   Intracellular diplococcus characteristic of Nisseria gonorrhea.

Sometimes male partners do not go for treatment because they do not have "symptoms." Education is one of the most important means of controlling the spread and extent of this disease.

Syphilis

<table>
<tr>
<td>Cause:</td>
<td>Treponema pallidum; a spiral, corkscrew-shaped organism. (See Figure 16-5.)</td>
</tr>
<tr>
<td>Influencing factors:</td>
<td>Spread by sexual contact.
May also be transmitted by casual contact with infectious lesions.
Improperly screened blood transfusions.
Use of unclean hypodermic needles.
Congenital syphilis transmitted to fetus in utero by infected mother.</td>
</tr>
<tr>
<td>Signs and symptoms:</td>
<td>PRIMARY
Chancre—a single, painless, clean-based ulcerated lesion appearing approximately two to three weeks after exposure.
Chancre appears at point of contact; frequent sites in female are cervix, vagina, labia; also may be found around anus, mouth or throat, and breast.

SECONDARY
Generalized rash involving entire body, including soles and palms; highly contagious in this stage.
Rash appears two to six months after appearance of chancre.
Rash is characteristically not itchy.
Occasional low grade fever and lymphadenopathy.
Sometimes large, broad-based, flat, wart-like lesions (Condyloma lata).
Patchy hair loss.

TERTIARY OR LATENT
Two-thirds of all infected people will remain asymptomatic for life.
Serious symptoms may not appear until ten to forty years after being infected.
Cardiovascular: Damage to heart and major blood vessels.
Neurological: Damage to brain and spinal cord causing paralysis and "insanity."</td>
</tr>
</table>

Diagnosis: PRIMARY
Dark field microscopic examination of serous fluid from
    chancre; motile spirochetes visible.
Serologic tests for syphilis: STS often negative for two to
    four weeks after exposure.

SECONDARY
Dark field microscope examination of scrapings of skin,
    condyloma, or mucous membrane surfaces.
STS can detect virtually 100 percent of cases.

TERTIARY OR LATENT
STS of blood and spinal fluid.

Treatment: CDC recommended schedule for PRIMARY, SECON-
    DARY, and LATENT of *less than one year duration* [14]
Benzathine penicillin G: 2.4 million units IM (1.2 million
    units in each buttock),
                   OR
Aqueous penicillin G: 4.8 million units IM (600,000 units
    daily for eight days),
                   OR
Tetracycline or Erythromycin: 30 gm total (0.5 gm qid for
    fifteen days).

LATENT of *more than one year* and *symptomatic* TERTI-
    ARY:
Benzathine penicillin G: 2.4 million units IM weekly, for
    three weeks (7.2 million units).
                   OR
Aqueous penicillin G: 600,000 units IM daily, for fifteen
    days (9 million units).
                   OR
Tetracycline or Erythromycin: 0.5 gm qid for thirty days
    (60 gm total).
Follow up treatment at any stage is extremely important.

Prognosis: PRIMARY
Chancre heals by itself and disappears in one to four
    weeks; if untreated, the disease continues to progress.
With adequate treatment, complete cure is achieved.

SECONDARY
If untreated, symptoms of this stage will resolve in two to
    six weeks while the disease continues to progress.
With adequate treatment, complete cure is achieved.

TERTIARY and LATENT of *less than one year:*
Adequate treatment results in complete cure.

TERTIARY and LATENT of *more than one year:*
Poor prognosis; usually fatal.

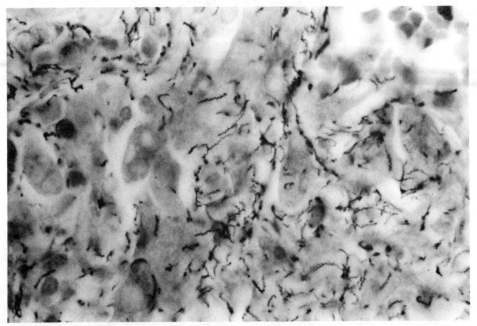

Figure 16-5.   Treponema pallidum spirochete, causitive agent of syphilis.

LABORATORY TESTS FOR SYPHILIS (BLOOD TESTS)

VDRL (Venereal Disease Research Laboratory). The VDRL is used for mass screening. It may be negative early in the disease so must be repeated in four to six weeks if a negative result occurs in a highly suspicious case. False positives may occur following a recent viral illness or immunization, following mononucleosis or infectious hepatitis, in lupus erythematosus, and rheumatoid arthritis. False positives are also found in drug addicts and pregnant women. Occasionally a woman may have a false positive VDRL throughout her lifetime [12].

FTA-ABS (Flourescent Treponemal Antibody Absorption). This test is more specific than the VDRL and is always done to confirm a positive VDRL. It is not used for mass screening because of its cost.

TPI (Treponema Pallidum Immobilization). This test is extremely accurate with few, if any, false positives. It is expensive and difficult to perform. Therefore, it is used where symptoms, medical history, and physical findings are confusing.

Cervicitis (Inflammation or infection of the cervix)

Cause: Numerous bacteria and viruses, including trichomonas, gonorrhea, herpes, and Chlamydia.

Influencing factors: Hormonal stimulation resulting in growth of the more fragile endocervical cells to the ectocervix; for example, pregnancy, oral contraceptives, or adolescence.

Lacerations from childbirth or gynecologic procedures make the cervix more susceptible to infections; trauma from mechanical forms of sexual stimulation.

Signs and symptoms: Persistent discharge which is sometimes malodorous.

Discharge may be clear or mucopurulent.

Cervix looks red and edematous.

Cervix may bleed on contact resulting in postcoital bleeding.

Pap smear may be abnormal due to inflammatory cell changes.

Diagnosis: Pap smear must be done to differentiate between cervicitis and cervical malignancy.

Colposcopy and biopsy if Pap smear is positive.

Identification of causative organism.

Treatment: Vaginal creams and suppositories may be helpful in mild cases.

Treatment specific to causative organism, if known.

Cauterization or cryosurgery may be necessary to destroy surface endocervical cells which remain a potential site of chronic or recurrent infection.

Prognosis: Usually cured with adequate treatment.

There is evidence that a chronically infected cervix places a woman at higher risk for developing cervical cancer.

Atrophic Vaginitis

See chapter 11.

Genital Herpes

The most serious implications of a genital Herpes infection are related to the involvement of the cervix and vagina. However, since the symptoms which are noticed by a woman occur on the external genitals, this infection will be discussed in chapter 17.

Condyloma Accuminata (venereal or genital warts)

Genital warts can be found within the vagina and on the cervix. However, since they are usually first noticed on the external genitalia, they will be discussed in chapter 17.

BENIGN CYSTS AND TUMORS

Benign cysts and tumors of the vagina are relatively uncommon and usually asymptomatic. Unless symptoms such as dyspareunia or pain with insertion of tampons or diaphragm occur, treatment is unnecessary.

Gartner duct cysts arise from vestigial remants of the Wolffian duct and thus are found on the anterolateral walls of the vagina. They are usually multiple and in a linear distribution. Unless they attain unusually large sizes they are left untreated.

Vaginal inclusion cysts result from episiotomy or vaginal surgery if a small bit of epithelium gets buried in the vaginal mucosa and becomes encysted. Subsequent degeneration results in the accumulation of a cheesy substance similar to that seen in a sebaceous cyst.

Endometriotic cysts develop from small implants of endometrial tissue. They are usually found in the posterior fornix. If they are composed of functioning endometrial tissue they can cause considerable pain and bleeding.

Adenosis refers to lesions which are composed of glandular epithelium and are often mucous secreting. They appear as reddish, polyploid areas and are usually found in the upper anterior or posterior vaginal walls. Although vaginal adenosis is rare, it occurs with a high degree of frequency in DES exposed women.

Symptoms may include vaginal discharge and abnormal vaginal bleeding, but it is often asymptomatic. Since evidence does not support the idea that these lesions progress to malignancy, no treatment is necessary. Periodic colposcopy is done to ensure that the natural healing process occurs without problems. For a description of colposcopy see chapter 24.

Cervical polyps generally arise from the endocervical tissue, but occasionally are found on the outer or ectocervix. The endocervical type are pedunculated and usually small. When they are large enough to protrude through the cervical os they appear as bright red growths occurring either singly or in clusters. Polyps on the outer surface of the cervix are usually broad based, firmer and paler in color.

Small polyps are asymptomatic, but as they grow, they usually cause intermenstrual or postcoital bleeding. Removal can usually be accomplished in an office procedure without much discomfort. Malignancy is rare, but the polyp should be sent for histologic examination.

Nabothian Cysts

Yellow or white translucent cysts are sometimes seen on the exocervix during a pelvic examination. They vary in size from pinhead to 0.5 cm or larger. Occasionally they are first noticed when a woman feels them while checking a diaphragm or IUD string. The cysts may be a result of chronic cervicitis or may occur as a result of the normal process of squamous metaplasia.

Cysts which result from infection are caused by bacteria, mucus, and cellular debris which become trapped in the crypts or "glands" of the endocervical tissue (see chapter 3). Nabothian cysts that occur in the absence of severe chronic cervicitis are a result of a significant eversion or "outgrowth" of endocervical cells to the exocervix. Squamous epthelium replaces this tissue in a gradual process called squamous metaplasia. The squamous epithelium "caps" the mucous secreting cells of the endocervical tissue and traps the fluid secretions, thus forming cysts.

Treatment is not necessary. The cysts frequently resolve by reabsorption of the fluid or spontaneous rupture. When a Pap smear is abnormal due to a chronic infection a colposcopy will be done and appropriate treatment recommended. Cryosurgery or cautery done as treatment for chronic cervicitis will also eliminate the Nabothian cysts.

MALIGNANCIES

Vagina

Fortunately, cancer of the vagina is extremely rare and accounts for only about 2 percent of all gynecologic malignancies. There are two types of vaginal cancer. Squamous cell carcinoma affects women between fifty to seventy years of age, while adenocarcinoma primarily affects women under thirty years. A noticeable rise in incidence of adenocarcinoma in the early 1970s has been related to in-utero exposure of the fetus to DES [5].

Symptoms: Painless vaginal bleeding is often the first symptom noted. This may be intermenstrual, postcoital, or postmenopausal. There is sometimes a vaginal discharge. Pain is seldom a symptom until the disease reaches its later stages.

Diagnosis: Lesions of vaginal cancer can easily be missed during a pelvic exam. They often occur on the posterior or anterior walls which are covered by the speculum. Pap smears are often the first indication of a problem. An abnormal Pap smear should be followed by biopsy of the lesion. Colposcopy can identify areas for biopsy in the absence of obvious lesions. For a description of this procedure see chapter 24.

An initial colposopy is recommended for all women who are known to have been exposed to DES. This should be done about the time of menarche, but no later than age fourteen. If results are normal, routine yearly pelvic exam and Pap smear follow-up is adequate.

Treatment: Vaginal cancer can be treated surgically or with radiotherapy. The method and extent of treatment depends on the stage of the disease and the age and condition of the woman. In addition to vaginectomy, hysterectomy and pelvic lymph node dissection may be necessary. Plastic reconstruction of the vagina has been successfully done thus ensuring the possibility of sexual activity.

Prognosis: Vaginal cancer carries a poor prognosis since it is usually asymptomatic until a late stage. An additional reason for the low survival rate from this type of cancer is that the thin walls of the vagina increase the potential for invasion of neighboring lymphatics and supporting tissues. The position of the vagina between the bladder and rectum results in a high incidence of involvement of these structures.

When the tumor is found in a very early, asymptomatic stage the cure rate approaches 90 percent [4]. In later stages, when penetration of the vaginal wall and invasion of nearby organs has occurred, the five-year survival rate drops to around 50 percent [5].

Cervix

Cervical cancer accounts for approximately 55–65 percent of reproductive tract malignancies. Squamous cell carcinoma generally occurs in women between fifty five to sixty-five years of age. It is the most common and accounts for about 95 percent of all cervical cancers. Adenocarcinoma arises from the columnar epithelium. Five percent or less of all cervical malignancies are of this type. Its highest incidence is found in women under the age of thirty who have been exposed to DES [2].

Some risk factors for squamous cell carcinoma have been identified. There is indication that it may be a sexually transmitted disease, but the exact mechanism of this is still unclear. Cervical cancer occurs rarely in celibate women but with high frequency in prostitutes and in heterosexual women with many sexual partners. However, evidence points to early age of onset of sexual activity being more important than the number of partners [10]. This may be due to the exposure of the more tender endocervical cells that grow out onto the cervix during the adolescent years.

Some sexually transmitted diseases have also been implicated as causes of cervical cancer. Strong evidence suggests that Herpes type II is linked in some way to this disease. Trichomonas vaginitis and chronic, untreated cervicitis are also suspected of contributing to the development of cervical carcinoma.

Symptoms: Early symptoms of cervical cancer are minimal and often go unnoticed or ignored. Occasionally a thin, watery, possibly blood-tinged discharge will be present. Postmenopausal spotting is usually more alarming to a woman than is spotting during the menstrual years. Thus older women with this symptom tend to seek earlier treatment. Symptoms of advanced disease are more dramatic. They include low back pain, dysuria, hematuria, rectal bleeding and constipation.

There is a slow progression of the disease process from its very early or premalignant phase to the invasive phase. The beginning of the process is with cervical dysplasia. This appears to be a precursor to malignancy and a large percentage of women with dysplasia later develop cervical cancer. These early stages of cervical cancer are often first detected with a Pap smear. Details of Pap smear procedure and interpretation of results can be found in chapter 23.

The other stages are carcinoma in-situ (CIN), microinvasive carcinoma and invasive carcinoma. The progression from dysplasia to invasive carcinoma may take fifteen to twenty years.

Diagnosis: The early diagnosis of cervical cancer is by cytology. Following a suspicious Pap smear report, biopsy of abnormal tissues should be done. Areas for biopsy can be detected by Schiller's Stain or colposcopy. (See Chapter 24.) If the disease has advanced to the invasive stage, clinically obvious lesions or palpable masses may be found during a pelvic examination.

Further tests may be needed to determine extent of disease. These may include a cone biopsy (removal of a cone-shaped section of the cervix and endocervix including the entire squamo-columnar junction), and a fractional curettage. Additional tests might include IVP, chest and skeletal X-rays, cystoscopy, proctoscopy or barium enema, and/or bone scan.

Accurate staging helps determine the mode of therapy and establishes a prognosis. The stages of cervical cancer are as follows:

Stage 0   Carcinoma-in-situ.
Stage I   Carcinoma strictly confined to cervix.
Stage II   Carcinoma extends beyond cervix, but not onto pelvic wall.
Stage III   Carcinoma has extended onto the pelvic wall.
Stage IV   Carcinoma has extended beyond the true pelvis. It may have in-
               volved the bladder or rectum or distant organs.

Treatment: If a woman desires future pregnancy, carcinoma-in-situ can be treated by conization of the cervix, deep cryosurgery, or laser therapy with very conscientious follow-up. A woman not desiring pregnancy should have a total hysterectomy.

Stage I and II invasive cervical cancers are treated surgically and/or by radio-therapy. Surgical treatment is radical, and includes dissection of all pelvic lymph nodes as well as removal of the uterus, tubes and ovaries. Radiation may be given by radium implants and/or external X-ray therapy.

Stage III and IV cervical carcinomas are not usually treated surgically except for palliative reasons. This surgery often includes removal of both rectum and bladder. The morbidity is high and the likelihood of already occurring distant metastases results in low survival rates.

Prognosis: The prognosis of Stage I and II cervical carcinoma treated by radiotherapy alone depends on the stage and responsiveness of the tumor as well as the radiologist. Survival rates following surgery approximate those following radiotherapy. Stage I has approximately a 20 percent mortality rate and Stage II a 35–40 percent [2]. Stages III and IV have a very poor prognosis. This reinforces the importance of early detection.

TRAUMA

Chemical

Chemicals used in douches and vaginal cleansing products are probably the main cause of chemically induced trauma of the cervix and vagina. Contraceptive foams, creams and suppositories occasionally cause irritations which can be quite severe.

Although routine douching is considered unnecessary, some women prefer to douche occasionally. If a douche is desired, a woman should be encouraged to use two tablespoonsful of white vinegar in a quart of warm water. This will not disturb the normal vaginal pH. A douche with Betadine solution is sometimes advised for vaginitis when other treatments are contraindicated.

A woman should douche while in a semi-reclining position. A bathtub is an ideal place for douching. The temperature of the solution should be warm, but not hot enough to burn. The douche nozzle can be inserted 2–3 inches with a gentle pressure. Hanging the douche bag more than 24 inches above the vaginal opening can cause the solution to enter the vagina with enough force to damage vaginal and cervical tissue. The labia should be held closed tightly around the nozzle in order to retain the liquid. When enough fluid has entered to cause a slight ballooning of the vagina, the flow can be stopped. It is desirable to retain the fluid for approximately one minute. The entire quart should be used in this alternate holding and releasing procedure. See Figure 16-6.

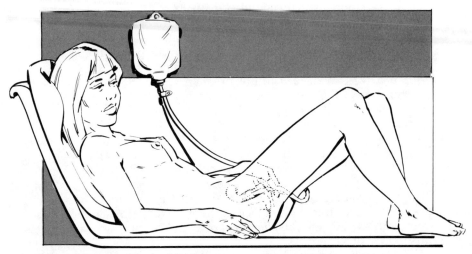

Figure 16-6.   Proper position for douching.

Intercourse

Bleeding from hymenal tears sometimes occurs with the first intercourse. This is less common in a woman who has used tampons than in one who has not. Bleeding and bruising of the introitus and surrounding area can sometimes be quite severe. Cold compresses to the area will help slow bleeding and reduce swelling. A woman who has been raped may also experience significant intercourse-related trauma. Very rarely a vaginal laceration occurs. It may bleed profusely and usually requires suturing under anesthesia.

Mechanical

Many women enjoy vibrators and other sexually stimulating devices as a regular part of their sexual practice. They may not be aware that these devices can cause damage to the vagina and cervix if not properly used. Women need to be informed of the early warning signs of unpleasant burning or tingling that precede tissue damage. If the device is being used for self-stimulation, she should stop at that point. If included as part of a hetero or homosexual experience, the woman should inform her partner of her discomfort before severe damage occurs.

REFERENCES

1. Cherniak D, Feingold A: V.D. Handbook. Montreal, Montreal Health Press, 1975
2. Frick H: Management of noninvasive carcinoma of the cervix. Surgical Clinics of North America, Vol. 58 No. 1, February 1978
3. Green T: Gynecology: Essentials of Clinical Practice. Boston, Little, Brown, 1977
4. Herbst A et al: Complications of prenatal therapy with diethystilbestrol. Pediatrics, Vol. 62 No. 6, December 1978
5. Hilgers RD: Squamous cell carcinoma of the vagina. Surgical Clinics of North America, Vol. 58 No. 1, February 1978
6. Kitai K et al: The changing trends of uterine cancer and cytology. Cancer, Vol. 42 No. 5, 1978
7. Novak E, Jones G, Jones H: Gynecology, 9th ed. Baltimore, Williams and Wilkins, 1975
8. Oriel JD: Infection of the uterine cervix with Chlamydia trachomatis. The Journal of Infectious Diseases. Vol. 137 No. 4, April 1978
9. Pheiffer TA et al: Nonspecific vaginitis. New England Journal of Medicine, Vol. 298 No. 26, June 1978
10. Sebastion J, Leeb B, See R: Cancer of the cervix—A sexually transmitted disease. American Journal of Obstetrics and Gynecology, Vol. 131 No. 6, July 1978
11. Schacter J: Chlamydial Infection Part 2. The New England Journal of Medicine, Vol. 298 No. 9, March 2, 1978
12. Tuffanelli D: False positive reactions part II: Normal individuals with chronic false positive (CFP) tests for syphilis. *In* Leslie N (ed): Sexually Transmitted Diseases. Springfield, IL, Charles C. Thomas, 1973
13. U.S. Department of Health, Education, and Welfare, Center for Disease Control: Recommended Treatment Schedules for Gonorrhea. Atlanta, GA, 1979
14. U.S. Department of Health, Education, and Welfare, Center for Disease Control: Recommended Treatment, Schedules for Syphilis. Atlanta, GA, 1976

17

External Genital Problems

Problems involving the external genitals are readily noticed because of their visibility and the extreme discomfort which many of them cause. Despite noticing these problems early, women do not always seek early treatment. The reason may be fear and embarrassment which accompanies genital problems. Some women associate these problems with uncleanliness and promiscuity further compounding their embarrassment. Giving non-judgmental information regarding infection, infestation, neoplasms and trauma of the external genitals may encourage prompt health care.

INFECTIONS

The preventive measures mentioned for vaginitis (chapter 16) are also helpful in preventing infection and inflammation of the vulva. As with the various forms of vaginitis and cervicitis, some of the following infections are sexually transmitted and some are not. Most of them cause considerable discomfort and some have serious implications.

Herpes Genitalis

Cause:

PRIMARY
Usually Herpes Simplex Virus, Type 2 (HSV-2) which is primarily genitally transmitted. Less commonly, Herpes Simplex Virus, Type 1 (HSV-1) which is transmitted by oral-genital contact.
Autoinoculation from oral to genital site may be possible.

RECURRENT
Virus becomes latent; recurs spontaneously under certain conditions despite circulating antibodies.
Stimuli for reactivation differ from one woman to another; may include sexual intercourse, fever, stress, or menstruation.

Signs and symptoms:

PRIMARY
Small vesicular eruptions on labia, at introitus, near urethral meatus or anus; lesions may be isolated or joined.

May be preceded by a tingling sensation or mild itching.
Vesicles break to form shallow, acutely painful ulcers.
Cervical lesions are not painful, but may cause discharge.
When examined, the cervix appears red, edematous, and raw, with ulcerated surface.
Enlarged lymph nodes in groin.
Fever.
Malaise.
Vulvar dysuria.
Symptoms appear two to ten days following contact and may last two to three weeks.

RECURRENT
Milder and of shorter duration.
Vesicles fewer; may be solitary; site is always the same.
Systemic symptoms usually absent.

Diagnosis:

PRIMARY
Most are diagnosed clinically by symptoms, onset, and appearance of lesions.
VDRL to rule out syphilis.
Confirmation is desirable and may be done in three ways:
A. Virus isolation by culture of vesicular fluid.
B. Pap smear to demonstrate morphological changes in cells and rule out cervical cancer.
C. Serologic evidence may be helpful; four-fold rise in antibody titer between acute and convalescent serum is considered significant.

RECURRENT
Usually by history and clinical findings.
Culture and Pap smear are seldom helpful since the virus is not easily recovered from recurrent lesions.
Serology is rarely helpful since a large percentage of adults have antibodies for herpes.

Treatment:

No cure or prevention of recurrences is available.
Directed at relief of symptoms; may include sitz baths, soothing ointments, analgesics, and antibacterial ointments to help prevent secondary bacterial infection.
Education.

Complications:

Urinary retention secondary to very painful urination which results from contact of urine with vulvar ulcers.
Disseminated infection or encephalitis in immunosuppressed patients (Hodgkins, renal transplants).

Prognosis:

Associated with an increased risk of cervical cancer; however, not considered a specific etiologic factor.

Approximately 50 percent of infants delivered vaginally when mother has active herpes will develop overwhelming, frequently fatal, systemic herpes infection [10].

The pain associated with a primary herpes infection is severe. Systemic symptoms of fever, malaise and enlarged, painful lymph nodes intensify the discomfort. In addition, the fact that it is often recurrent, that it may be associated with cervical cancer, and that it may have serious consequences during pregnancy contribute to the depression and "hopelessness" felt by many women with herpes.

Treatments such as heterocyclic dyes followed by exposure to light, ether application, smallpox vaccine, zinc applications, and herpes-specific vaccines have so far proved either sporadically effective, ineffective, or harmful. Application of a cream containing 2-deoxy-D-glucose is one of the more recent treatments being used for herpes. L-Lysine taken by mouth in doses from 300–1000 mgm per day also seems to be helpful in decreasing the severity of symptoms and preventing recurrences. Results of double-blind, placebo controlled studies are still needed to prove the effectiveness of these treatment regimes.

When dysuria is present, a woman may find that urinating in the shower or in a bathtub full of water is helpful. Pouring water over the genital area while urinating can also help reduce the discomfort caused when urine contacts the open lesions. Because of the dysuria, women frequently drink less in order to urinate less often. This, of course, causes the urine to become more concentrated and consequently more irritating. Therefore these women should be encouraged to increase their fluid intake.

Loose fitting clothing is essential to avoid pressure on the painful ulcers. Sitz baths assure cleanliness and prevent secondary bacterial infection. Drying with a hair dryer avoids trauma from rubbing with a towel. A perineal wash with Betadine solution is also helpful in reducing secondary infections. A woman may need medication if pain is severe.

Concerns of women with herpes are generally focused on four areas:

Fear of recurrence. Perhaps as many as 50 percent of infected individuals will never have a recurrence. When herpes does recur, symptoms are much milder and less severe than the initial episode. When a woman becomes familiar with the stimuli that reactivates lesions, she can try to avoid them whenever possible.

Concern about transmission. Transmission is usually by direct contact with a lesion. It is wise to abstain from intercourse or to use a condom while active lesions are present and for a few days following disappearance of lesions. When warning signs are recognized, preventive measures can be started before actual appearance of the lesions. Oral-genital contact should also be avoided since both HSV-1 and -2 can cause disease of both the oropharynx and genitals.

Concern with relationship of herpes to cancer. A very high percentage of women with cervical cancer have HSV-2 antibodies in their serum. Conversely, women with a history of genital herpes have a higher than average incidence of cervical cancer. In addition the virus itself has been found in tumor cells. Although this evidence points to a strong *link* between the two diseases, there may be other factors which play a part. As noted in chapter 16, the progression from cervical dysplasia to invasive carcinoma is a slow one. Women should be encouraged to be conscientious in obtaining a yearly pelvic examination with Pap smear to detect any premalignant or malignant lesions in their earliest stage. Some clinicians advise Pap smears twice a year for women with a history of herpes.

Concern surrounding implications for pregnancy. If genital herpes is present at the time of a vaginal delivery the risk of the infant developing neonatal herpes is 40–60 percent. More than half of these infants will develop severe or fatal disease [9]. A Cesarean delivery can significantly decrease this risk particularly where membranes are unruptured or ruptured less than 4 hours before delivery. A woman can be reassured that her doctor will be able to check her for evidence of herpes as she approaches full term. A Cesarean section may be necessary, but with it chances of having a healthy baby are good.

Women with genital herpes are in need of reassurance, emotional support and education. Sound information and advice as well as up-dates on current herpes research are available in a quarterly newsletter published and distributed by HELP/ASHA (Herpetics Engaged in Living Productively/American Social Health Association). Information can be obtained by writing to HELP/ASHA , P.O. Box 100, Palo Alto, California 04302.

Vulvitis

Cause:	May be secondary to irritation from discharge of a specific vaginitis. Underlying systemic disease such as diabetes. Dermatological disease. Poor hygiene. Inflammatory reaction to underlying malignant lesion.
Symptoms:	Itching. Erythema. Swelling of labia. Soreness with pressure from clothing. External pain with urination (vulvar dysuria).
Diagnosis:	Identification of underlying cause by wet smears, skin scraping, biopsy, or culture. Medical tests to rule out underlying systemic disease.
Treatment:	Treatment of underlying cause.
Prognosis:	Depends on cause.

Condyloma Accuminata

Cause:	Human Papilloma Virus.

Influencing factors:	Primarily sexually transmitted.
	Concurrent vaginal infection.

Symptoms: Warty growth at introitus, on vulva, or around anus; occasionally on vaginal walls and cervix.

Lesions are usually narrow-based, pedunculated; large lesions have cauliflower appearance.

Usually painless; discomfort with intercourse, sexual stimulation, tampon use, or bowel movement may occur with increasing size.

Diagnosis: Clinical appearance and history of contact.

Biopsy will differentiate between condyloma and malignant vulvar tumor.

VDRL is done to rule out condyloma lata of secondary syphilis.

Treatment: Application of 20–25 percent Podophyllin in Tincture of Benzoin to all lesions, applied at one week intervals.

Cautery.

Surgical excision.

Spontaneous regression frequently occurs.

Prognosis: Genital warts do not appear to have serious consequences.

Sometimes very difficult to eradicate; recurrence rate is high.

When partners are treated simultaneously, recurrence is less.

Since warts have a preference for warm, moist areas the problem is usually more severe in the female than in the male. There is often a prior vaginitis and the discharge presumably creates a good environment for the wart virus to grow. Sexual partners should be checked and treated if necessary. A condom should be used with intercourse until all lesions have disappeared.

Podophyllin treatments sometimes need to be repeated weekly for many weeks. Some people become extremely irritated by Podophyllin so care should be taken to avoid touching normal tissue. A thin coating of vaseline to surrounding areas is often helpful. It is important to instruct a woman to wash off the Podophyllin two to four hours after the initial application. If it is well tolerated it can be left on four to six hours after subsequent treatments. Podophyllin should *not* be used during pregnancy or on intravaginal lesions.

Warts have more nuisance value than medical significance. However, since they can become painful and do spread, most women want thorough and prompt resolution of the problems. Cautery or surgical excision can be used if the lesions are extensive, intravaginal, or resistant to Podophyllin. Treatment of a co-existing vaginitis and/or venereal disease will hasten a cure. Preventive techniques listed in chapter 16 are applicable to condylomata accuminata.

Molluscum Contagiosum

Cause: Large "pox" virus usually transmitted sexually.

Symptoms: Separate, raised, umbilicated lesions; orange-pink with a
                       pearly, opalescent top.

Diagnosis: Clinical appearance.
                       Contents of lesion can be expressed and viral body
                       viewed microscopically.

Treatment: Curettage.
                       Lesion opened with a sterile needle or scalpel and the
                       firm, viral-containing core is expressed; this may be
                       followed by application of 30 percent aluminum chlor-
                       ide.

Prognosis: No serious consequences.
                       Recurrence common if sexual partner is not treated.

INFESTATIONS

Pediculosis Pubis (Crabs)

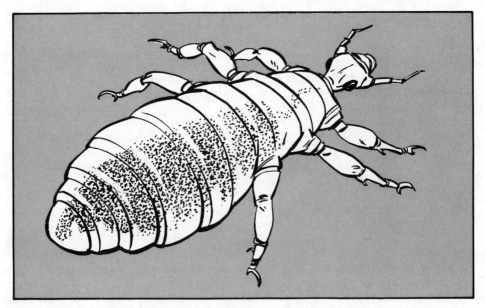

Figure 17-1.   Pediculosis Pubis.

Cause: *Phthirus Pubis*, a parasite 1–2 mm in length and resembling a crab.

Influencing factors: Primarily transmitted through direct contact.
                    Can be transmitted via infected clothing, towels, bedding, and toilet seats.

Signs and   Intense itching in pubic area.
  Symptoms: Oval, grey nits (eggs) can be seen attached to hair shafts.
                    Adult lice can sometimes be seen.
                    Occasionally, there will be excoriated papules on skin.
                    Small black specks are often noted in underpants from excreta of lice.

Diagnosis: Microscopic findings of lice or nits.
                    By visualization of adult lice, nits, or black specks in underwear.

Treatment: 1 percent gamma benzene hexachloride (Kwell, Gammene).
                    Nits that adhere to hair after treatment can be removed by applying a 1:1 solution of white vinegar and water; follow by shower and combing of pubic hair with a fine-tooth comb.
                    DO NOT USE KWELL DURING PREGNANCY. Eurex cream can be used in place of Kwell or Gammene.
                    Organisms cannot survive high temperatures; dry clean or machine wash all bed linen, towels, and clothes worn next to the skin.

Prognosis: Treatment is generally effective if contacts are treated and instructions followed for washing clothing.
                    No serious implications.

Scabies

Cause: *Sarcoptis scabiei*, a mite transmitted by direct contact.

Signs and   May be asymptomatic for four to eight weeks; however,
  Symptoms: can be transmitted during that period.
                    Itching, especially at night.
                    A burrow which appears as a wavy, dark line with a minute papule at the end is the initial lesion; burrows may vary from a few mm to 1 cm in length.
                    Burrows usually found in webbed areas of fingers, along bra lines, in axilla or groin.

Intense scratching may result in secondary inflammatory lesions.

Diagnosis: Microscopic visualization of mite, egg, larvae, or feces on mineral oil wet mount.
Burrow is scraped and prepared as above.

Treatment: Kwell or Gammene lotion.
Launder towels, sheets, and clothing worn next to body.
Eurex cream or lotion during pregnancy.

Prognosis: Reinfection, unless contacts are also treated. No serious sequelae.

Women are seldom more upset than when their problem is diagnosed as "crabs" or scabies. Many people assume that these infestations are always associated with uncleanliness. Although poor hygiene and crowded conditions foster the spread of these parasites, they by no means happen only to "dirty" people.

FOLLICULITIS

Infection of the hair follicles in the pubic area is common. Often it is due to pressure of tight clothing combined with the natural warmth and moisture of the genital area. Treatment consists of hot soaks and wearing of loose, nonrestrictive clothing. The lesions should not be squeezed! If the problem is extensive or recurrent in nature, underlying disease such as diabetes should be considered.

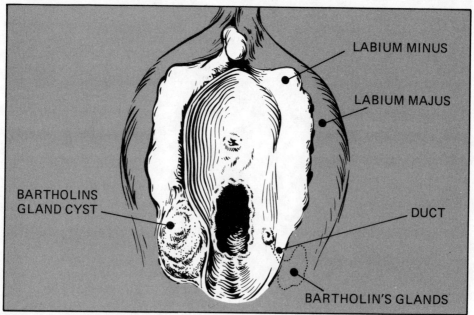

Figure 17-2.   Bartholin's gland cyst.

BENIGN TUMORS

Bartholin's Cyst

This condition is a result of obstruction of the Bartholin's gland duct with entrapment of glandular material. It follows an inflammation which is often, but not always, due to a gonococcal infection. Occasionally it is found in conjunction with atrophic vaginitis.

The size of these cysts can vary from being barely detectable to orange-sized. They are quite prone to secondary infection and abscess formation. When this happens, they become extremely painful. Pain may become so severe that walking, sitting, and even wearing underclothing becomes almost impossible.

Diagnosis and treatment of the underlying infection is the initial step in resolving this condition. If the cyst is small and there is no indication of abscess formation, hot moist soaks applied three to four times a day will sometimes resolve the problem.

Surgical incision and drainage becomes necessary when the abscessed cyst becomes large and painful. The enlargement of the gland and fibrosis of the duct often result in chronic cyst and abscess formation. Surgical excision is effective, as is marsupialization.

Inclusion and Sebaceous Cysts

Sebaceous cysts due to blockage of the sebaceous ducts are quite common on the vulva. Epidermal inclusion cysts may follow episiotomy or other trauma of the vulva or introitus. Neither of these conditions requires treatment unless they become infected or attain sizes large enough to become annoying. Should that happen, they can be incised and drained.

VULVAR MALIGNANCIES

Vulvar carcinoma is relatively uncommon and accounts for only 4 percent of all gynecologic cancers [3]. This disease primarily affects elderly, postmenopausal women with the highest incidence being after age sixty. Although it is a slow-growing malignancy, until recent years it has had a very low survival rate.

The historically poor prognosis of cancer of the vulva is due in part to the delay in making a correct diagnosis. The older woman often delays seeking medical attention because of embarrassment, inadequate knowledge of the severity of the problem, or inaccessibility to health care. Another contributing factor is failure on the part of the clinician to recognize the problem and carry out appropriate diagnostic tests and treatment.

Leukoplakia, a benign skin condition precedes vulvar carcinoma in a high percentage of cases. It is characterized by gray-white, thick, patchy lesions which are often edematous, fissured or excoriated. Symptoms are usually very bothersome, and include itching, soreness and vulvar dysuria. Women with such symptoms, particularly in the postmenopausal age group, should have very careful follow-up to detect a malignancy in its earliest stages.

Symptoms of vulvar carcinoma, similar to leukoplakia, include intense itching, local pain, and tenderness. In addition, there may be an awareness of a lump or ulcerated lesion and sometimes an irritating discharge. These are also symptoms of benign, less serious diseases. Therefore, if a woman in an older age group has a presumed minor condition that fails to respond to appropriate treatment, it should be investigated for vulvar carcinoma.

Diagnostic tests consist of biopsy of any obvious lesion. When the vulva appears diffusely abnormal without any obvious lesions or tumors, staining with toluidine blue stain will reveal areas for biopsy. Colposcopic examination of the vulva is also helpful. (See chapter 24.) A pelvic and rectal examination can help determine the extent of the disease. Many women with this disease are elderly and have additional medical problems that make them poor surgical risks. However, at the present time, surgery seems to be the most effective treatment for cancer of the vulva. Carcinoma-in-situ (Bowen's Disease) and intra-epithelial carcinoma are treated with a total vulvectomy. When invasive carcinoma is present the pelvic lymph nodes are also removed. Radiotherapy and chemotherapy for cancer of the vulva have not been found to be effective.

Five-year survival rates depend upon the stage of the disease, age, and condition of the woman when diagnosed. When the pelvic lymph nodes are involved the survival rate is lower. With adequate surgical treatment overall cure rates can approach 75 percent [10]. Reconstruction of the vulva in the sexually active woman is of great benefit to her postoperative adjustment.

TRAUMA

The vulva is subject to trauma from chemicals as well as to mechanical injury. Common causes of injury to the vulva in children are sudden stops while bicycling or from straddle falls on monkey bars and see-saws on the playground. Adult women are also subject to straddle injuries. In addition, vibrators and mechanical sexual stimulators account for many vulvar injuries in an adult woman. When improperly used, these devices can cause bruising, lacerations and abrasions.

Chemicals in the form of bubble baths, harsh soaps, contraceptive preparations, ointments used in sexual foreplay and feminine hygiene products can cause allergic reactions and burns. Non- irritating substances such as a waterbased lubricating jelly or plain vegetable oils can be advised if added lubrication is desired with intercourse.

REFERENCES

1. Aurelian L: Genital herpes update. The Female Patient, November 1979
2. Azzan BB: Bartholin's cyst and abscess: A review of treatment of 53 cases. The British Journal of Clinical Practice, Vol. 32 No. 4, April 1978
3. Benedet JL et al: Squamous carcinoma of the vulva: results of treatment 1938-1976. American Journal of Obstetrics and Gynecology, Vol. 134 No. 2, May 1979
4. Edwards MS: Veneral herpes: A nursing overview. Journal of Obstetric, Gynecologic and Neonatal Nursing, Vol. 7 No. 7, September/October 1978

5. Felman Y, Nikitas J: Genital herpesvirus infections. New York State Journal of Medicine, Vol. 79 No. 8, July 1979
6. Green T: Gynecology: Essentials of Clinical Practice. Boston, Little, Brown, 1977
7. Harahap M: Asymptomatic gonorrhea among patients with condyloma accuminata. British Journal of Venereal Disease, Vol. 55 No. 6, December 1979
8. Keith L, Brittain J: Sexually Transmitted Diseases, Aspen, CO, Creative Infomatics, 1978
9. Kibrick S: Herpes Simplex infection at term. Journal of the American Medical Association, Vol. 243 No. 2, January 1980
10. Krupp P. Cancer of the vulva. Surgical Clinics of North America, Vol. 58 No. 1, February 1978

18

Menstrual Irregularities

The change in a previously established pattern of menstrual periods or the failure to establish a cyclic menstrual pattern is usually extremely upsetting to a woman. When a woman's menstrual periods attain cyclic regularity she often assumes that this will continue unchanged until menopause. Yet most women will have one or many periods of unusual uterine bleeding during their menstruating years. In most cases, this will occur in the absence of any pathology.

Disturbances of bleeding and alteration of bleeding patterns probably account for one of the largest groups of problems seen in gynecology offices and clinics. A menstrual history will help with evaluation of a menstrual problem. Important questions to ask are:

At what age did your periods begin?

> A normal range is age nine to sixteen with the most common time being between eleven and fourteen. Onset of menstruation outside of this range may indicate underlying abnormalities.

What is the usual interval between periods?

> Normal variation is between twenty-one to forty days. A woman's age needs to be considered, since variation is more common at the beginning and end of the menstrual years. In addition, each individual woman's period may vary from cycle to cycle.

How long do your periods last?

> The usual range is three to seven days. However, one to nine days is considered normal if this does not represent an unusual change.

How many pads or tampons do you soak on your heaviest day or days?

> Complete soaking of one pad or tampon per hour is considered heavy bleeding. Bleeding at this rate for more than six to eight hours would be considered excessive.

Do you normally have clots and of what size?

> Clots greater than 1–2 cm are not normal and may indicate excessive bleeding.

What was the date of your last menstrual period and the one previous to it?

> This information assists in evaluating the usual cycle length. It also helps in determining what phase of her cycle the woman is in and/or length of gestation if pregnancy is suspected.

259

If contraception is used, what type?

Irregular bleeding is sometimes associated with oral contraceptives and IUD's. This may or may not be normal.

Are you taking any medications?

Some medications such as Librium, Dilantin, Mellaril and oral contraceptives can cause irregular or absent menses.

Have you been ill recently or do you have a chronic disease?

Debilitating systemic diseases such as tuberculosis or uncontrolled diabetes can cause alterations in endocrine function. High fevers interfere in follicular development. Blood diseases such as leukemia may first be manifested by abnormal uterine bleeding.

Have you had a recent weight change?

Both obesity and rapid weight loss are associated with amenorrhea.

Have there been any recent periods of significant stress?

Stressful situations in a person's emotional and physical environment influence menstruation on the hypothalamic level.

Was the onset of the problem sudden or gradual and what is its duration? Is it accompanied by breast secretions or changes in body or facial hair pattern?

Sudden onset of amenorrhea may mean pregnancy whereas a gradual lengthening of cycles may indicate an endocrine problem or approaching menopause. Similar clues can be obtained in regard to onset of abnormal bleeding.

Have you had a recent full term delivery, abortion or gynecological procedure?

Answers to these questions may indicate possible causes for abnormal bleeding patterns.

Do you jog or participate in regular, sustained hard physical exercise?

Ballet dancers and athletes often experience long periods of oligomenorrhea. Apparently the ratio of muscle mass to body fat affects the blood level of estrogen[1].

Although the menstrual history alone can often give enough information to reach a reasonably accurate diagnosis, a pelvic examination is essential. This is necessary in order to eliminate the possibility of either a pregnancy or a reproductive tract abnormality as the cause of the problem. Diagnostic procedures can then be determined on the basis of the pelvic findings and the information elicited in the history.

As has been stated, disturbances in established menstrual patterns can be extremely frightening. An understanding of some of the most common causes of menstrual irregularities will enable the nurse to educate a woman as to a possible cause of her problem. This can be reassuring and may help to reduce anxiety. However, education and reassurance are not intended to dissuade a woman from seeking medical attention and follow-up.

INFREQUENT OR ABSENT MENSTRUAL PERIODS

Oligomenorrhea

Infrequent menstrual periods with intervals greater than forty to forty-five days is called oligomenorrhea. In some women periods occur as much as two to three months apart with menstruation occurring only three to four times a year. If ovulation can be documented by the basal body temperature (BBT) method, then the infrequency probably results from an unusual lengthening of the proliferative phase of the menstrual cycle.

The cause of this condition is not always clear. Generally the problem originates at the hypothalamus resulting in a disruption of the hypothalamic-pituitary-ovarian axis. Some recognized but poorly understood causes are obesity, malnutrition, emotional factors, and systemic disease. A more specific cause is polycystic ovary disease. This is a clinical syndrome where oligomenorrhea or amenorrhea may be present along with hirsutism, obesity, and a high incidence of infertility.

There are two potentially serious consequences of persistent anovulation. The first is decreased fertility. The second is that the effect of steady, unopposed secretion of estrogen by the ovaries places these women at higher risk of endometrial cancer [4].

Treatment: When oligomenorrhea is due to emotional problems, nutritional factors or systemic disease, treatment is aimed at correcting the underlying cause. This frequently results in a more normal menstrual pattern.

Women who wish to become pregnant can usually do so by carefully plotting their BBT and timing intercourse to coincide with ovulation. Induction of ovulation can often be achieved by a medical approach. The most commonly used preparation is clomiphene citrate (Clomid). Side effects from this drug are minimal but may consist of vasomotor flushes, abdominal distention, or nausea and vomiting. There is also a higher incidence of multiple births reported following use of this drug.

A surgical method can also be used to restore ovulation in a woman with polycystic ovary disease. A bilateral wedge resection of the ovary may be successful, although results are usually temporary. Operative risk and subsequent development of adhesions, which in themselves decrease fertility, make this treatment less desirable than the medical approach.

For a woman who does not desire pregnancy, therapy is directed toward interruption of the steady effect of estrogen on the endometrium which may lead to premalignant cell changes. Oral progestins given daily for five days will insure withdrawal bleeding, thus preventing endometrial hyperplasia. Treatment in this manner can be given at two to three month intervals.

Another approach would be to use a low dose oral contraceptive which will also cause endometrial sloughing. However, there is some concern that future fertility may be compromised by suppressing ovulation in one who ovulates so infrequently. If she does not want to use an oral contraceptive a woman choosing to postpone pregnancy should be urged to use another effective method. Ovulation may be unpredictable and result in an unplanned and possibly unwanted pregnancy.

Amenorrhea

The absence of menstrual periods is called amenorrhea. This can be either primary or secondary. The following criteria define primary amenorrhea:
- No menstrual period by age fourteen and the absence of growth and development of secondary sexual characteristics.
- No menstrual period by age sixteen regardless of the presence of secondary sexual characteristics.

Secondary amenorrhea is the cessation of menstruation in a previously menstruating woman. It is generally considered to be significant when menstruation has been absent for three consecutive cycles or six months [4].

Speroff's approach to the classification of factors causing amenorrhea provides a useful framework. He describes four compartmental systems on which regular menstruation depends. Diagnostic workup is aimed at determining which compartment contains the disorder [4].

Compartment I—Disorders of the uterus
- Infection
- Asherman's Syndrome is a condition in which there is significant destruction of the endometrium. This is often the result of overly vigorous curettage and may be found post abortion or post D&C.
- Müllerian abnormalities
- Testicular feminization

Compartment II—Disorders in this compartment involve the ovaries themselves as in Turner's Syndrome.

Compartment III—Problems in this compartment are due to disorders in the function of the anterior pituitary. The most common cause of this is a benign pituitary adenoma.

Compartment IV—Disorders in the CNS or hypothalamus are responsible for problems in this category. Hypothalamic amenorrhea is the most common type and is diagnosed by exclusion. It is frequently associated with stress, weight loss or obesity or following the use of oral contraceptives. (See Figure 18-1.)

Treatment: Specific therapy of amenorrhea can be decided upon only after the cause has been determined. Disorders of Compartments I and II are perhaps the most complicated. Fortunately these disorders are also the most rare. They can be handled surgically or medically or by a combination of therapies.

Chromosomal disorders and congenital anomalies of the reproductive organs need individual, personalized approaches. Therapy is usually geared towards preserving sexual functioning and reproductive capability if it is present. Supportive therapy for these women and their families is directed towards reinforcing their gender identity and enhancing their self-concept.

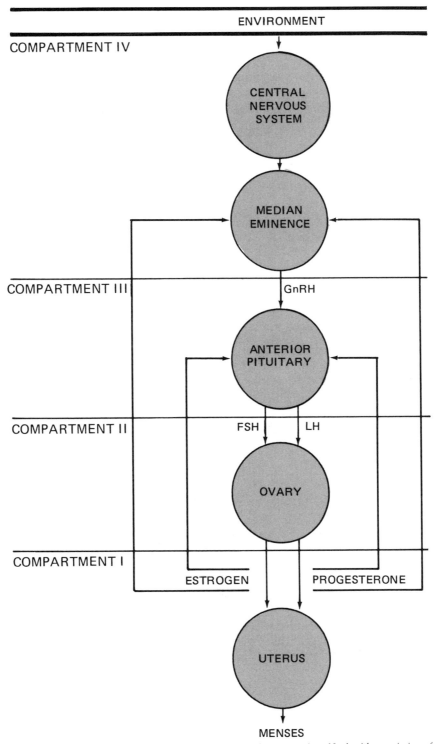

Figure 18-1. Compartmental systems involved with regulation of menstruation. Used with permission of Leon Speroff from Clinical Gynecologic Endocrinology and Infertility. Baltimore, Williams and Wilkins Co., 1978.

Pituitary tumors are surgically removed if they attain large sizes, cause visual disturbances or headaches, or if pregnancy is desired and drug-induced ovulation fails. In both pituitary and hypothalamic amenorrhea, periodic sloughing of the endometrium is desired to interrupt the constant estrogen stimulation. This is done by administering oral progestins or intramuscular progesterone at two to three month intervals.

DYSFUNCTIONAL UTERINE BLEEDING

Dysfunctional uterine bleeding (DUB) is abnormal endometrial bleeding in which organic lesions of the reproductive tract cannot be found [2]. There are numerous causes for abnormal uterine bleeding. As stated previously, abnormal bleeding patterns are usually caused by hormonal imbalance rather than by underlying pathology. However, it is important for health care providers to be aware of organic causes and to check for them when it seems appropriate. These include:

- Disorders of early pregnancy.
- Thyroid or other underlying endocrine disorders.
- Blood disorders and abnormal bleeding tendencies.
- Pelvic inflammatory disease.
- Functioning ovarian tumors.
- Polycystic ovary disease.
- Endometriosis.
- Fibroids and polyps.
- Cancer.

Most of the above problems can be detected by a pelvic examination and appropriate laboratory tests. A routine Pap smear and gonorrhea culture are simple and inexpensive screening techniques. Therefore, at a minimum, these should be done on every woman whose chief complaint is abnormal menstrual bleeding.

Abnormal Bleeding Associated With Ovulatory Cycles

Midcycle spotting: Some women may have spotting or light bleeding for one or two days at the time ovulation occurs. Most women will experience this at least a few times during their menstrual years. It is probably due to the slight drop in estrogen at that time which produces a relative estrogen deficiency. It can be documented by the BBT, ferning, and the fact that a menstrual period begins fourteen days later. Treatment consists of education and reassurance.

Premenstrual spotting: This is thought to be due to corpus luteum failure to some degree. There is a resultant fluctuation and gradual decline in estrogen and progesterone levels. This is in contrast to the normal sharp decline which causes the abrupt onset of menstruation. If it becomes very bothersome, an oral estrogen-progestin preparation can be given during the last five days of the cycle to support the endometrium.

Polymenorrhea: By definition polymenorrhea is bleeding at intervals of less than eighteen days. It is fairly common during premenopause and in the months following menarche. Although treatment is seldom necessary, a three month course of birth control pills often is corrective. This treatment would not be available for women over forty or women who would be at risk when taking estrogen.

Hypermenorrhea: Profuse or prolonged bleeding that occurs at regular intervals is termed hypermenorrhea. This is sometimes hard to document because "heavy bleeding" is a subjective symptom. However, any change from a normal pattern must be viewed as significant. A hemoglobin and hematocrit can help document the severity of the bleeding. A D&C will usually help determine the diagnosis and, interestingly, often corrects the problem.

Abnormal Bleeding in the Absence of Ovulation

Women who have extended periods of anovulation will usually, sooner or later, experience episodes of acyclic, heavy, often lengthy menstrual bleeding. Prolonged estrogen stimulation produces continued endometrial proliferation. Eventually the uterus can no longer support this endometrial growth and resultant sloughing and bleeding occurs.

Therapy is usually aimed at correcting the underlying problem which is causing the anovulation. When systemic disease or endocrine disorders are found to be the cause, adequate treatment of them will usually correct the dysfunctional bleeding.

As has been noted, most women will have a Compartment IV or hypothalamic cause for anovulation. These are usually transient episodes and may be due to emotional influences, travel, medication, nutrition, or illness. Counseling, reassurance and support for adequately coping with situational crises are helpful.

It is the lack of ovulation and the resulting progesterone deficiency that is the cause of the prolonged, irregular bleeding. Therefore, providing progestins orally or progesterone intramuscularly will promote normal maturation of the endometrium with subsequent complete shedding. Bleeding usually stops within a few days of administration of the hormone. It is then followed at an interval of a few days to two weeks by a withdrawal bleeding. Women should be told to expect this because it can often be frightening and may be mistaken for a return of the initial problem. Acute bleeding episodes may require D&C.

REFERENCES

1. Dale E et al: Menstrual dysfunction in female distance runners. Medicine and Science in Sports, Vol. 11 No. 1, Spring 1979
2. Kistner R: Gynecology: Principles and Practice, 3rd ed. Chicago, Yearbook Medical Publishers, 1979
3. Novak E: Textbook of Gynecology, 9th ed. Baltimore, Williams and Wilkins, 1975
4. Speroff L, Glass RH, Kase NG: Clinical Gynecologic Endocrinology and Infertility, 2nd ed. Baltimore, Williams and Wilkins, 1978
5. Treolar A et al: Variation of the human menstrual cycle through reproductive life. International Journal of Fertility, Vol. 12 No. 1, January-March 1967

19

Dysmenorrhea

Janet Stearns Wyatt, Gail M. Woodall and Sandra L. Tyler

Most women look forward to the beginning of menstruation because it is a clear sign that they are normal females. However, for some women, it marks the onset of a monthly pattern of predictable discomfort which may continue for more than forty years. Each woman experiences this discomfort in a unique way, although there are similar patterns.

The problems associated with menstruation are diverse. It helps to loosely group them into three categories: those associated with fluid retention such as breast tenderness and irritability; G.I. symptoms such as nausea, vomiting and diarrhea; and, lastly, pain and cramping. These symptoms may be experienced anytime following ovulation up to the onset of menses (premenstrual syndrome) or after menstruation starts (dysmenorrhea).

Dysmenorrhea has traditionally been categorized as Primary and Secondary. Primary dysmenorrhea refers to difficult menstruation of unknown etiology. Secondary dysmenorrhea is difficult menstruation that can be traced to an underlying pathological condition. The two types differ in respect to age of onset, nature and duration of pain, and associated symptoms. (See Table 19-1.)

Table 19-1. Summary of Primary and Secondary Dysmenorrhea.

	Primary	*Secondary*
Age of onset	Within a few months after establishing pattern of regular, ovulatory cycles.	Varies according to etiology (onset at young age with imperforate hymen; later adulthood with endometriosis, fibroids, or PID).
Nature of Pain	Sharp and colicky; may radiate to lower back and thighs; usually coincides with onset of menses; rarely lasts more than twenty-four hours.	From dull to sharp depending on etiology; may be unilateral, bilateral, radiating or non-radiating; onset may precede menses and often lasts through entire period.
Associated Symptoms	Nausea, vomiting, diarrhea, syncope.	Specific to etiology (fever with PID; heavy bleeding with fibroids and IUD's).

Primary Dysmenorrhea

Historically, the specific research undertaken to discover the cause of primary dysmenorrhea has mirrored the popular medical practices of that period. In the 1900s surgery was popular, so surgical treatment was recommended. Unfortunately, this often resulted in unneeded surgical correction for such normal anatomic variations as a retroflexed or "tipped" uterus, and a "tight" or stenotic cervix. Presacral neurectomy was another form of surgical "cure."

Various other conditions that were considered to be causes of primary dysmenorrhea were faulty posture, heavy flow with clotting, obesity, and physical inactivity. Treatment recommendations were based on the supposed cause.

When these treatments proved unsuccessful, scientists in the 1930s and 40s began postulating theories concerning an imbalance in the female hormones which had been discovered. These theories, primarily describing an estrogen excess or progesterone deficiency, became difficult to prove. The menstrual cycle itself weakened these ideas since it demonstrated a precise endocrine function even in dysmenorrheic women [14].

Pregnancy, with the resultant cessation of ovulation, was often recommended as the best way to break the monthly cycle of discomfort until the final cure of menopause arrived. Many women noticed that following even one pregnancy their symptoms of dysmenorrhea were lessened or absent for many years. However, this really wasn't a practical or acceptable "cure" for all women.

Interest in psychological aspects of disease was popular in the 1960s. Along with this trend, behavioral research created a psychology of menstruation. Clinicians began looking for behavioral explanations for primary dysmenorrhea. Women were sometimes told that dysmenorrhea represented a rejection of womanhood or was a result of conditioning by their mothers.

These psychological studies did identify some negative behavioral changes which occasionally were seen in association with menstruation:

• An increase in irritability and pessimism, including a reported increase in violent activity.

• An increase in passive behavior and a change in self-confidence and self-esteem, which has been associated with a reported increase in female suicides, and suicide attempts.

• A decrease in work and testing performance which has been correlated to a reported increase in female accident rates.

It doesn't seem surprising that negative behavior would be noted in connection with dysmenorrhea. Most people in pain do exhibit negative behavior.

Based on these observations, treatment methods originated which are still in use to some degree today. These include psychotropic drugs and strong narcotics. At times psychotherapy was recommended. Some doctors even recommended that during difficult menstruation women should refrain from travel, elective surgery, and participation in competitive activities.

Although psychological influences do have a bearing on one's perception of pain, it does not necessarily follow that these influences cause the pain. Yet most of the prescribed treatments were directed at the symptoms as if they were the underlying cause. Primary dysmenorrhea remained a syndrome of unknown etiology.

Understandably, when a woman's periods stopped during pregnancy and following menopause so did her dysmenorrhea. However, when oral contraceptives became available, many women who started taking them and who had previously had dysmenorrhea, stopped having pain even though their periods continued. Many physicians immediately adopted the Pill as their primary mode of treatment.

Although at the time, the underlying mechanism was not understood, the Pill represented the first treatment aimed directly at the underlying cause of dysmenorrhea. The synthetic estrogen and progestins in the Pill halt ovulation and limit endometrial growth. We now know that the normal pattern of ovulation and subsequent endometrial growth and shedding are the crucial elements which contribute to the experience of primary dysmenorrhea.

The discovery of a special lipid extract from menstrual blood has contributed much to the growing knowledge about primary dysmenorrhea. These lipids are menstrual prostaglandins which are specialized hydroxy-fatty acids. They are responsible for increasing the contractile action of the smooth muscle of the uterus. Thus when prostaglandin levels in the endometrium are high, contraction of the uterus is increased [8, 12].

Scientists were able to recreate symptoms of dysmenorrhea simply by administering exogenous prostaglandins to female patients. When prostaglandins were given, uterine contractions occurred and blood supply to pelvic structures was compromised [9]. The uterine ischemic reaction created is now thought to contribute to the pelvic and abdominal pain associated with menstruation [3]. (For additional details, see chapter 3.)

Many women who received prostaglandins also experienced diarrhea, nausea, flushing and syncope [9]. These systemic effects, characteristically associated with primary dysmenorrhea, are thought to be due to the release of prostaglandins into the extra-pelvic circulation [3, 9]. Further study into the circulatory effects of the prostaglandins may continue to yield information that will better explain the complexities of this disorder.

With the research data now available, clinicians have begun to make changes in their treatment and management of patients with primary dysmenorrhea. Many gynecologists are now recommending the use of prostaglandin inhibiting substances as an initial form of treatment.

Perhaps the most common prostaglandin inhibiting substance known today is aspirin. Other substances that inhibit prostaglandin action include indomethacin, (Indocin), ibuprofen (Motrin), and naproxen (Naprosyn) [1, 2]. Not only are these drugs highly effective for relief of dysmenorrhea, but they are also relatively free of side effects [3].

As initially mentioned, symptoms other than pain and G.I. problems may be associated with menstruation. Symptoms of fluid retention such as abdominal bloating, peripheral edema, weight gain, and breast changes may occur. Although usually associated with the premenstrual syndrome, they often continue during menstruation. Research has demonstrated a positive correlation between estrogen levels and aldosterone secretion. Since aldosterone plays a vital role in sodium regulation, it seems likely that estrogen may in some way be linked to fluid retention [4, 9].

Thus two normal physiological mechanisms have been implicated as contributing to primary dysmenorrhea. This means that now treatment can be specifically directed at the cause whether it be estrogen or prostaglandin induced. Consequently, most women can now be free from the pain of primary dysmenorrhea.

Not all women experience premenstrual problems and dysmenorrhea severely enough to require medication. There are other measures that can be taken to provide relief. A heating pad or hot water bottle will increase vasodilation and relieve ischemia. Exercise and good posture help insure normal circulation to the pelvic area. A well balanced diet with reduction of foods which are high in sodium will minimize fluid retention and maintain normal G.I. functioning. Many women find that curling into a knee-chest position brings relief.

Secondary Dysmenorrhea

There are many etiologies for secondary dysmenorrhea. These include endometriosis, pelvic infection, endometrial or endocervical polyps, fibroids, cervical stenosis following surgical procedures or instrumentation, congenital abnormalities such as imperforate hymen, and the use of an IUD. All of these conditions except for endometriosis have been discussed in other chapters. The remainder of this chapter will be devoted to a review of endometriosis.

Endometriosis is the location of functioning endometrial tissue in places other than the uterus. The most common sites for endometrial implants are the ovaries, the uterosacral ligaments and the peritoneum of the cul-de-sac. Less commonly, sites of implants are found in the bladder, rectum, lung, and incisions from surgery such as Cesarean section and episiotomy.

There is more than one theory to explain the origin of endometriosis. However, the most popular theory states that viable fragments of endometrium are regurgitated with menstrual blood in a retrograde fashion through the oviducts. This tissue subsequently implants on the ovaries, cul-de-sac or other nearby organs. Another theory explains implants in distant sites such as the lung as occurring from metastases through lymphatic or blood channels. Transplantation at the time of surgery may be an explanation for incisional sites of endometrial tissue [6].

One of the primary symptoms of endometriosis is an acquired dysmenorrhea. This usually occurs after a number of years of pain-free periods. However, a woman with primary dysmenorrhea may only notice an increased intensity and duration of symptoms as she develops endometriosis. The pain often precedes the onset of the menstrual period and may last throughout its entire course. It may be felt in the pelvic area or as sacral backache. Dyspareunia is a common complaint. The degree of pain that a woman experiences does not seem to correlate with the severity or number of endometrial implants.

When a pelvic exam is done some typical signs may be present. These include nodular growths particularly in the cul-de-sac and along the uterosacral ligaments, a fixed, retroverted uterus (from adhesions), and enlarged ovary or ovaries (endometrioma). Many women with endometriosis also have a history of infertility. This may be due to impaired ovarian function, adhesions that distort the tube or to some as yet unidentified factor.

A diagnosis can be accurately made only by visualization of the endometrial implants at the time of surgery. Laparoscopy has greatly facilitated the diagnosis of endometriosis in patients with suspicious pelvic findings and typical history. A high index of suspicion should be raised when a woman complains of acquired, progressive dysmenorrhea, deep dyspareunia, sacral backache and infertility.

Treatment for endometriosis is either surgical or hormonal. A woman with mild symptoms and few pelvic findings can often be treated with a combination estrogen-progestin oral contraceptive. This controls the pain and seems to retard the progression of the disease. This may be due to the inhibition of ovulation and the resultant reduction of cyclical endometrial stimulation. It also has the advantage of providing contraception if desired.

A relatively new treatment with danazol, a synthetic anti-gonadotropic steriod, has been highly successful. This inhibits FSH and LH and does not have any stimulatory effect on the endometrium. It produces a pseudo-menopausal state and allows for regression of the endometrium both intra and extra-uterine. Its advantages are a high degree of alleviation of symptoms, prompt resumption of ovulation when discontinued, and good post-treatment fertility rates. Its disadvantages include distressing menopausal symptoms such as hot flushes, mild depression and irregular bleeding. Widespread use of danazol is limited by its high cost and suspicion that endometriosis recurs when treatment is discontinued [5].

Surgical treatment in a young woman desiring pregnancy can be difficult and painstaking. Endometriomas of the ovaries must be meticulously excised with care to preserve some ovarian tissue. Separation of adhesions and cauterization of endometrial implants may reduce symptoms and enhance fertility. In a woman who does not desire future pregnancies, a total abdominal hysterectomy with bilateral salpingo-oophorectomy is often performed.

Painful menstruation affects more than half of all women in their reproductive years and is the greatest single cause of lost school and working hours among young women. For a condition of this magnitude, it has received very little attention and research until recent years. A woman who must look forward to predictable often incapacitating pain for one or more days each month deserves a careful and thorough investigation of the cause.

With the recent growth in understanding of the possible role of prostaglandins in the etiology of primary dysmenorrhea, we can now offer most women a solution to the pain accompanying a previously poorly understood syndrome. Similarly, advances have been made in surgical and medical treatment for conditions which may contribute to secondary dysmenorrhea. Therefore, nurses can assure women with either type of dysmenorrhea that relief of their symptoms is possible.

REFERENCES

1. Budoff PW: Use of mefenamic acid in the treatment of primary dysmenorrhea. Journal of the American Medical Association, Vol. 24 No. 25, June 22, 1979
2. Dingfelder JR: Do prostaglandins cause dysmenorrhea? Contemporary OB/GYN, Vol. 8 No. 1, July 1976
3. Dingfelder JR: Patient guide—Q and A about dysmenorrhea. The Female Patient, August 1977

 4. Field PA, Funke J: The pre-menstrual syndrome: Current findings, treatment, and implications for nurses. Journal of Obstetric and Gynecological Nursing, September-October 1976
 5. Greenblatt R, Vassilious T: Danazol treatment of endometriosis: Long-term follow-up. Fertility and Sterility, Vol. 32 No. 5, November 1979
 6. Kistner R: Gynecology Principles and Practice, 3rd ed. Chicago, Yearbook Medical Publishers, 1979
 7. Morrison JC, Hennings JC: Primary dysmenorrhea treated with indomethacin. Southern Medical Journal, Vol. 72 No. 4, April 1979
 8. Pickles VR et al: Prostaglandins in endometrium and menstrual fluid from normal and dysmenorrhoeic subjects. Journal of Obstetrics and Gynecology, No. 72, 1965
 9. Reichman KW: Menstrual Products, Chapter 16, Handbook of Nonprescription Drugs, 5th ed. Washington, DC, American Pharmaceutical Association, 1978
10. Round Table Discussions: Endometriosis: New views, new therapies, Patient Care, Vol. 12 No. 9, November 1978
11. Rubin RT et al: Postnatal gonadal steroid effects on human behavior, Science, Vol. 211 No. 4488, March 20, 1981
12. Speroff L, Ramwell PW: Prostaglandins in reproductive physiology. American Journal of Obstetrics and Gynecology, Vol. 107 No. 7, August 1, 1970
13. Ylikorkala O, Dawood Y: New concepts in dysmenorrhea. American Journal of Obstetrics and Gynecology, Vol. 130 No. 7, April 1978
14. Wentz AC, Jones GS: Office gynecology—managing dysmenorrhea. Postgraduate Medicine, Vol. 60, July 1976

20

Urinary Tract Infection

Urinary Tract Infection (UTI) can occur in the urethra, the bladder, or the kidney. Infection of the kidney (pyelonephritis) is by far the most serious of the three. Cystitis and urethritis, although not serious in themselves, occasionally result in pyelonephritis if they are not adequately treated. Although the kidney can also become infected by blood or lymphatic spread of bacteria, the most common route is thought to be by ascending infection from the lower urinary tract. Therefore cystitis and urethritis deserve prompt and adequate treatment with careful follow-up.

Females are much more susceptible to urinary infections than are males. This is due in part to anatomy. The short female urethra positioned close to the vagina and anus makes introduction of bacteria relatively easy. In contrast, the long urethra of the male and its greater distance from the contaminated rectal area makes the introduction of bacteria less likely. When bacteria do gain access to the male urethra, there is a good chance that they will get flushed out during urination before they reach the bladder.

Even in childhood UTI is more common in females than in males, but its incidence increases dramatically at puberty and with the onset of sexual activity. It persists at a high level into the menopause and post menopause ages. It is estimated that at least half of all women will have at least one UTI before the age of sixty-five [7].

Because of the prevalence, discomfort, and possible complications of urinary tract infections, it is important for a nurse to understand the symptoms, treatment and prevention. This chapter will discuss urinary tract infection with the emphasis placed on cystitis. A brief discussion of pyelonephritis will be given first.

Pyelonephritis

Pyelonephritis is a bacterial infection of the kidney. It is characterized by abcesses that usually begin in the renal pelvis and spread through the medulla and cortex. The process of inflammation and resultant scar formation secondarily involves the glomeruli, tubules and blood vessels. If the acute process evolves into a more chronic condition, significant kidney damage may result.

Acute pyelonephritis is often characterized by symptoms of bladder irritability such as frequency, urgency, and dysuria. However, sometimes these symptoms are not present. Typically a patient will have fever, chills, nausea and vomiting, and complaints of back or flank pain. During examination tapping over the costovertebral angle results in extreme pain. Pyuria, hematuria and proteinuria are often, but not always, present. Urine cultures will be positive for bacteria.

Treatment consists of appropriate antibacterial preparations determined by the culture and sensitivity. Additional tests such as IVP, cystogram, BUN, and creatinine may be necessary to investigate the possibility of structural damage or abnormalities.

Cystitis

Cystitis is an infection of the bladder. Bladder infections are almost always due to gram-negative bacilli. By far the most prevalent causative organism is E. coli. However, other organisms that may gain access to the bladder and cause cystitis include Klebsiella, Proteus, Pseudomonas, Staphylococcus, Streptococcus, trichomonas and even yeast.

The short length of the urethra and its position near the vagina and rectum facilitate the entrance of bacteria into the urethral meatus. The warmth and moisture of the genital area also fosters the growth of bacteria. A high growth of bacteria on the vaginal vestibule seems to predispose a woman to bladder infections [6]. Apparently, most women have a defense mechanism that prevents the growth of pathogenic bacteria on the perineum. If the defense mechanism is inadequate, the number of bacteria is unusually high, or other contributing factors are present a bladder infection may result. Conditions which may contribute to bacterial invasion of the bladder are poor hygiene, trauma (from instrumentation, sexual activity, motorcycling and bicycling), chemical irritation (from bubblebaths), pregnancy and diabetes.

If there is an underlying abnormality that prevents complete emptying of the bladder, the residual urine provides a good growth medium for bacteria. Incomplete emptying of the bladder may result from structural or congenital defects such as bladder neck or urethral strictures. The cause may also be neurogenic such as following spinal cord injuries. Habitual voluntary "holding-back" of urine may also lead a child or older woman into problems of cystitis.

There is one type of cystitis, the so-called "honeymoon cystitis", that may not always be associated with bacteriuria. Its name comes from the fact that the onset of symptoms usually occurs shortly after the first sexual experience, increased frequency or vigor of sexual activity, or resumption of sexual activity after a long period of abstinence. The thrusting of the penis can cause a considerable amount of trauma to the urethra and the base of the bladder in the area of the trigone. This in turn leads to tissue trauma, edema, capillary rupture and inflammation. This condition, which may also be called trigonitis, can lead to the unpleasant symptoms of cystitis with or without the presence of bacteria.

Symptoms and Signs. The discomfort of a bladder infection is remembered long after the problem has been resolved. The three classic symptoms of cystitis are frequency, urgency and dysuria. At times there are the additional symptoms of nocturia, hematuria and inability to retain urine. Some women will also have a lower abdominal aching pressure or "dragging" feeling. When examined, there may be supra-pubic tenderness.

A woman with cystitis will often be bothered most by the symptom of urgency.

There is the feeling that she must urinate immediately, but when she does she voids very small amounts of urine with considerable pain. The passing of bloody urine is extremely frightening.

Fever is *not* a symptom of lower urinary tract infection. A woman with fever and flank pain may have pyelonephritis. Because of its more serious prognosis, the possibility of kidney infection should always be investigated and ruled out when fever is present.

Diagnosis. A diagnosis by symptoms alone is inadequate. A urinalysis and urine culture and sensitivity must always be done. The following urinalysis findings are generally accepted as presumptive evidence of UTI:

- WBC's—more than 5 per high powered field.
- RBC's—more than 0–3 per high powered field.
- Proteinuria and presence of bacteria.

The only accurate means of diagnosing infection is by urine culture. A colony count of 100,000 (10^5) or more bacteria per milliliter of urine is considered strong evidence of urinary infection. A finding of less than 10,000 colonies (10^4) bacteria per milliliter indicates absence of bacteriuria. There is a gray area between these two numbers. If two consecutive cultures fail to result in counts above 100,000, the chances of infection are not great. The reason for the presence of bacteria in these circumstances is thought to be from external contamination.

Catheterization is not routinely employed for urine culture because of the risk of introducing infection. A clean-catch, mid-stream urine culture is generally utilized. It is important for a woman to receive clear instructions for obtaining the specimen in order to decrease the chance of contaminating the urine. She should be told the following:

- Wash hands.
- Open the sterile container and do not touch either the inside of the bottle or its cover.
- Sit on the toilet with legs spread wide apart.
- Spread the labia and hold open with one hand.
- Using cotton balls or gauze squares soaked in water or soap solution, wipe from front to back over the urethral meatus; this should be done three times using a new gauze each time; soaps containing hexachlorophine and solutions such as aqueous zephiran should not be used since they may render the urine sterile and result in false-negative culture results.
- If soap was used, rinse well in the same manner.
- Begin urinating and let the first few drops go into the toilet.
- Catch some of the mid-stream urine being careful not to touch the container to the vulvar area.

Insertion of a tampon during specimen collection may be helpful in preventing contamination from a vaginal discharge or menstrual flow.

If a woman has symptoms of vaginal infection, appropriate tests should be done. A gonorrhea culture should be included since the irritating discharge and occasional infection of the Skene's gland can cause symptoms of cystitis. Trichomonas and yeast may cause similar symptoms.

Treatment. Treatment for infection is based on the results of sensitivity testing of the organism. While waiting for culture results, most clinicians will begin therapy with a sulfa drug such as sulfasoxazole (Gantrisin) or sulfamethoxazole (Gantanol) since most of the organisms responsible for cystitis respond to that drug. Resistance to sulfa by the organisms found in the intestinal flora usually develops. Therefore, a re-infection may not respond to this therapy. If the organism is not sensitive to sulfa, other drugs that are often effective include Ampicillin, tetracycline, nitrofurantoin, trimethoprim + sulfamethoxazole (Bactrim or Septra) or cephalosporin.

A high fluid intake of eight to ten glasses per day is essential. An acidic drink such as cranberry juice is often recommended. Coffee, tea and cola drinks are sometimes irritating and if so should be avoided.

If symptoms are very severe, a urinary tract analgesic such as phenazopyridine HCl (Pyridium) can be used along with the anti-microbial medication for the first few days. This provides symptomatic relief only. It turns the urine bright orange which may be alarming if the woman has not been warned of this in advance. With Pyridium symptoms generally disappear rapidly. Women need to be encouraged to complete all of the medication since incomplete treatment is one of the most common causes of recurrence of a urinary tract infection.

Treatment for the symptoms of cystitis when no bacteriuria is present are aimed at correcting the underlying cause. For heterosexual women with "honeymoon cystitis" a period of abstinence may be necessary. Sometimes a change in coital position may be helpful. Positions where deep thrusting is more likely, such as woman-superior, may need to be avoided. If pressure from the rim of a diaphragm seems to be contributing to the problem, a different size or rim style may be helpful. Occasionally a different birth control method will be necessary.

Prevention. Prevention is directed towards decreasing the amount of bacteria in the perineal area as well as eliminating or minimizing contributing factors. Youngsters should be taught to wipe from front to back after a bowel movement to prevent the spread of bacteria from the rectal to the urethral area. Older women should be encouraged to do the same which may require changing a previously formed habit. Avoiding the use of nylon underwear, pantyhose and tight clothing will minimize the warmth and moisture of the area and help prevent infection. A highly susceptible woman may need to bathe in the shower rather than the tub since bacteria from the rectal and vaginal areas that are washed into the water may enter the urethral meatus.

A susceptible woman must also take some special precautions with sexual activities. Showering before lovemaking may help reduce the number of bacteria present. Emptying the bladder before and after sexual activity decreases the amount of trauma it receives and may help flush out any bacteria that are in the urethra. In the face of recurrent UTI's additional treatment may be necessary and referral to a urologist should be made. A commonly used guideline for referral is if a woman has three or more UTI's within one year.

Women should be encouraged as youngsters to empty their bladders soon after the urge to urinate is felt. It seems that children often postpone urinating to avoid using public toilets or because of a reluctance to ask permission to leave class during early school years. This then becomes a habit which is hard to break.

Urethritis

An infection of the urethra without involvement of the bladder is much less common in women than in men [1]. The resultant dysuria may be caused by a vaginal or cervical discharge. A woman with dysuria without significant bacteriuria should be checked for other infections such as gonorrhea, trichomonas, yeast and herpes. Appropriate treatment can be instituted according to the cause.

When a woman has the distressing symptoms of dysuria, frequency and urgency, and there is no bacteriuria and no apparent contributing factors, the term "urethral syndrome" has frequently been employed. This is a general term applied to a symptom complex which is poorly understood. Women with such problems should be referred to a urologist for evaluation.

REFERENCES

1. Bowie W: Urethritis and infections of the lower urogenital tract. Urologic Clinics of North America, Vol. 7 No. 1, February 1980
2. Cooper J: Urinary tract infections: Cause and prevention. Hospital Formulary, Vol. 12 No. 2, February 1977
3. Fine M: How to manage urinary tract infections: Part I—Recognition and workup. Consultant, Vol. 17 No. 7, July 1977
4. Kaye D: Urinary Tract Infection and Its Management. St. Louis, C. V. Mosby, 1972
5. Martin L: Health Care of Women. Philadelphia, J. B. Lippincott, 1978
6. Stamey T: Urinary Infections. Baltimore, Williams and Wilkins, 1972
7. Stefan R, Klaus B: Urinary tract infections. Nurse Practitioner, Vol. 3 No. 5, September/October 1978

21

Crisis and Its Intervention

It is important to distinguish between stress and crisis. Although these two concepts interact, intervention for each has a different focus. Stress results in a physical response while a crisis is a psychological reaction to a stressful situation.

Stress

Selye defines stress as being anything which increases energy consumption by the body. In turn, the body mobilizes its various defense mechanisms in an attempt to reduce the threat and "cope." If the stress is not reduced or is too much for the body to handle, the individual will reach a stage of exhaustion and collapse. If intervention does not become available at some point, the person will die [8].

In a general way, stress is always present in each of us. In fact, a review of the definition shows that we could not live without some stress. At a somewhat higher level, stress motivates us to grow and accomplish in both a physical and psychological sense. Even more specifically, when an individual confronts a change or threat to an otherwise balanced life, the stress response is intensified and coping mechanisms are mobilized by the individual.

Selye describes three phases which the body goes through when dealing with intensified stress. Briefly summarized, these stages are:

1. Alarm—during this phase, general resistance falls below normal.
2. Resistance—the body mobilizes coping mechanisms and resistance rises above normal. This phase uses a great deal of energy.
3. Exhaustion—resistance again falls below normal due to depletion of energy sources.

No one can be prepared for every intensely stressful experience which life will bring to them. If previous, similar stressful situations have been experienced it may be easier to handle a new, difficult situation. If a way to cope cannot be found, an individual may experience a crisis.

Crisis

The basis for our English word, crisis, is the Greek "Krisis" which means point of decision. Everyone approaches a crisis or turning point many times in life. When this happens, some people are able to mobilize resources, cope, and use the situation as a transition episode. For others, the experience may be perceived as difficult or seemingly impossible to resolve, thereby precipitating a crisis. Caplan defines a crisis as being:

A psychological disequilibrium in a person who confronts circumstances that for him constitute an important problem which he can for the time being neither escape nor solve with his customary problem solving resources [5].

It is important to remember that an event is not a crisis. The stress created by an event, no matter how high, also does not constitute a crisis. A crisis is an individualized, internal experience, a "psychological disequilibrium" which occurs in relation to the stress created by one or more external events.

Characteristics of a Crisis

A crisis has certain identifying criteria which separate it from situations that require more traditional types of therapeutic approaches. These include:
- *Precipitating Event.* An event occurs which increases the individual's stress state to an intolerable degree. Remember, the event is not the crisis, instead, its role is that of precipitating the crisis.
- *Personal Experience.* A crisis, that is, the "psychological disequilibrium" exists within the person. If an individual defines a situation as being a crisis, it is. The person's experience is what determines whether a crisis exists.
- *Limited Time Span.* A crisis covers a relatively short time span and lasts anywhere from three to six weeks. A period of psychological disequilibrium which lasts less than two to three weeks is more accurately referred to as an event or episode [5]. A situation lasting longer than six weeks is more likely a psychological problem which will require more extensive professional intervention [5].
- *Self Limited.* The individual who is in crisis is experiencing a great deal of emotional pain. This pain is usually of such intensity that it cannot be tolerated very long and so the person will end the crisis in one way or another.

Balancing Factors

There are three factors which determine an individual's vulnerability to a crisis. These balancing factors are also related to the extent or severity of a crisis. They are as follows:
1. The individual's *perception of the event*—How does the person expect this situation to affect other aspects of life?
2. The available *situational supports*—Including family, friends, and religion.
3. *Internal coping mechanisms*—Variables may include the number of stressors being faced, the duration of the stress situation, and past experiences.

Categories of Crisis

There are two categories of crisis. *Maturational crises* occur as a result of the expected, normal changes in a developing individual. A person experiencing difficulty in relation to changes of puberty or menopause is experiencing a maturational crisis. *Situational crises* occur in response to unexpected or accidental events which are imposed on an individual. Examples of situational crises are those caused by natural disasters, rape, or a sudden devastating illness.

Development and Resolution of a Crisis

Initially, the individual recognizes a stressful situation and experiences a rise in tension. There will be attempts to use known problem-solving techniques. When there is a lack of success in coping with the stress, many different coping mechanisms are tried and discarded. As the stress level continues to rise, tension and discomfort become more severe.

As tension continues to increase, the person will mobilize as many internal and external problem-solving techniques as are available. At this point one of four things will happen. The person may:

1. Solve the problem,
2. Redefine the problem,
3. Avoid the problem by giving up the goal or becoming resigned to the situation, or
4. Experience a major psychological disorganization because the problem can be neither solved nor avoided.

Intervention and/or resolution at any point in this precrisis state may act to abort the crisis. If none of the first three alternatives occur, the individual will go to the crisis stage of disequilibrium. Once this happens, the individual will move through three phases:

- *Impact*. This stage is characterized by bewilderment, confusion, denial, i.e., "This can't be happening to me."
- *Turmoil*. In this stage the individual experiences anxiety, depression, anger, guilt, shame, and withdrawal. There may be psychosomatic complaints. A great deal of meaningless activity may be exhibited with greatly reduced efficiency. Physical and mental tension is high.
- *Resolution or adaptation*. During the third phase, the tension is reduced or satisfaction is found in some way. A crisis *cannot* continue for any extended length of time without something being done to abort it. It is too painful for a person to continue in a crisis state.

The most drastic resolution which may be chosen is suicide. On a less drastic level there will be a range of resolution as follows:

- The individual will break down psychologically and move to a lower level of mental functioning.
- The individual will abandon the problem and return to the precrisis level of functioning.
- The individual will learn new ways of coping and become stronger.

Figure 21-1 gives a diagrammatic representation of these levels of resolution.

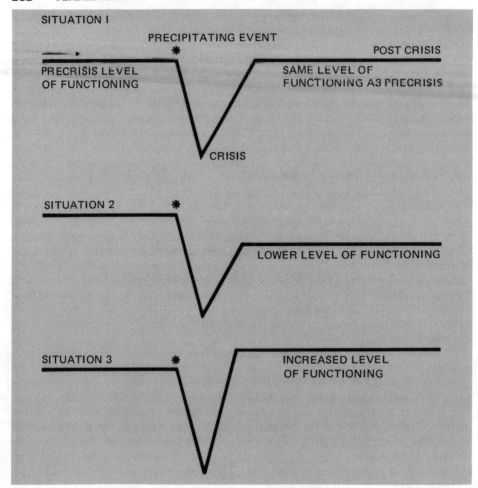

Figure 21-1.   *Schematic representation of changes in the level of functioning following a crisis.*

Crisis Intervention

People who are experiencing a crisis are very vulnerable, psychologically. They need a solution and nothing that they know of or have tried seems to be working. This makes them open to help and learning new ideas and new behaviors. The intervenor needs some understanding of biopsychosocial processes, although not to the extent of a formally trained therapist. Crisis intervention can be very competently done by nonprofessional people with a minimum of training.

The *individual* approach to crisis intervention involves assessment of the interpersonal processes of the person in crisis. The unique needs of the person must be considered in order to arrive at a solution that deals with that particular situation. This approach assumes a one-to-one interaction between client and intervenor.

The *generic* approach focuses on the characteristic course of a particular kind of crisis. Specific intervention is designed to be effective for all members of a given group rather than being aimed at individuals. This is based on the idea that there are common, recognized patterns of behavior that occur in most crises which are precipitated by a similar event. An example of a paradigm which has been developed utilizing the generic approach is Kubler-Ross' four grieving stages.

The generic and individual approaches are not exclusive. Rather, they bring complementary perspectives to the process of crisis intervention. The situation and the client will determine the emphasis of approach.

In addition to choice of an approach, some key points will facilitate the intervention process.

• In contrast to the passive role of intervention used in most traditional types of psychotherapy, crisis intervention assumes that the intervenor is actively involved.

• The goal is to restore the individual at least to the prior level of functioning.

• Coping is the key to resolution and the individual in crisis is open to learning new ways of coping.

• Time for intervention is short due to the self-limiting, painfully high anxiety levels which characterize a crisis.

• Communication must be clear, specific, direct, and open. High anxiety creates a reduced attention span and great possibility for misunderstanding.

• The client needs acceptance and encouragement to express feelings. The exception is if the client, nurse, or others are in danger (that is, suicide, homicide).

• Flexibility and availability of the intervenor are a must. If for any reason a nurse feels incapable of intervention, referral must be made and a clear explanation given to the client. However, the client must *NOT* be abandoned until the new contact is established. The basic responsibility is first to ensure the client's safety and then to obtain help.

Aguilera suggests using the four-part problem solving approach to crisis intervention. Because it parallels the nursing process, it is a familiar and comfortable approach for nurses whose work often places them in positions which call for crisis intervention. The familiar steps of assessment, planning, implementation, and evaluation serve as an organizer to help guide the process of crisis intervention.

Assessment: During crisis intervention it is extremely important to keep the definition of crisis in mind. Because of the client's high anxiety level, assume nothing. A careful check of relationships between seemingly random thoughts and ideas as the client presents them will help maintain clarity and prevent misunderstandings for both the nurse and client.

Define the problem, separate it from the crisis, and determine what has already been done. This helps to establish a base of information. Essential items to include are:

• What is the precipitating event?

• What is the client's perception of this event and what are other contributing factors (additional stress, past experience)?

• What coping methods were or are being used?

• Why are the usual coping methods not working?

• What support system is available? Has it been used?

• How long has the crisis existed?

• How is this crisis affecting the client and other people who are significant to the client?

- If the crisis were to continue, what consequences are anticipated? Is there a possibility of suicide or homicide?

NOTE: If the answers to direct questions about suicide or homicide are "yes" or "maybe," ask if the person has a plan. If there is a plan, ask for details. For continued follow-up, details of name, address, phone numbers, friends or family to contact, and other identifying data are needed. This is especially important if the client has called and not come for help in person.

Although assessment continues throughout the entire process of intervention, this data will give some basis for immediate planning. The client needs activity and mobilization of resources in order to resume daily functioning. An awareness of the intervenor's concern and involvement as well as an immediate response and assistance may provide hope and initiate the client's resumption of coping.

Planning: Once enough data has been collected and the problem is clearly identified, the planning stage begins. The intervenor and the client work together closely making sure that the goals "belong" to the client instead of the intervenor. Major guidelines include:

- Determine the strengths and weaknesses of the client.
- Establish the existing alternatives.
- Explore new alternatives and activities.
- Choose a solution and set short-term realistic goals.

Implementation: This step, like the others, is ongoing. It is important for the intervenor to first separate and then attempt to shift the focus from the external event to the internal, emotional event. Some suggestions for the intervenor in this stage include:

- Be reliable, consistent, and available.
- Provide consistent, relevant feedback and reinforcement.
- Provide open, genuine communication.
- Encourage expressions of feelings, and practice of new coping methods. Monitor this process so that the client feels safe and things won't "get out of hand."
- Be a role model expressing such feelings as humor, hope, realism, self-awareness, and self-investment.
- Encourage the mobilization of available, external resources.
- Keep the focus on the current crisis.
- Allow for dependency and assist when the client cannot take the initiative.
- Assign tasks and provide a sense of immediate action.
- Know what social resources are available and refer when necessary.

The client needs to be actively involved in "doing." However, when new coping behaviors are being learned, a safe environment is needed for practicing. Time must also be allowed for practicing and adopting new ways of coping.

The client must make a cognitive connection between the internal crisis and the precipitating event before an understanding of what happened is reached. This understanding will be demonstrated when the client can give a logical, acceptable explanation of what happened without rationalizing, intellectualizing, or projecting. In addition, feelings such as anger or fear will be recognized and acknowledged.

Evaluation: Once the crisis is resolved, the client's growth will be strengthened by reviewing what happened. In addition, further growth of the skills of the intervenor are dependent upon a review of the crisis intervention process and feedback from the client. Both the client and intervenor need to consider their strengths and weaknesses, as well as what was learned and how to improve. Important evaluative components to consider include:

- A summary of what was learned.
- What still needs to be done and how it will be done.
- How this new learning can be projected and used in future situations.
- Was the outcome satisfactory and why?

FEMALE CRISES

In most cases, maturational and situational crises are precipitated by the same kinds of events for both men and women. Examples of such crises may include puberty, aging, divorce, alcoholism, or death or disablement of a mate. Primarily because of cultural factors, intervention of a given type of crisis may assume a somewhat different perspective for a man than that given for a woman. Although general crisis intervention techniques are used in all situations, some situations may call for specific, additional guidelines.

Female crises that occur in response to normal developmental processes are described in other chapters and so will not be discussed here. Two events in particular which happen to women and nearly always precipitate a situational crisis are unplanned pregnancy and rape. Some basic suggestions for intervention with these situations follows.

Unplanned Pregnancy

Many women would not be upset, and, in fact, may be pleased to discover that they are unexpectedly pregnant. Their life situation is such that they can deal with and be excited about such news. Needed adjustments are made with minimal difficulty. For other women, this is not the case and they experience a crisis.

The purpose of intervention with an unplanned pregnancy is to help the woman review alternatives, choose one, and then act on that choice. Before the alternatives can be reviewed, the date of the last menstrual period and probable length of gestation must be determined. If the woman is more than twenty-four weeks pregnant, she must continue the pregnancy. If fewer than twenty-four weeks have elapsed, the alternatives available to the women include:

- Continue the pregnancy and relinquish the baby for adoption.
- Continue the pregnancy and keep the baby.
- Obtain an abortion. This will be done by suction D&C if less than sixteen to seventeen weeks gestation, although under twelve weeks is preferable. Saline abortion is recommended when gestation is between seventeen and twenty-four weeks.

Information which must be discussed during the decision-making process includes religious and personal beliefs about pregnancy and abortion, other current factors in the woman's life situation (age, work, school), economic resources, involvement and wishes of the partner, and available economic and emotional support from family and friends.

The woman must be allowed to make her own choice without pressure from the intervenor. However, she must be assisted in considering the implications of each choice as, of course, each choice presents pro and con arguments. If abortion is a potential choice, she must be informed of her time limitations and helped to make a final decision as quickly as possible.

Once the initial choice regarding pregnancy or abortion is made, referral is in order. If the woman wishes to continue the pregnancy, prenatal care from an obstetrician or midwife will be necessary. If the woman chooses abortion, she will need help in choosing a reputable clinic or physician to provide the health care which is desired and needed.

In either case, sensitive and caring attitudes on the part of physicians, nurses, and other staff members are of invaluable help to the woman. The final decision must remain with the woman. After careful consideration of all of the alternatives, she must know on a long-term basis that *her* choice was best for this situation at this time. The health care provider's role is to give support while that decision is being made. Hopefully, through follow-up and evaluation, the woman will be taught new coping mechanisms and be able to avoid a repeat of this crisis.

If the woman elects to continue her pregnancy and keep the baby, she may or may not need additional referrals (such as to social services) depending on available help and support from her partner, family, and friends. If adoption is chosen, it may be arranged through reputable adoption agencies and social services. Many times an obstetrician will assist with this referral. The woman may need continued emotional support during the pregnancy. Sources of this support in the form of friends, family, or professional help should be identified and utilized.

If the woman elects abortion, she should be told what to expect. This should include cost, laboratory tests, a description of the procedure (see chapter 24) and length of time she should expect to be at the clinic or hospital. She should know what to expect both emotionally and physically following the abortion. After the procedure, further counseling and review of feelings are in order. A review of contraception and/or perhaps a change of method is also needed at this time.

A woman who finds that she is unexpectedly pregnant must make many crucial decisions. These decisions are, at best, extremely difficult. If the situation is compounded by a developmental crisis, it is even more difficult to resolve. It is a rare woman (at any age) who will treat these decisions casually. She often feels threatened, guilty, angry, conflicted, and alone. Even though she may have the support of her partner, the woman is still the one responsible for the final decision. She, in particular, must deal with the repercussions whether she decides to carry the pregnancy or have the abortion.

Nurses are in a unique position to help women define these assorted feelings, review the alternatives, and choose a plan of action. They can provide referrals for safe, needed medical care. Finally, education and sensitive guidance from nurses may help women in this situation to grow a great deal as a result of this crisis.

Rape

For most women, rape will precipitate a crisis. Many times women who have been raped will immediately approach the health care system for help, especially if physical trauma is involved. However, some women will suppress the event and not speak of it for a long period of time. Whether the rape occurred recently or some time in the past, these women need a great deal of sensitivity, understanding and caring.

Because laws vary from one locale to another, history and examination procedures must be checked against local requirements. In any case there are some basic procedures which must be done.

A woman who has been raped must be examined to insure that vaginal and/or anal tissues are intact. Cultures from these areas and the throat (depending upon the areas of attack) must be done for gonorrhea. If the woman had no contraceptive protection (IUD or oral contraceptives), she may wish to take DES or similar drugs to protect against pregnancy.

Although she may not be able to decide at the moment, the woman may wish to prosecute later. In that eventuality, evidence of the rape will be needed. Details of any physical injuries or bruising must be carefully described and recorded. Specimens of semen and pubic hair from the offender will become important evidence.

Although a pelvic examination must be done as soon as possible following the rape, this may be an emotionally difficult procedure for the woman to submit to at this time. The lithotomy position and/or a male examiner may cause the woman to reexperience the fear and vulnerability which she felt during the rape. She needs to understand the importance of this examination to her, and be given help to differentiate the procedure from the rape. Allow her time and do not force her to do anything. Wait until she is ready. Above all, the nurse should *stay with her.*

The initial psychological reaction to rape may be of hysteria, shock, denial, guilt, fear, or disgust. Often a woman will begin to review what she "did" or "could have done." She may even blame herself. Although she has been taught to assume a passive role in a male-female dyad, she may feel guilty because she did not "fight" [3]. Friends and family may be of little help and, in their own shock, may even reinforce these ideas.

Many women who have been raped assumed at the time that they would also be killed. The fear, lack of control of the situation, intrusion into their most private self, disregard of their humanness, and a feeling of total vulnerability is a very difficult combination of feelings with which to deal. For many women, these feelings will persist for an extended length of time [1, 3].

Crisis intervention involves helping the raped woman to deal with both her physical and legal needs as well as her psychological trauma. Some important points include:

• Stay with the woman at all times including during the examinations and until she feels that she wants or can handle some time alone. If police are involved, stay with her during the questioning.

• As stated before, do not force her to do anything. Wait until she is ready for examinations or calls to friends or family members.

• Help her with decisions by giving clear explanations and showing understanding of her reactions.

• Assure her that her responses are normal. Tell her that her actions during the rape had to do with self-preservation and survival.

• Help the woman begin to identify a support network that she can call upon.

• Make calls for her when she is ready if that is her preference.

• Assure her that she is safe.

- Establish a plan with her for somewhere to stay or someone to stay with for a few days if she lives alone. Many women are afraid that their attacker will find them and kill them.
- Be available to the woman so that she can continue to work through her feelings and fears until the crisis is resolved and she is able to function again.
- Advise her to avoid making sudden, important decisions during this time. For example many women will break off a relationship with a boyfriend, fearing he will not "want" her now. She may be afraid to talk with him about the rape. Should a boyfriend or husband react with anger or rejection, the woman will need additional support to deal with this. Often the man's reaction is temporary and represents his inability to deal with the crisis. If at all possible, involve a partner in the intervention process as soon as the woman will allow it. See that support is provided for him as he begins to work through his feelings.
- The nurse who becomes involved but feels uncomfortable handling such a situation should stay involved only until an appropriate referral which will insure sensitive, caring help for the woman can be made. DO NOT ABANDON HER! Many communities have rape crisis centers, some law enforcement agencies provide excellent rape-crisis counseling and support, and many women's organizations will provide immediate response and help.

As with any other type of crisis, the aim is to help the women return, at the least, to her precrisis level of functioning. If the woman had difficulties with sexuality prior to the rape, this may be an even more severe crisis episode for her. It may also be that effective intervention and problem-solving will help her find a way to deal with her other difficulties as she resolves this crisis.

REFERENCES

1. Aguilera DC, Messick JM: Crisis Intervention Theory and Methodology, 2nd ed. St. Louis, C.V. Mosby, 1974
2. Brownmiller S: Against Our Will: Men, Women, and Rape. New York, Simon and Schuster, 1975
3. Burgess AW, Holmstrom LL: Rape: Crisis and Recovery. Bowie, MD, Robert J. Brady Co., 1979
4. Cain A: Crisis theory and intervention, Mississippi RN, November 1973
5. Caplan G: Principles of Preventive Psychiatry. New York, Basic Books, 1964
6. Ewing CP: Crisis Intervention as Psychotherapy. New York, Oxford University Press, 1978
7. King JM: The initial interview: Basis for assessment in crisis intervention. Perspectives in Psychiatric Care, Vol. 9, 1971
8. Selye H: The Stress of Life, 2nd ed. New York, McGraw-Hill, 1976

22

Sexual Function

KATHRYN J. HENDERSON AND GAIL M. WOODALL

In the United States there is an overwhelming awareness of and preoccupation with sexuality. It is evident in our advertising, our movies, books, and popular music. Educational systems from elementary schools through college levels offer courses on sex and family life. Many churches offer sexuality seminars and marriage enrichment workshops. Books on the subject range from solid research on sexual response and sexual dysfunctions to do-it-yourself manuals on how to overcome your own and others' sexual inhibitions. *Playboy, Penthouse, Playgirl,* and similar publications proclaim the pleasure of the sensual.

This is quite remarkable when one considers that as recently as 1948 Alfred Kinsey shocked and outraged a large proportion of the American people with the publication of his now classic work, *Sexual Behavior in the Human Male.* The outrage was compounded in 1953 when *Sexual Behavior in the Human Female* made its appearance. Although many proclaimed such interest in sexual behavior to be immoral and the subject unfit to be considered for serious research, his books were apparently widely read—perhaps by some who protested most loudly. In 1966, almost twenty years after Kinsey's publication, William H. Masters and Virginia E. Johnson published their book, *Human Sexual Response.* In it, they reported the results of many years of scientific study which demonstrated four physiological phases which comprise male and female sexual response cycles. They had succeeded in placing the study of human sexual behavior and physiology on a firm scientific basis, but they too were criticized.

Much of the criticism of their work was generated from the concern that they had reduced a heretofore emotional act of love to scientific analysis. Their critics proclaimed that study of the various parts of the sexual response cycle would cause people to become preoccupied with what was happening to individual body parts instead of being "caught up" in the passion and love of the total act. One wonders about the rationality of this deduction.

An understanding of the physiology of respiration does not cause us to concentrate on oxygen and carbon dioxide exchange with each breath. An understanding of the action of the urinary sphincters does not result in analyzing each set of muscle responses during urination. Similarly, an understanding of the various stages of the sexual response cycle does not prevent lovemaking from being done joyfully and with abandonment.

The present climate of comfort with sexuality and freedom of sexual expression is a welcome change from the repressiveness of the past hundreds of years.

However, religious, cultural, and family values do not always keep pace with social change. Thus, we have men and women who are conflicted and being pulled in one direction by traditional teachings of church, family, and community and in another direction by the "new sexual freedom."

Anxieties concerning sex and sexual functioning are prevalent. According to Kaplan, anxiety is the common denominator in the etiology of sexual dysfunction [4]. Societal pressure to be sexually aware, sexually free and sexually competent often contrasts sharply with traditional values and the traditionally female passive role. In addition, ignorance about sexual matters often leads to fear, misunderstanding, and poor sexual functioning. Although misconceptions and myths regarding sex are disappearing, they are still present.

As more was discovered about the physiological aspects of sexual intercourse, its biphasic nature became apparent. In other words, the sexual response does not comprise a single entity but rather consists of two distinct components. The first is a genital vasoconstrictive reaction which produces erection in the male and vaginal lubrication and genital swelling in the female. The second component is reflex muscular contractions which constitute orgasm in both male and female. A third phase has been described as the desire phase. This is an extragenital phase and can be thought of as a sexual appetite or drive. At present, it is unclear to what degree desire is biological or instinctual and to what degree it is a learned response. However, it does appear that desire (libido) is a complex interaction of the two. Kaplan refers to the triphasic concept of human sexuality as being comprised of desire, excitement, and orgasm [5].

Having identified these phases it became apparent that problems could exist in any one of them or in a combination of two or more phases. Prior to defining the phases, male dysfunctions were lumped together under the catch-all phrase "impotence." Female dysfunctions were referred to as frigidity. Both of these terms are extremely negative.

Dysfunctions can now be classified according to the phase in which they occur. For example, disorders of the desire phase, disorders of arousal (failure to achieve erection in the male or lubrication-swelling in the female) and orgastic disorders (premature or retarded ejaculation in the male or lack of orgasm in the female). Sex therapy can be more specifically directed and adjusted to fit the problem as well as its level of severity.

FEMALE SEXUAL RESPONSE CYCLE

Masters and Johnson have divided the sexual response cycle in both males and females into four stages. Certain physiologic events have been observed in both genital and extragenital locations. These events follow a natural progression from one stage to another but will vary in duration and intensity from one individual to another. They will vary according to circumstances such as partner, physical environment, mood, and health to mention only a few. Each stage can be interrupted, in which case progression to the next stage will not occur [8]. The physiologic response is the same for both heterosexual and homosexual individuals.

Excitement Phase

The excitement phase can be initiated by sight, sound, touch, or smell of a sexual stimulus. It can sometimes be initiated by thought or fantasy alone. The physiologic response is caused by vasoconstriction. Vaginal lubrication is the first sign. This fluid is a transudate and results from the congestion of the blood vessels supplying the vaginal wall. Contrary to previous thoughts, the Bartholin and cervical glands play an insignificant part in this phenomenon.

The second vaginal characteristic of this phase is the ballooning or tenting phenomenon. The inner two-thirds of the vagina distends and the uterus rises up into the false pelvis resulting in expansion of the upper vagina. There is also a darkening of vaginal color caused by the vasocongestion.

Organs other than the vagina also exhibit changes during this phase. The shaft of the clitoris increases in diameter. There is also an increase in size of the labia minora while the labia majora tend to flatten and retract from the mid-line. The nipples of the breast become erect and breast size generally increases. The effects of vasocongestion can also be seen superficially in the form of a "sex flush." This resembles a measles rash, and is most prominent on the chest. Finally, there is an overall increase in muscle tension.

Plateau Phase

The plateau phase is actually a continuation and intensification of the excitement phase. The walls of the lower one-third of the vagina now become so engorged with blood that the canal actually constricts. At the same time, the labia minora further increase in size. These two events form a tension reaction which Masters and Johnson have termed the "orgasmic platform." In addition to a size increase, the labia minora undergo further color changes.

The shaft and glans of the clitoris retracts from its normally exposed position to become completely covered by the clitoral hood. It is still capable of being stimulated, but stimulation is now indirect through the clitoral hood.

The breasts become further engorged and the sex flush may spread to the abdomen, thighs, and back. Muscle tension also increases and heart rate and blood pressure increase.

Orgasmic Phase

The subjective experience of orgasm is extremely variable from woman to woman. Some women describe a mild, tickling sensation in the pelvic area that is only briefly felt. Others describe an intense, sometimes almost pleasurably unbearable throbbing. Between these two extremes an almost infinite variety of sensations are reported.

The physiological process starts with strong muscular contractions in the "orgasmic platform." These contractions are rhythmic and occur at 0.8 second intervals. The number of contractions range from three to fifteen and vary from woman to woman or from one orgastic experience to another. The inner two-thirds of the vagina does not undergo changes at this time, but uterine contractions occur. The heart and respiratory rate reach a peak during orgasm. Changes in sex flush, breast size, labia, and clitoris do not occur.

One of the most important results of this research has been that it finally ended the controversy over the superiority of the vaginal versus the clitoral orgasm. We now know that all female orgasms consist of a reflex series of involuntary rhythmic contractions of the structures comprising the orgasmic platform. This reflex is triggered by stimulation of the clitoris which acts both as a receiver and transformer of sexual stimuli [8]. The quality of an orgasm from clitoral stimulation alone does not differ from one which results from vaginal stimulation. In fact, penile thrusting brings about orgasm by exerting indirect pressure and traction on the clitoris. Many women find vaginal stimulation alone is seldom enough to cause orgasmic release. Freud described such women as infantile and sexually immature having failed to transfer their eroticism from the clitoris to the vagina. We now know from Masters and Johnson's research that clitoral stimulation to bring about orgasm is not only normal but necessary [8].

Resolution Phase

Following orgasm there is a gradual return to the pre-excitement state. The vasocongestion of the outer third of the vagina disperses rapidly. The inner two-thirds of the vagina shrinks to its unexpanded state and the uterus descends back into the true pelvis. The labia minora change back to their normal color and size and the labia majora resume their position close to the midline. The clitoris resumes its normal position protruding from the clitoral hood. Breast size returns to normal and the sex flush disappears. Heart rate, blood pressure, and muscle tension rapidly return to normal.

SEXUAL DYSFUNCTION

In order for the phases of the sexual response cycle to occur and progress smoothly from excitement to orgasm the genital organs must be intact and physiologically able to respond. General health status must be such that the neurological and endocrine systems can interact to bring about sexual release. In addition an individual must be mentally receptive to sexual stimuli and free from psychological impediments to good sexual functioning.

Sexual problems can have biological or psychological determinants. Estimates of sexual dysfunctions with primarily biological components vary from 10–20 percent [4]. In addition many biologically-caused dysfunctions will produce psychological complications. For example, a woman may develop painful intercourse as a result of a poorly repaired episiotomy. After successive painful, unpleasant experiences, she may well begin to develop a dislike or fear of intercourse. This may cause problems in her sexual response long after the physical problem is resolved.

Some biological causes of sexual dysfunction include illness, depression, gynecological problems such as a septate vagina, injuries related to childbirth or resulting from gynecological surgery, and drugs. There are a wide range of drugs which may alter sexual response including sedatives, hormones (such as estrogen and progestins), amphetamines, antihypertensives, and antidepressants. Alcohol is one of the most widely used drugs which may adversely affect sexual functioning.

There has been disagreement over the years regarding psychological determinants of sexual dysfunctions. The psychoanalytic theory holds that they are rooted in the unconscious and arise from conflicts derived from childhood experiences. These may be an unresolved Oedipal conflict, penis envy, or deep seated guilt arising from verbal or nonverbal expression of negative attitudes about sex by the child's parents or "significant others."

Family and marital therapists focus on interpersonal conflicts and destructive behavior as the etiological factors of sexual dysfunction. Such things as power struggles between partners, lack of trust, and lack of communication are blamed.

Behavior therapists have demonstrated that milder anxieties and more immediate concerns can impair sexual functioning. Learned anxieties such as performance fears, overconcern with performance, and simple lack of sound sex information have been implicated.

Kaplan believes that sexual dysfunctions are due to both remote and immediate causes. A woman with an inability to experience orgasm may have a pervasive sense of guilt and shame instilled by her parents, a disabling inability to allow herself to experience pleasure, or a severe problem in her relationship with her partners. On the other hand it may be that she is simply trying too hard to achieve orgasm, "spectatoring" or watching herself, or trying so hard to please her partner that she is unable to experience the abandonment necessary to allow the reflex of orgasm to happen.

Treatment: The first step in any treatment approach is assessment. It is important to know which phase of sexual response is disrupted. There is often an overlap but one or more phases may be intact. For example, treatment of disorders of the desire phase differs from treatment of disorders of orgasm.

A sexual problem history should include information about when the problem began, under what circumstances it occurs, with whom it occurs, and if it occurs with masturbation. Information regarding sexual lifestyle, marital status, type of job, number of children, and living arrangements may help in defining the problem.

A general health survey is also important since debilitating diseases may interfere with sexual function. Since drugs can interfere with sexual desire, excitement, or orgasm, it is important to know if the person is on any therapeutic drug regimen or is an alcohol or drug abuser.

Injuries related to childbirth, or incisions and scarring from gynecological surgery may cause pain which in turn leads to sexual problems. A thorough pelvic examination should be part of the initial assessment of a woman with a sexual problem. Although physiologic causes of sexual dysfunction are far less common than psychologic causes, they must be ruled out.

Once a biologic cause for dysfunction has been eliminated, psychologic therapy can be started. This type of therapy grew out of Masters and Johnson's work and is widely and successfully practiced today. Approximately 80 percent of sexually dysfunctional individuals can be relieved of their symptoms in this manner [4].

A well qualified sex therapist will be alert to signs of deeper disturbance, either intrapsychic or interpersonal, that may impede progress. Many, but not all programs use co-therapists of different gender. All programs prefer to have couples together in therapy, but if an individual does not currently have a partner, they will not be denied treatment. The basic goal of therapy is to increase sexual pleasure and awareness of sensations as well as to decrease fears or anxiety surrounding performance. This is accomplished by assigning sexual tasks or exercises.

Masters and Johnson begin the therapy with a period of orgastic abstinence i.e., coitus and orgasm are prohibited. During this time the couple engages in mutual stimulation of erotic areas, excluding the genitals, with the emphasis on giving and receiving pleasure. These non-demand, pleasuring exercises are referred to as "sensate focus." Later, genital stimulation is included but orgasm is still discouraged. The goal of these experiences is to heighten the couple's awareness of sensuous pleasure, free from demand.

When this goal has been achieved, exercises are prescribed which are designed to relieve symptoms for specific problems. Some examples of these will be given with the description of the female dysfunctions. Again, the goal is relief of the sexual symptom. If deeper problems exist which impede progress, they will need more intensive therapy.

In addition to specific suggestions such as sensate focus and prescribed sexual tasks, Annon describes a treatment model with four different levels. The first two levels can be used in relatively unstructured settings with minimal time and do not require formal sex therapy training. Basic therapist prerequisites should include a comfort with sexuality, an ability to listen, the ability to refrain from imposing one's own value system on the client and a willingness to say "I don't know." Annon's PLISSIT model contains the following elements [1]:

P = PERMISSION. Many times people need reassurance that they are normal and not perverted or deviated. They may be bothered by a concern that what they are doing is "wrong" or "abnormal." If they can be reassured that their behavior is normal they may be able to prevent a small problem from becoming significant.

Areas where permission to engage in certain activities can be helpful are masturbation, sexual thoughts, fantasies, and dreams. Receiving permission for normal feelings such as sexual arousal while nursing an infant or from horseback or bicycle riding can relieve guilt. Permission for having intercourse as frequently as desired or for practicing a variety of types of sexual stimulation may be needed. Permission may also be needed *not* to engage in certain behavior or feelings. Needless to say, permission giving must be done within the context of the professional's own value system.

LI = LIMITED INFORMATION. Providing factual information that is specifically related or limited to the client's sexual concern can be extremely effective as prevention or treatment of problems. Such information is especially helpful in dispelling myths. Many women are concerned because their genitals "do not look like the picture" and are relieved to learn that there is a great amount of variation. Concerns about the harmful effects of masturbation can be corrected by giving some factual information about the numbers of women who report masturbating. References such as the Kinsey report and the Hite report are useful resources [6,3]. Information regarding penis and vagina size can be very useful. Many women voice concern that their vagina is too small or too big to accommodate their partner's penis. The fact that the vagina is a potential space capable of great expansion and that an erect penis will vary little in size from one man to another can dispel or minimize her fear.

SS = SPECIFIC SUGGESTIONS. This level corresponds to the suggestions already described. (Sensate Focus Exercises.)

IT = INTENSIVE THERAPY. This level of treatment would generally be provided by psychiatrists or psychologists. Recognition of the need for referral is extremely important for successful outcome.

Sexual Dysfunctions Specific to the Female

General Sexual Dysfunction. A disorder of a general nature usually involves both a lack of desire (desire phase disorder) and a lack of arousal (excitement phase disorder). On an emotional level, the woman may exhibit feelings ranging from disinterest in sexual matters to revulsion which leads to avoidance of any sexual encounter. On a physiological level, there is usually very little vasocongestive response to sexual stimulation with little or no vaginal lubrication. Disorders of this type seem to be the most complex, the least understood, and the most difficult to treat successfully. Illness, depression, and drugs or alcohol abuse can result in general sexual dysfunction. Treatment of the underlying problem may result in improvement.

Behavioral treatment usually follows the format previously described beginning with orgastic abstinence and progressing to sensate focus, genital stimulation, and finally coitus. However, the lack of desire and deeper personal or interpersonal conflicts often interfere with progress and frequently result in avoidance of the prescribed tasks. Psychotherapy or couple counseling are usually helpful adjuncts in the treatment of women with a problem of this nature.

Orgasmic Dysfunction. Orgasmic difficulties are probably the most prevalent female sexual problem. They are also the most easily and successfully treated. A woman is considered to have primary orgasmic dysfunction if she has never experienced an orgasm. Secondary orgasmic dysfunction is the inability to achieve orgasm after a period of time without problems. This may be absolute (no orgasm under any circumstances) or situational (orgasm only with certain partners, only with masturbation, or only with oral stimulation, etc.).

Examples of the application of different levels of therapy may be useful. *Permission* may be given to such a woman "to be a sexual being," "to accept as well as to give pleasure," "to have an orgasm before or after her partner," "to show her partner what stimulation feels good and what does not."

Information can be given regarding the physiology of the orgastic response which will help her to understand the need for clitoral stimulation. An explanation can be given that by watching her own performance ("spectatoring") and "willing" an orgasm to occur she interferes with the reflex. It is similar to the difficulty experienced when trying to swallow on demand.

Specific suggestions might include the use of fantasy to break the "spectatoring" habit and to promote abandonment and enjoyment of the sensuous feelings. Successful treatment of orgastic problems often includes teaching a woman to masturbate to orgasm. This is initially done manually but often progresses to the use of a vibrator. Once a woman is able to achieve orgasm alone, the therapy moves to the achievement of orgasm with her partner. Again, the progression is from "sensate focus" to coitus using a non-demand approach.

In the absence of severe mental or physical illness or serious relationship problems, all women seem able to learn to respond sexually and to have orgasms. Using the methods described above, many women become orgasmic with coitus alone. However, a large number of women require more direct clitoral stimulation either by manual or oral means. It is quite important to help such couples realize that this does not mean that the woman is neurotic nor does it imply that she is sexually inadequate or that her partner has failed. Kaplan has speculated that perhaps failure to reach orgasm by any means but clitoral stimulation is within the bounds of normal female sexuality. [4].

Vaginismus: Vaginismus is the involuntary spasm of the muscles surrounding the introitis whenever an attempt is made to insert an object into the vagina. This is usually a conditioned response resulting from the association of pain or fear with attempts at penetration. The pain may be real or fantasized, physical or psychological. If early experiences with intercourse (or pelvic examination) were physically painful or psychologically traumatic, then subsequent attempts may be avoided or guarded against by vaginal spasm. Although vaginismus is frequently associated with a general sexual dysfunction or orgasmic disorders, some women report high levels of sexual interest, arousal, and even orgasm from clitoral stimulation.

Physical causes of pain may include a rigid or tight hymenal ring, painful hymenal tags, vaginitis, endometriosis or pelvic inflammatory disease. Psychologic causes include fear of pain, fear of pregnancy, guilt, and shame surrounding the sexual act, or sometimes early traumatic sexual experiences such as rape, incest, or sexual molestation.

Sex therapy is aimed at correcting the immediate cause of the disorder. More remote causes and interpersonal or intrapsychic conflicts are dealt with only as they interfere with therapy. Before proceeding with the therapy any physical cause of pain should be corrected. However, removing the cause of pain does not always correct the vaginismus since often a phobic response has developed.

Permission can be used in the initial interview with a woman with vaginismus. Permission can be given to "be sexual," "to enjoy intercourse" or "to communicate negative feelings to her partner."

Information giving is an extremely effective level of intervention in vaginismus. The pelvic examination done with the woman observing can be an effective tool for imparting this information. Information can also be used to reassure the woman that no harm or damage will occur when an object enters the vagina. Ignorance of her own genital anatomy is sometimes the basis for the fear of penetration. The partner's presence during the examination is often helpful in dispelling misconceptions which he or she may have.

Specific suggestions are given in an attempt to overcome a woman's fear of entry. Masters and Johnson's plan involves the insertion of graduated catheters or dilators into the vagina. The woman may begin with one that may be no larger than the string of a tampon. As each one is comfortably tolerated a slightly larger one is used. Intercourse is not attempted until a dilator the size of a penis can be introduced and retained for some time without discomfort or fear.

The woman is instructed to insert the dilators herself. This gives her control over the situation which helps to reduce anxiety. First attempts at intercourse are also controlled by the woman with insertion of the penis guided by her. Since some women may have a negative response to a device such as a dilator, some therapists prefer to instruct the woman to use her own or her partner's fingers to dilate the introitus.

At first only the tip of one finger will be inserted. When that task can be accomplished she progresses to full insertion of the finger and then proceeds to two. When two fingers can be comfortably inserted, coitus can be attempted. When discomfort and anxiety are experienced the woman is encouraged to "stay with it." This helps her face and overcome the problem rather than flee from it.

Excellent treatment results occur with this approach to sex therapy for vaginismus. Masters and Johnson have reported 100 percent cure rates without relapse in a series of patients treated with this method. It has also been successful when used by gynecologists.

The new approach to behavioral treatment of sexual problems certainly seems to offer "cures" that are as good or sometimes better than psychotherapy and couple counseling. It cannot completely overcome all problems nor does it always work without the help of other disciplines. As with other areas of health care one can find unethical practices occurring. Couples with a sexual problem would be well advised to ask a trusted source for a referral to reputable sex therapists. They can then proceed to work through their problems knowing that improvement is a probable outcome.

REFERENCES

1. Anon JS: Behavioral Treatment of Sexual Problems: Volume 1, Brief Therapy. Honolulu, Enabling Systems, Inc., 1974
2. Barbach LG: For Yourself: The Fulfillment of Female Sexuality. Garden City, NY, Anchor Press/Doubleday, 1976
3. Hite S: The Hite Report. New York, Macmillan, 1976
4. Kaplan HS: The New Sex Therapy. New York, Brunner/Mazel, 1974
5. Kaplan HS: The New Sex Therapy, Volume II: Disorders of Sexual Desire. New York, Brunner/Mazel, 1979
6. Kinsey AC et al: Sexual Behavior in the Human Female. New York, Pocket Books, 1970
7. Kolodny R, Masters W, Johnson V: Textbook of Sexual Medicine. Boston, Little, Brown, 1976
8. Masters W, Johnson V: Human Sexual Response. Boston, Little, Brown, 1966
9. Pengelley ET: Sex and Human Life, 2nd ed. Reading, MA, Addison-Wesley, 1978

Section VII

APPROACHES TO CARE

23

The Gynecologic Examination: Breast and Pelvic

Amazingly, many women still think that pelvic examinations are unnecessary unless they are ill, about to be married, need a contraceptive method, or are pregnant. From infancy on, we are accustomed to the ritual of the yearly physical check-up and routine dental examination. Women who are quite conscientious when it comes to other routine preventive health care tend to put off having their pelvic exams. The reasons for this are numerous and not always fully apparent.

Parents often equate their daughter's need for a pelvic exam with her growing up and becoming sexually active. Therefore, her exam may be delayed because they discourage or prohibit it. Women postpone their own first pelvics because of feelings of fear and embarrassment. For some women, religious and cultural reasons are given for delaying a pelvic exam. All too often a pelvic is requested as an unavoidable means to an end, such as obtaining a contraceptive method or treatment of vaginitis.

Ideally, a routine pelvic examination is a preventive health measure. It is best started about the time of puberty, but certainly no later than twenty years of age. Thereafter a repeat pelvic exam on a yearly basis is advisable. It should be done whether or not a woman is sexually active, but if intercourse begins earlier than puberty, so should the annual pelvic exam. Postponing an exam until there is an urgent need prevents the relaxed atmosphere desired for a positive learning experience.

The American Cancer Society announced new recommendations regarding routine cervical–vaginal cytology in March 1980. Following two normal Pap smears taken at a one year interval, they feel subsequent smears may be done every three years unless the woman is at high risk for developing cervical cancer. Their recommendations differ from those of the American College of Obstetricians and Gynecologists in the frequency with which an asymptomatic woman should be examined. The latter group still advocates yearly Pap smears. Controversy over these conflicting positions does exist and it may take health care providers some time to evaluate the merits of the two positions in their own practices.

Women have many and varied feelings surrounding the procedure which they are about to experience. If it is their first pelvic exam there is fear of the unknown. If they have had previous pelvics which have been uncomfortable, the fear is well founded. Most women know very little about their bodies and in particular about their pelvic anatomy. It is little wonder then that they are fearful of what is going to be done and *how* it will be done.

Embarrassment is also a common feeling. From early childhood on, women are overtly as well as subtly discouraged from touching or looking at their own or others' nude bodies. Therefore it is uncomfortable, and sometimes very threatening, to be required to expose oneself. When there is little preparation of the woman for the experience, her feelings of fear and embarrassment may be heightened.

A woman may bring with her worry about a physical symptom. She may just carry the concern "Am I normal?" She may want to discuss sexuality and not know how to bring it up. On the other hand, she may come with a positive attitude, but be confused about how to ask her questions or communicate her needs. In particular, lesbians may be uncomfortable discussing their sexual concerns.

A nurse can have a positive influence on the varied feelings that women bring with them to the exam. She can use her knowledge, attitude and actions as tools to effect change. For this reason the following chapter has two objectives. First, it can serve as a guide to the nurse who is asked for information. Second, some suggestions will be offered for the nurse who may be assisting with or performing the exam. Hopefully this will maximize the potential for the gynecologic exam to be a positive, relaxed, learning experience.

Routine gynecologic exams vary according to local practices, individual clinician, and office or laboratory facilities. However, certain elements should always be included to some extent. These are preliminary education, laboratory tests, history taking, the exam itself, and whatever follow-up is indicated.

A woman should be told that if she inserts anything of a chemical nature into the vagina twenty-four hours prior to her examination, it may interfere with test results. This includes douching, medication, and contraceptive creams and foams. Intercourse is not precluded. However, if a barrier method necessitating spermicidal agents is used for contraception, abstinence would be advisable. It is best to try to avoid scheduling an examination during a menstrual period. However, if her period does begin a woman should check with her clinician before cancelling an appointment.

Preliminary laboratory tests often include a routine urinalysis, hemoglobin or hematocrit. Sometimes a Rubella titer as well as a routine VDRL are done. Blood pressure and weight are also included.

A gynecologic history will be taken. It is well if a woman comes prepared with important information such as age of menarche, date of last menstrual period (and sometimes the previous menstrual period), intervals between periods, length and nature of flow, and presence and nature of pain with periods. She will also be asked questions regarding contraception including types of methods previously used, problems, if any, and desire for initiation or continuation of a method. Dates and outcomes of any pregnancies will be asked.

Along with collecting gynecologic information, the health care provider will ask for additional history. When taking a sexual history, it is helpful to determine whether the woman is heterosexual, bisexual, or homosexual. Frequency of sexual activity and any associated pain or problems are important pieces of information. Personal and family history of any diseases such as diabetes, hypertension, heart disease, or epilepsy are also important information needed to plan an individual's health care. In recent years we have also become aware of the need to document in-utero exposure to diethylstilbesterol (DES). If a woman knows in advance that these questions will be asked it will help her feel more relaxed.

THE BREAST EXAM

Hopefully, each woman will be asked if she knows and does breast self examination (BSE). The importance of early detection in the outcome of breast cancer has been well documented. Although there are variations in technique for doing this, it is helpful and less confusing to a woman if she is taught basic principles of BSE. These can then be reinforced by giving her detailed printed instructions to take home. Excellent patient education brochures are available [1,4,7].

As the examiner checks the breasts the woman can be reminded of the following (See Figure 23-1):
- Check breasts monthly AFTER a menstrual period when the breast tissue is less irregular and less confusing to feel.
- If no longer menstruating, or if periods occur only a few times a year, pick a specific date to do this exam each month.
- Inspect the breasts in front of a mirror for changes in skin color, texture, or any dimpling or puckering.
- Palpate the breasts. This can be done in the shower, but should also be done lying down with a hand under the head on the side being checked. This spreads the breast tissue out and makes a lump more apparent.
- Be methodical. Do not be concerned with trying to remember exact technique. Follow a plan so no area of the breast is missed.
- Feel with the balls (not tips) of the fingers.
- Include the nipple in the exam. Squeeze it *gently* to check for discharge.
- Feel carefully in the axillary areas.
- Regular examinations increase skills enhancing the likelihood of early recognition of changes.
- Remember! 80 percent of lumps are benign [7]. Report any change from normal to your physician.

INSPECTION OF THE EXTERNAL GENITALIA

The examiner will begin by observing such things as amount and distribution of pubic hair, appearance of labia majora, labia minora, clitoris, and vaginal and urethral orifices. The appearance of the external genitalia varies as much from one woman to another as does facial appearance. An experienced examiner, however, will be able to detect any obvious departure from the norm. This may be due to congenital defect, infection, or injury.

INSPECTION OF VAGINA AND CERVIX

In explaining the purpose of the speculum exam to a woman, it is helpful to describe the vagina as a *potential* space with the walls normally lying against one another. The vaginal speculum is an instrument which enables the examiner to separate the vaginal walls and thereby inspect the vagina and cervix. The vagina is capable of tremendous expansion, and within reason, accommodates whatever is placed within it. This may range from a regular tampon to a full term infant.

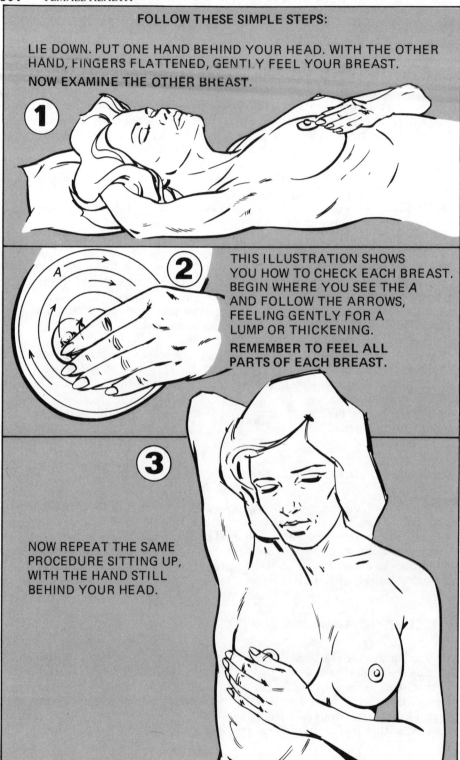

FOLLOW THESE SIMPLE STEPS:

LIE DOWN. PUT ONE HAND BEHIND YOUR HEAD. WITH THE OTHER HAND, FINGERS FLATTENED, GENTLY FEEL YOUR BREAST.

NOW EXAMINE THE OTHER BREAST.

1

2

THIS ILLUSTRATION SHOWS YOU HOW TO CHECK EACH BREAST. BEGIN WHERE YOU SEE THE *A* AND FOLLOW THE ARROWS, FEELING GENTLY FOR A LUMP OR THICKENING.

REMEMBER TO FEEL ALL PARTS OF EACH BREAST.

3

NOW REPEAT THE SAME PROCEDURE SITTING UP, WITH THE HAND STILL BEHIND YOUR HEAD.

Figure 23-1.   Steps to follow when doing a monthly breast self examination.

The vaginal opening with its hymenal ring of tissue may not be quite as accommodating as the vagina in a woman who has never had intercourse. However, if a woman is accustomed to using tampons, the hymen has undoubtedly been stretched sufficiently to allow comfortable entry of the speculum. (Since this instrument comes in different sizes there is usually no problem.) If the vaginal introitus is too tight to admit one finger, it is unlikely that the examination can proceed until that has been changed. Methods for dealing with this situation will be discussed under "Special Considerations." (See Figure 23-2.)

Inserting the speculum obliquely avoids undue pressure on the anterior vaginal wall and prevents painful pressure on the urethra. Advise the woman to breathe normally and try to relax the abdominal and perineal muscles. These methods will help her be more comfortable. Terms most often used by women to describe what is felt during this part of the examination are "stretching" and "pressure" rather than "pain." See Figure 23-3.

With the speculum inserted and opened, the examiner will inspect the vaginal walls and cervix. Color, texture, presence of lesions or irregular contours should be noted. The amount, color, consistency, and odor of any discharge present are also important observations. Before removing the speculum, some routine laboratory tests will be done. These include the Pap smear and gonorrhea culture.

Pap Smear

Dr. Papanicolaou would be amazed to know how frequently used the term "Pap test" or "Pap smear" has become. Even women who do not have any idea of

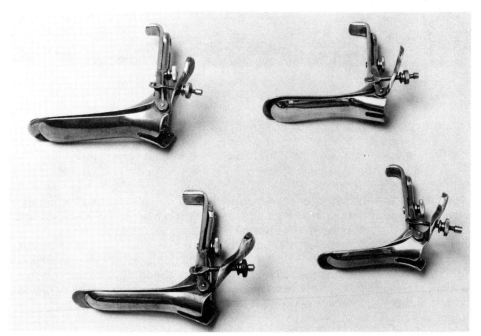

Figure 23-2.   Various sizes of vaginal speculums.

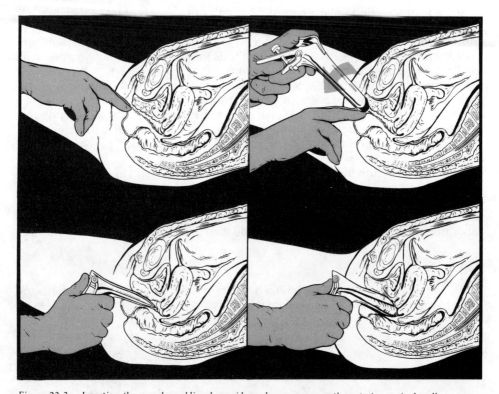

Figure 23-3.   Inserting the speculum obliquely avoids undue pressure on the anterior vaginal wall.

what this test is, know that it is important for them to have it done on a regular basis. The term has almost become synonymous with "cervical cancer test." This is not entirely accurate, since the test can be used in many other ways.

It is true that the Pap smear is primarily used to detect malignant or pre-malignant changes in the cells of the cervix. However, it can also be used to determine changes in cells from sites elsewhere in the body such as evaluation of breast secretions. In addition to screening for malignancy it can detect inflammatory cell changes and the presence of viral inclusion bodies such as might be seen with herpes. When there is concern about whether the vaginal tissue is receiving adequate estrogen stimulation, the pathologist will describe the cell maturation.

The technique for doing the Pap smear varies from one clinician or institution to another. It is sometimes partly determined by guidelines given by the particular laboratory that will be reading the slides. Since there is no "one best" way some general descriptions follow.

Cervical and endocervical cells can be obtained by aspirating a small amount of cervical mucus with a bulb syringe and then transferring this material to a slide.

Another method is to insert a cotton tipped swab into the endocervical canal and/ or rotate a spatula on the surface of the cervix. The cells are then spread thinly onto a slide. It is important that the slides be sprayed with, or dipped into, a fixative solution *immediately* as drying distorts the cells and results in inaccurate readings. Additional points of concern are that the slides be accurately labeled and carefully packaged for transporting to the pathologist.

Although laboratories vary somewhat in the terminology employed in reporting Pap smear results, the following guideline can be used as an example.

Class I—Negative.

Class II—Atypical cells which are benign; not suspicious.

     IIA—mild cellular atypia.

     IIB—moderate to severe atypia.

Class III—Atypical cells with dysplasia noted; inconclusive for malignancy.

Class IV—Suspicious for malignancy.

Class V—Definite malignant cells noted.

A Class II Pap smear may occur as a result of a vaginal or cervical infection producing inflammatory cells which appear as atypical. Many physicians recommend treatment of the infection followed by a repeat Pap smear in four to six weeks. (For details of vaginal and cervical infections, see chapter 16). When the repeat smear is not Class I or when a Class III, IV, or V is reported, colposcopy and biopsy are recommended to determine treatment. See Figure 23-4.

Since cervical cancer is a slowly developing disease, a yearly Pap smear is usually considered adequate. More frequent screening may be necessary in women at high risk. There may be some difference of opinion among health care providers as to what constitutes "high risk." Some place women over forty and those on oral contraceptives in this category and others do not. The most important point for nurses to emphasize is that widespread use of this important health screening test has contributed to the decline of deaths from cervical cancer over the past forty years [5].

Gonorrhea Culture

Unfortunately, the gonorrhea culture is not done as routinely as the Pap smear. Most clinics that serve a high risk population do gonorrhea cultures routinely each time a speculum is inserted. However, in many private practices this is not generally done. Unfortunately, a woman who thinks she may have been exposed is then put in the awkward position of having to request a gonorrhea culture. Since many women with gonorrhea are asymptomatic in the early stages, a routine culture can be an important means of reducing both the spread and morbidity of the disease.

The test is done by inserting a sterile Q-tip into the endocervical canal. It should be left in place a full thirty seconds to ensure proper absorption of the mucus. The material is then streaked onto a chocolate agar medium.

Since the gonococcus cannot grow in the presence of oxygen, the plates are incubated in CO_2 for forty-eight to seventy-two hours. An alternate procedure uses "transgrow" bottles. These small bottles contain chocolate agar and CO_2. They are usually available through state health departments.

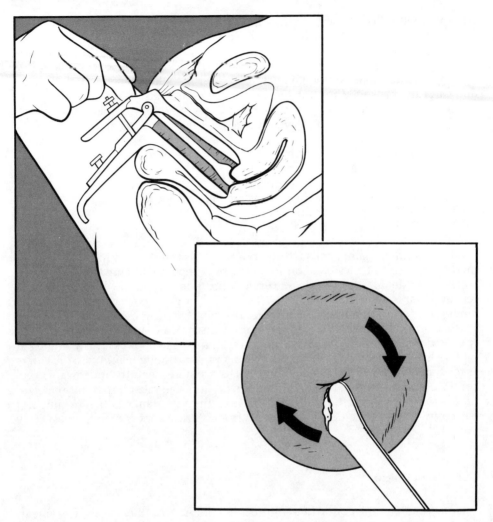

Figure 23-4. Spatulas are shaped in such a way that both exo- and endocervical cells are obtained.

THE BIMANUAL EXAMINATION

Following removal of the speculum, the examiner will proceed to the part of the examination that utilizes palpation. Each step should be explained to the woman before proceeding. This will ensure her comfort and an accurate exam.

The posterior aspects of the labia majora are palpated between the thumb and index finger at four and eight o'clock positions. Swelling or tenderness in these areas may indicate a Bartholin's duct cyst or abcess. The index finger is gently but firmly drawn along the anterior wall of the vagina in the area of the urethral meatus. This "milking" action will elicit a discharge if there is an infection involving Skene's glands. While depressing the perineum and asking the patient to cough or bear down, the examiner notes any perineal relaxation, cystocele, rectocele or prolapse.

The examiner then inserts two fingers the full length of the vagina, palpating the walls and the cervix as the fingers are moved along. The uterus is elevated by pushing up with two fingers under the cervix. With the other hand pushing down

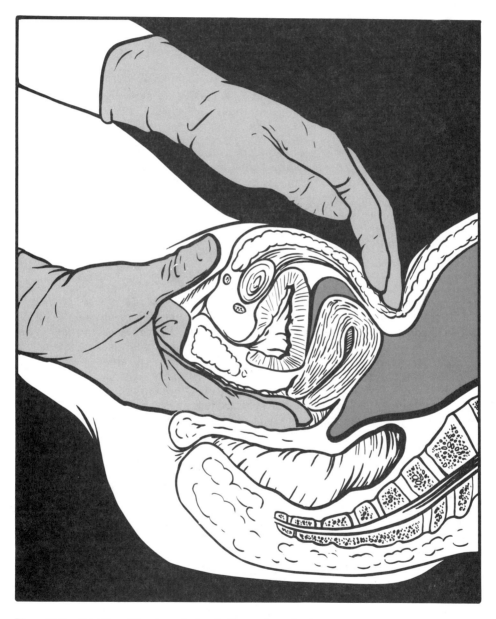

Figure 23-5.   Palpation of the uterus during the bimanual examination.

over the pelvic area, the examiner can palpate the uterus. Uterine position, size, and contours can be checked by this technique. This part of the exam usually causes a feeling of pressure and occasionally the desire to urinate. Since a full bladder can give misleading results and be uncomfortable, a woman should always urinate before her exam. See Figure 23-5.

Following palpation of the uterus, the ovaries are examined. They can be trapped between the two hands and checked for size and any unusual tenderness. Normally ovaries are about the size of unshelled almonds and regular in contour. They are sensitive when squeezed and women can be forewarned to expect a "twinge" of discomfort.

Finally, recto-vaginal examination may be performed. This involves palpation of the recto-vaginal septum and posterior aspect of the cervix and uterus through the rectal wall. It is usually done with one finger in the vagina and one in the rectum. In addition to uterine problems, any rectal swelling or tenderness can be noted.

Many examiners do not go beyond performing the technical aspects of the exam. This technical approach may create a barrier between women and the health care system and may reinforce the fear and embarrassment that they sometimes bring with them. The result may be that these women may avoid preventive health care in the future.

HUMANIZING THE EXPERIENCE

There are numerous ways to create an atmosphere which communicates a caring attitude. Cheerful color schemes, attractive pictures, and posters or mobiles on the ceiling over the examining table are a welcome relief from a stiff, sterile, medical environment. The use of oven potholder mitts or socks on the stirrups add to the patient's comfort, are easy to launder and frequently are ice-breakers which help relax a nervous woman. A small, screened off area for undressing avoids adding to her embarrassment.

The traditionally elaborate method of draping a woman for a GYN exam reinforces the feeling that it is shameful to be exposed. It effectively separates her from both the exam and the examiner. Giving the woman a sheet to place over her lap while waiting for the examiner is often adequate. Also the possibility that some women may feel comfortable without a drape sheet should be considered. If asked their preference, many women would trade the drape sheet for fuller involvement in the examination process. See Figure 23-6.

How the equipment is used can also communicate a concern for comfort. A warm speculum is particularly appreciated. Methods used to warm speculums may include putting a heating pad in the drawer where they are stored or holding them under warm running water. Allowing the woman to see and handle equipment whenever possible removes some of the fear.

One of the most worthwhile pieces of equipment to have available is a simple hand mirror. By holding the mirror herself, a woman can watch what is being done. She can even be helped to see inside the vagina and glimpse her own cervix if the examiner adjusts the light. If there is a deviation from normal it can be pointed out to her. On follow-up visits she can note any changes. This is an excel-

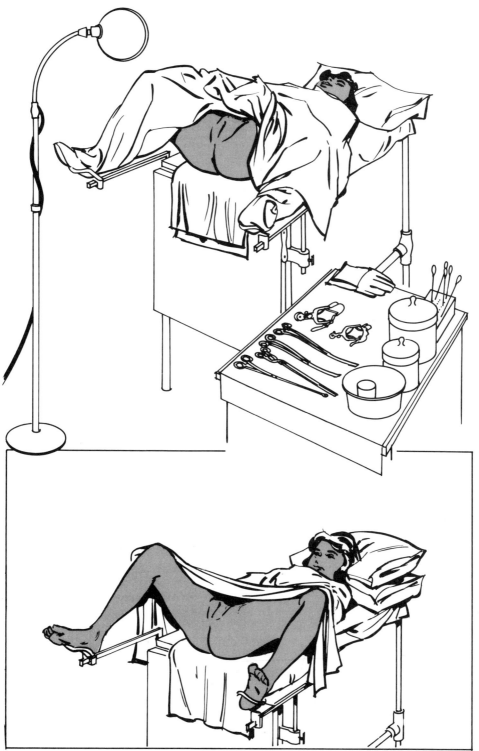

Figure 23-6. Traditional method of draping for a gynecologic examination versus the method encouraging client involvement.

lent way of teaching a woman about her body. Although pictures, charts, and models are helpful, they cannot replace first-hand knowledge of her own body.

These are only a few suggestions. They are all inexpensive and easy to incorporate into the exam. Expenditure of time is minimal and results are usually gratifying.

Remember, each woman has unique feelings and needs. If gynecologic health care is delivered in a thoughtful, caring, and considerate manner, the physical surroundings become secondary in importance. The ongoing education and the manner in which the exam is performed are of primary importance.

SPECIAL CONSIDERATIONS

The "Virginal" or Tight Hymen

The myth of the hymen is that it is a covering over the vaginal introitus. The woman retains her "virginity" until her hymen is broken or penetrated. Textbook pictures often misrepresent the appearance of the hymen and thus perpetuate the myth. Although the hymen may cover the introitus, usually it is nothing more than an elastic ring of tissue encircling the introitus. (See chapter 3.)

Widespread use of tampons has possibly been one of the reasons that pelvic exams and experiences with first intercourse are much easier physically now than thirty or forty years ago. Inserting tampons and removing them after they have been expanded by the menstrual flow probably helps stretch the hymen, allowing easier entrance of the speculum and a more comfortable first intercourse experience.

Some women have a relatively inelastic hymen. The extreme of this is the imperforate hymen. This is often undetected until menarche when medical complications arise from the inability of the menstrual blood to flow from the vagina. This situation needs surgical intervention. A hymen that will not allow entrance of a finger tip will also probably need surgical intervention before a pelvic exam can be done. However, these are rare occurrences.

A more frequently encountered problem is that of a woman arriving for her first pelvic exam having never had intercourse and having never used tampons. Sometimes in this case the hymen may be too tight to admit even the pediatric speculum. If it will admit the examiner's index finger, the woman can be taught how to stretch the hymen.

After first determining that the woman can touch her genital area without extreme anxiety, some helpful instructions include:

● Relaxing in a warm tub of water is a helpful place to do the following exercises. If a tub is unavailable, any private spot will do.

● One finger should be inserted into the vagina until slight discomfort or a burning sensation is felt. The woman will feel a rubber band-like constriction around her finger at that point.

● Using a circular motion, she should push against this "band" of tissue. Continue doing this for five to ten minutes.

● Continue this daily until one finger can be inserted completely.

● Repeat the same steps using two fingers.

By the end of two or three weeks, most women will have sufficiently stretched the opening to allow a relatively comfortable pelvic to be done. This is also extremely helpful in preparing such a woman for her first experience with intercourse. A routine pelvic exam is not an emergency. It can be postponed and the time better used for teaching.

Vaginismus

Vaginismus is the involuntary constricting of the perineal muscles to prevent entry of the penis during intercourse or the speculum during a pelvic exam. True vaginismus is usually a result of a negative sexual experience such as rape or incest. It can also stem from strict religious or moral sanctions against the enjoyment of sexual pleasure. For more detail, see chapter 22.

Proceeding with a pelvic exam under conditions that would cause pain is unjustified. A woman with true vaginismus should be referred to a well qualified and trusted counselor. Close communication between therapist, patient, and clinician will allow for re-scheduling of the pelvic exam when the woman has solved the underlying problems.

Occasionally the term vaginismus is used to describe the response of a woman who is too frightened to relax, and therefore difficult to examine. Educating her before the exam and explaining what is being done as the examiner proceeds often "cures" the problem, although this may take more than one visit. Establishing trust is usually more important than finishing the exam in one session.

The DES Exposed Woman

Much has been written in the past ten years about the effects of in-utero exposure to DES on the vaginal and cervical tissue. The purpose of this section will be to give the nurse some basic information to help her adequately answer the questions that a concerned woman may direct towards her.

What is DES?

Diethylstilbesterol is a synthetic estrogen preparation.

Why and when was it given?

It was administered to pregnant women who had a history of previous spontaneous abortions, women who were threatening to abort, or to diabetics. It was given to help maintain the pregnancy. This drug was used from the early 1940s through the late 1960s. Its peak use was in the 1940s and 1950s.

Were other drugs used for this purpose?

There were many DES type drugs used for this purpose. Exposure to any of them should be followed up in the same manner as DES exposure. A listing of these drugs can be found in an excellent pamphlet on DES published by the Department of Health, Education, and Welfare, *Questions and Answers About DES Exposure During Pregnancy and Before Birth*.[7]

What effect did use of these hormones have?

DES type drugs were found to be ineffective in prevention of miscarriage and so their use was discontinued. Since then it has been demonstrated that a small number of female offspring who were exposed to these drugs have developed an extremely rare form of vaginal cancer called clear-cell adenocarcinoma.

Although very few DES exposed women have developed this cancer, most will have some type of abnormality. The resulting abnormalities are usually not cancerous, but they need to be followed closely to detect any early signs of malignant changes. The most critical time of in-utero exposure is during the first five months of the pregnancy.

What type of examination and follow-up is recommended?

Beginning at menarche, a routine pelvic and Pap smear should be done. In addition to the routine tests, the examiner may also stain the vaginal and cervical tissue with an iodine solution. In the event of abnormal staining, a colposcopy and biopsies will be done. The frequency of follow-up examinations may vary from every three months to once a year. If no abnormalities are found on the initial visit, no special follow-up is necessary beyond the annual gynecologic exam.

Are there any symptoms or signs of DES exposure?

There may be abnormal bleeding patterns or an excessive amount of vaginal discharge. This results from misplaced glandular tissue on the cervix and in the vagina. The examiner may notice an abnormal appearance of the cervix. However, since many women will have no symptoms at all, it is important that all known or suspected DES exposed women be checked by the procedure which has been described.

REFERENCES

1. ACOG Technical Bulletin: The frequency with which a cervical vaginal cytology examination should be performed in gynecologic practice. No. 29, February 1975
2. American Cancer Society: Cancer of the Breast. 1972
3. American Cancer Society: How to Examine Your Breast. 1975
4. Kistner RW: Gynecology: Principles and Practice, 3rd ed. Chicago, Yearbook Medical Publishers, 1979
5. New York State Department of Health: DES, The wonder drug women should wonder about. Albany, NY, 1979
6. U.S. Department of Health, Education and Welfare, Center for Disease Control: Criteria and techniques for the diagnosis of gonorrhea. Atlanta, GA, 1974
7. U.S. Department of Health, Education and Welfare, DESAD Project, National Cancer Institute: Que ..ons and answers about DES exposure during pregnancy and before birth. DHEW Publication No. NIH 80-1118, Bethesda, MD, Office of Cancer Communications, March 1980
8. U.S. Department of Health, Education and Welfare: Breast exams, what you should know. DHEW Publication No. NIH 80-2000, Bethesda, MD, Office of Cancer Communications, 1980
9. Wells G: Reducing the threat of a first pelvic exam. American Journal of Maternal Child Nursing, Vol. 2 No. 5, September/October 1977

24

Gynecologic Procedures

There are many gynecologic procedures that can be done in an office or outpatient setting. They range from simple tissue staining techniques to biopsy. The obvious advantages to an office procedure rather than one done in the hospital are both the reduced cost and the shorter length of time lost from normal activities. A less apparent advantage is that a procedure done in an office setting seems to carry with it less of an aura of dread or fear than one done in a hospital.

In either case, preparation and education of the woman is of primary importance. The problem necessitating the procedure may be causing her discomfort, pain, or abnormal bleeding. She may have some very real concerns and fears regarding the outcome of the test she is about to have. Even if the results have a very good chance of being normal or benign she may have some apprehension concerning the procedure itself.

The descriptions that follow will provide the nurse with information regarding technique and preparation for the procedure. Communicating this information to a woman in advance may help allay her anxiety. An additional benefit is that a well informed woman is often better able to relax. The procedure thus goes more smoothly and quickly with a resultant decrease in discomfort. Accuracy of test results is sometimes enhanced under these conditions.

A printed handout is a helpful adjunct to a verbal description of a procedure. Attention span and amount of information absorbed are limited when anxiety is high. A printed sheet should include any risks associated with the procedure. It can also include instructions for follow-up self care as well as signs of possible complications.

It is helpful to provide a woman with a list of phone numbers which may be used in case of complications. The printed matter is best used to reinforce the verbal explanation and is not intended to be a substitute for it. The greatest advantage to a verbal explanation is the opportunity it affords a woman to ask questions and communicate special concerns.

SCHILLER'S STAIN

Schiller's stain is an iodine solution and is used to identify abnormal tissue on the cervical and vaginal mucosa. It is helpful in identifying suspicious areas which may not be visible to the naked eye such as carcinoma in situ, microinvasive carcinoma, leukoplakia, and vaginal adenosis. Glycogen-containing cells of normal cervical and vaginal tissue take up the stain and produce a mahagony-brown color. Any nonstaining areas will require biopsy.

The woman assumes the lithotomy position with her feet in stirrups and a speculum is inserted into the vagina. Secretions must be gently wiped away from the cervix in order to lessen chances of contact bleeding which would interfere with test results. It is important for the examiner to visualize and note the location of the squamo-columnar junction. (Columnar cells do not stain and if their presence on the ectocervix has not been noticed they may be mistaken for abnormal tissue.) The Schiller's solution can then be poured into the vagina or swabbed on to the cervix and vaginal walls. As mentioned before, nonstaining areas are abnormal and indicate sites for biopsy. See Figure 24-1.

TOLUIDINE BLUE STAIN

The toluidine blue stain does for the vulva what Schiller's stain does for the cervix and vagina. It is used to identify areas of abnormality on the vulva which are then biopsied. Conditions in which this diagnostic test is useful include leukoplakia, various chronic inflammatory processes, carcinoma in situ, or early invasive cancer.

The woman is asked to assume the lithotomy position with her feet in stirrups. A one percent aqueous solution of toluidine blue is applied to the entire vulva staining it a deep blue color. After drying, the skin is sponged with a one percent acetic acid solution. All normal areas will become decolorized. Any areas that retain the blue stain represent abnormal epithelium and will need biopsy.

COLPOSCOPY

Colposcopy is yet another method for identifying areas of abnormality on the cervix and vagina. It can be used in place of the staining techniques or in addition to them. Its use remains somewhat limited by the expense of the equipment, the special training and experience needed by the examiner, and the time involved in carrying out the procedure. It is not used for mass routine screening. It is, however, an invaluable diagnostic aid for follow-up of patients with abnormal staining tests, abnormal Pap smears, DES exposure, and other proven atypical cervical, vaginal, or vulvar changes.

A colposcope is a binocular instrument that allows visualization of cervical and vaginal tissue under magnification (10–20 times). The woman assumes the lithotomy position and a vaginal speculum is inserted. A three percent acetic acid solution is applied to accent the morphologic features of the tissue. The examiner then carefully scans the tissues through the colposcope and identifies any areas that appear abnormal. Pictures can be taken to be used for comparison to previous or subsequent colposcopy findings. Abnormal areas thus identified can be biopsied.

The colposcopy itself is no more uncomfortable than a pelvic examination. However, the lithotomy position does become tiresome and the procedure often takes as long as 30 minutes or more. In addition, if a biopsy is needed, the woman will experience mild discomfort. As previously mentioned, colposcopy is fairly expensive due to the cost of the equipment and the additional training required for its use. Women with insurance will probably find that most of the cost will be

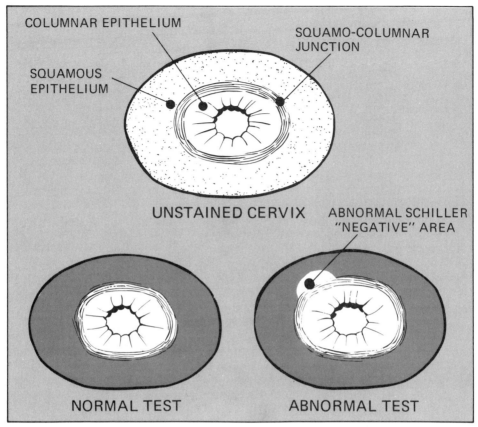

Figure 24-1. Appearance of a normal and abnormal cervix after staining with Schiller's solution contrasted with an unstained cervix.

covered. Women without medical insurance can often receive the examination at little or no cost in special colposcopy clinics held at large teaching hospitals in many cities. See Figure 24-2.

CRYOSURGERY

Cryosurgery is a procedure which destroys abnormal tissue by freezing. Carbon dioxide or nitrous oxide is used to cool a disc or special tip. This cold tip is then placed against the abnormal tissue, freezing and destroying it. Healing then restores normal tissue.

Conditions in which cryosurgery is utilized for treatment include persistent or chronic cervicitis and cervical dysplasia. During the procedure a woman may experience some mild to moderate cramping and a feeling of pressure. Following treatment she may have an increased vaginal discharge for one to two weeks.

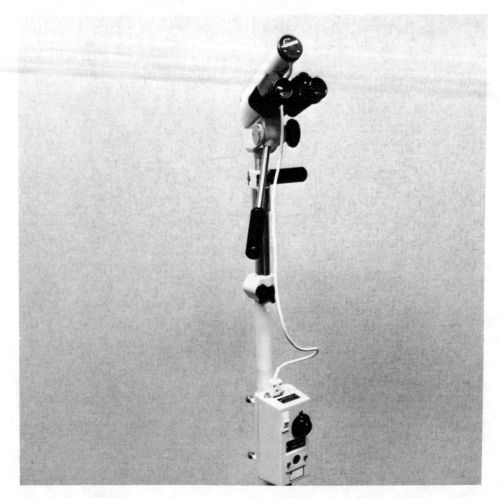

Figure 24-2.   Colposcope.

BIOPSY

Cervical

Biopsy of the cervix is done with a punch biopsy instrument. It can be done in the office since discomfort is minimal. Most women complain of a cramp-like pain as the tissue sample is obtained. The biopsy site may be cauterized with a silver nitrate stick. Placement of a tampon in the vagina for a few hours following the procedure acts as a pressure dressing and also absorbs the slight oozing which may occur. If the biopsy was unusually deep, a suture may be needed.

Breast

In the past, biopsy of breast masses was almost always done under general anesthesia, particularly if there was a high index of suspicion for malignancy. It

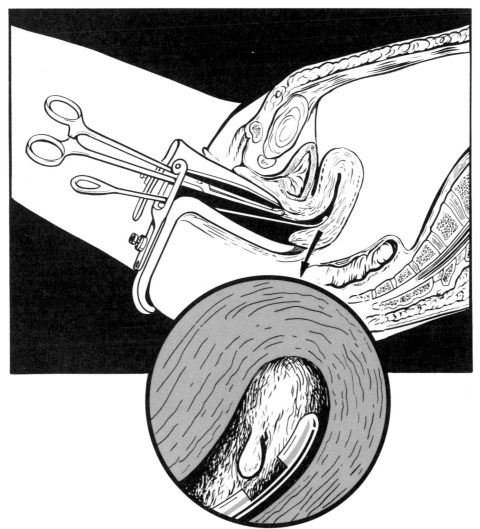

Figure 24-3. Endometrial biopsy.

was not uncommon for a woman to submit to breast biopsy not knowing whether she would wake up in the recovery room with or without a breast. The shock, anger, depersonalization and feelings of helplessness that resulted are discussed in chapter 25. At present, biopsy as an outpatient under local anesthesia is becoming the rule rather than the exception.

If a cyst is suspected a needle aspiration of the fluid will be attempted. If the tumor is large, a section will be removed and prepared for histological examination (incisional biopsy). An excisional biopsy is done on tumors that can be totally removed in such a setting. No matter how benign a tumor appears grossly it must be sent for examination by the pathologist. Mammography often precedes a biopsy to help determine which area or areas need sampling.

Following a breast biopsy, a pressure dressing is applied and arm and shoulder activity on the affected side should be limited for a few days. A mild analgesic such as aspirin is usually sufficient to control any discomfort.

Endometrial

A sample of endometrial tissue can be helpful in diagnosing functional menstrual disorders, infertility problems, and malignant or benign lesions. A positive report for malignancy establishes the diagnosis in a woman suspected of having such a problem. However, if her symptoms strongly suggest malignancy and the test is negative, a diagnostic dilatation and curettage (D&C) should be done.

The woman assumes the lithotomy position with feet in stirrups and a vaginal speculum is inserted. The cervix is cleansed with an antiseptic solution and a tenaculum applied to its anterior lip. Women vary in their response to the tenaculum. Some perceive it as a mild cramp and some as a sharp pain. A uterine sound is next passed to determine the length and direction of the endocervical canal and endometrial cavity. A curved endometrial-biopsy curette is passed into the uterus, pressed firmly against the anterior, posterior, or lateral wall of the fundus and is then withdrawn. The cupped, spoonlike end removes a strip of endometrium. A woman should be warned to expect moderate to severe cramping from the uterine sounding as well as from the curetting. See Figure 24-3.

Some physicians feel that suctioning the endometrium with a suction or aspiration-biopsy instrument is preferable to using the curette. They feel that obtaining more of the endometrium provides increased accuracy of diagnosis. The procedure is similar to that described above except that in place of the curette a slim, flexible plastic cannula is inserted and attached to a suction device. The woman experiences mild to moderate cramping during the 2–3 minutes it takes to "vacuum" the uterus clean. This procedure is often referred to as an office D&C.

MAMMOGRAPHY

Mammography is a technique in which x-rays of each breast are taken and developed on photographic film. Xeroradiography is a variation of mammography. The source of radiation remains the same, but instead of being recorded on film, it is recorded on paper using a Xerographic process. See Figure 24-4.

Mammography can detect breast cancers before there is palpable clinical evidence of a lump. It can also show changes in the structure of the breast which may point to very early cancer or a precancerous condition. Therefore, mammography has become recognized as an invaluable tool in the diagnosis and early detection of breast cancer. It can also be used as an adjunct in treatment of breast masses by determining areas for biopsy and screening the "unaffected" side when a malignant mass has been found in one breast.

However, since radiation is known to have carcinogenic potential, there is concern about what degree of risk may result from repeated exposure to mammography. Most new equipment and techniques have reduced the rads received by each breast during a procedure to less than one. (A rad is a "radiation-absorbed dose.") At these low levels of exposure, it has been estimated that a woman

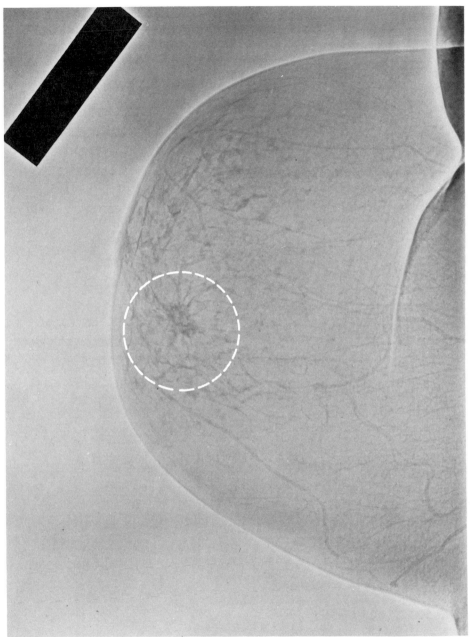

Figure 24.4.   Xerogram of breast showing abnormal tissue. Courtesy of Radiology Department, Washington Hospital Center, Washington, D.C.

would need fifteen consecutive examinations to increase her risk of developing breast cancer to eight percent. Without x-ray exposure, the risk is seven percent [5].

Since the carcinogenic potential of radiation is thought to be cumulative, it is difficult to accurately establish the risk of low-dose exposure. For this reason, the National Cancer Institute, the American Cancer Society, and the American College of Obstetricians and Gynecologists have all developed guidelines for the use of mammography for routine screening of asymptomatic women. Mammography guidelines can be found in chapter 13.

When a woman has a mammography she will be asked to undress completely from the waist up. Two views at right angles to each other are taken of each breast. One view is taken from the top of the breast with the woman in a sitting position and her breast lying on the radiographic plate. Compression of the breast improves the image and is sometimes provided by the arm of the equipment itself and sometimes by a strong inflated balloon exerting pressure. The second view is filmed with the woman lying on her side with the outer aspect of the breast on the plate. See Figure 24-5.

The entire procedure usually takes 30 minutes or less. After reading the films, the radiologist will send a report to the woman's physician. She should be advised that she will not receive test results at the time of the procedure.

THERMOGRAPHY

During thermography infrared heat waves emitted from the skin of the breast are transferred into visual patterns which can be photographed thus producing a record of the heat pattern of the breast. It has been found that hot areas frequently correlate with carcinoma. This is presumably due to the increased metabolism of the malignancy.

This technique is not highly accurate. There are non-malignant causes for an increase in heat and conversely, some cancers do not result in increased heat in the skin overlying them. Therefore, at present, thermography is not considered appropriate for mass screening if used alone. However, it is a very valuable method if used in combination with clinical examination, breast self examination, and mammography.

A woman having thermography should be advised that her breasts need to be cooled to 19-21°C for a period of 10-15 minutes prior to the procedure. This is accomplished by having the woman undress from the waist up and sit with her arms raised and away from her body in an air conditioned room. This allows equal, symmetrical cooling of both breasts. Both frontal and oblique pictures are taken of each breast. The procedure involves no discomfort and no special preparation other than that described. An advantage of thermography is that its safety allows it to be done as often as desired. See Figure 24-6.

ULTRASONOGRAPHY

Although ultrasonography is used in many specialties of medicine as a diagnostic aid, it is of particular usefulness in the practice of obstetrics and gynecology. It is hoped that it may prove to be a means of detecting early breast cancer. However, at the present time its usefulness remains limited since it cannot detect lesions much before they become palpable.

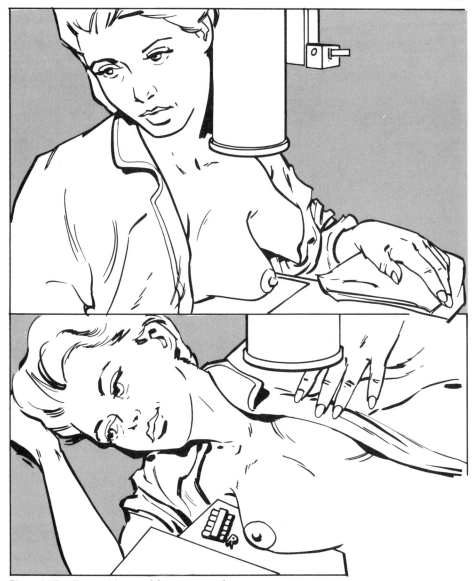

Figure 24-5. Two positions used for mammography.

The technique of ultrasound employs a system of sound reflection. Pulsed sound waves of high frequency (greater than 20,000 cycles per second) are transmitted from a transducer or scanner to the area being studied. In the case of pelvic ultrasound the abdomen and pelvis are scanned in a linear fashion. Tissue interfaces cause some of the sound to be reflected back and the transducer then becomes the receiver. The transducer receives these echos and displays them on an oscilloscope screen. Different tissue density is shown by different shades which vary from light to dark. A summation of these echos produces a cross-sectional picture which can then be recorded on film.

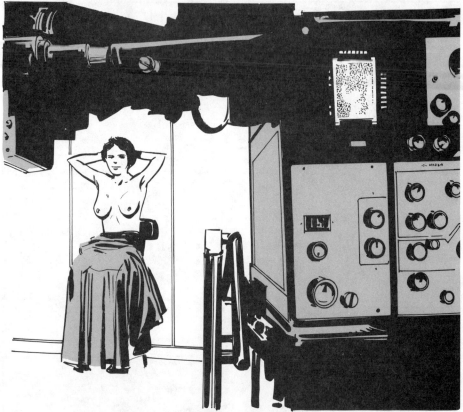

Figure 24-6. Woman prepared for thermography.

Ultrasound can outline and define soft tissue masses and can usually distinguish between solid and cystic tumors and between free fluid such as ascites and encapsulated fluid. It is particularly useful in the diagnosis of pelvic masses. It can be used to monitor the response of masses being treated by radiotherapy or the growth or regression of fibroids. It can often help in pinpointing the location of pelvic abcesses and IUD's. The gestational sac can be visualized as early as five to six weeks and, in addition, it is very useful in diagnosing multiple pregnancies or in determining fetal age and presentation.

Although ultrasonography of most areas of the body does not involve special patient preparation, pelvic ultrasound does. The woman is instructed to empty her bladder one hour before the procedure. She must then drink one quart of liquid and not void again until the ultrasound is completed. This can be extremely uncomfortable for some women, particularly during the later stages of pregnancy. The purpose of the full bladder is to help delineate the pelvic organs and to raise the intestine away from them.

The procedure itself is not uncomfortable. The woman lies on a table. Her abdomen is exposed and mineral oil is liberally applied to the skin. This ensures good contact between the transducer and the skin and prevents an air gap which would reflect sound. The procedure usually does not take more than 30-45 minutes. The radiologist interprets the results and passes on the information to the woman's physician.

FIRST TRIMESTER ABORTION

Termination of pregnancy during the first trimester is done by means of suction D&C and is similar to the procedure described under endometrial biopsy. Once a decision to terminate her pregnancy has been made, a woman will want to know how the procedure will be done and what risks are associated with it. The situation may precipitate a crisis for some women.

A therapeutic abortion can be performed by means of suction D&C up to 15-16 weeks from the first day of the last period under special circumstances. However, most free-standing clinics performing first trimester abortions do not do them past 12 weeks from the last menstrual period (LMP). If there is a question regarding the date of the last *normal* period or if the length of gestation cannot be determined by pelvic exam, a sonogram may be required prior to performing the abortion.

Most clinics that perform abortions follow a similar routine. This includes pre-operative laboratory work and counseling. The laboratory tests include a pregnancy test, hemoglobin, blood type, and Rh factor. Following the abortion Rho-GAM serum is given to Rh negative women. Counseling may be done in small groups or individually. During the session the nurse or counselor explores the circumstances underlying this unwanted pregnancy, feelings surrounding the pregnancy and abortion decision, and plans for future contraceptive practice.

Following a pelvic examination, a local anesthetic is given by injecting Xylocaine into the cervix. A tenaculum will be applied to the cervix in order to stabilize and properly align the uterus. The cervical os is then dilated to accommodate the diameter of the suction catheter. After passing the catheter the suction machine is turned on and the uterine contents are thus removed. A final exploration of the uterine cavity may then be done by curettage.

Most women feel mild, moderate, or severe menstrual-like cramps during the dilation of the cervix as well as during the suctioning. It is difficult to accurately predict for any one woman just how much discomfort to expect. However, the type of pain will be familiar to most women since it is similar to strong menstrual cramps.

Following the procedure a woman will be asked to remain under observation for one to two hours. During this time she can be given instructions for self care and guidelines for medical follow-up. She may be asked to take her temperature for four to five days to check for early signs of infection. Bleeding may range from none to amounts consistent with a normal period. A foul smelling, purulent vaginal discharge is abnormal. Heavy bleeding with large clots also indicates a need for medical evaluation. Bleeding and cramping of a severe degree may be signs of an incomplete abortion.

Since incomplete abortions are more common under six to eight weeks from the LMP, many clinics will not perform them until after the eighth week. Therefore the newer blood tests that can determine pregnancy within a few days after conception may not always be advantageous. Even though the pregnancy can be confirmed, a woman may not be able to terminate it until eight weeks following her LMP. In most cases women will prefer to wait until two weeks after the missed period when a less expensive urine determination can be done.

The main risks associated with therapeutic suction abortion are infection, hemorrhage, uterine perforation, and incomplete abortion. Women should be completely informed of these risks prior to undergoing the procedure. Since we do not yet have conclusive evidence about long-term effects of abortion on future pregnancies, women should be encouraged to use an effective contraceptive in order to avoid any unwanted pregnancy.

A follow-up examination is recommended two or three weeks following a first trimester abortion. Most clinics and private physicians recommend that a repeat pregnancy test be done at that time. A thorough pelvic examination is done to determine the size of the uterus, presence or absence of adnexal masses, characteristics of vaginal discharge, appearance of the cervix and cervical os, and the presence or absence of pelvic tenderness.

In addition to physical assessment it is important to determine how well the woman has adjusted to the emotional impact of the abortion experience. Grieving seems to be a common, although transient, aspect of most women's post abortion recovery period. Reassurance that this is normal is often helpful. Indications that a woman may be experiencing a more severe emotional response might include disturbances of sleep, appetite changes (either anorexia or excessive eating), unexplained bouts of crying, difficulty concentrating, or problems in previously good relationships with family or friends.

A nurse can often intervene simply by allowing a woman to ventilate her feelings surrounding the abortion experience and its aftermath. Education regarding normal post abortion recovery is often reassuring. However, the nurse should also be alert for signs of deeper disturbance and make appropriate referrals for counseling when necessary.

MID TRIMESTER ABORTION

Therapeutic abortions done by suction curettage are performed up until the seventeenth or eighteenth week from the last normal menstrual period in some facilities. Such procedures are done in the same way as first trimester abortions.

Abortions done later in the second trimester are performed by infusion of saline or prostaglandins into the amniotic sac. The substance which is instilled causes intrauterine fetal death and precipitates labor. Protocols for this type of abortion differ from one locality or from one physician to another. An example of a typical protocol is as follows:

The woman is admitted to the hospital and routine laboratory studies including complete blood count, urinalysis, and electrolytes are done. An intravenous drip of D_5W with addition of an antibiotic such as cephalothin sodium (Keflin) is started. Following preparation of the abdomen, 100–200cc of amniotic fluid is withdrawn and replaced by an equal amount of 20 percent saline or prostaglandin $F_2\alpha$ in solution. Occasionally a combination of these substances will be used. The saline or prostaglandin may be instilled as a drip over a period of 10–20 minutes.

Prior to admission the woman is instructed to have nothing to eat or drink for 12 hours. Following the infusion she may be ambulatory and is placed on a regular diet until labor contractions begin. Labor may begin anywhere from 12–24 hours following the infusion. Some physicians prescribe prostaglandin suppositories every four hours to speed up the onset of labor thus decreasing the hospital stay.

When this is done it is helpful to have an order for prochlorperazine (Compazine) or Lomotil® to be used if nausea, vomiting, or diarrhea occur.

The woman may be discharged from the hospital approximately 24 hours after delivery. The average hospital stay varys from 48–72 hours depending upon how rapidly labor progresses. Discharge orders are similar to those following a full term delivery. Orders include avoidance of strenuous activity and no sexual intercourse, tub baths, or tampon use for four weeks. A prescription is given to suppress lactation since breast changes associated with pregnancy are well underway.

Major physical complications include heavy bleeding or hemorrhage, infection, uterine rupture, and incomplete abortion which may result in the need for an operative procedure such as a D&C or hysterotomy. The emotional impact of a late abortion is often much greater than one done earlier in a pregnancy. Not only have many physical changes taken place making a woman acutely aware of her pregnant state, but also enough time has passed to allow for an emotional attachment to the fetus. The pain and discomfort experienced during labor and delivery intensify the feelings of loss.

Following a mid trimester abortion a woman should be encouraged to seek counseling if she experiences feelings of depression that she has difficulty handling. A framework for crisis intervention can be found in chapter 21. An important aspect of this for the nurse is an awareness of when a referral is indicated. Referral sources may include mental health professionals as well as clergy.

REFERENCES

1. Egan R: Mammography, 2nd ed. Springfield, IL, Charles C. Thomas, 1972
2. Evans K, Gravelle TH: Mammography, Thermography and Ultrasonography in Breast Disease. London, William Clowes & Sons, Ltd., 1973
3. Green T: Gynecology: Essentials of Clinical Practice, 3rd ed. Boston, Little, Brown, 1977
4. Wolfe J: Xeroradiography of the breast. In Grundmann E, Beck L (eds): Early Diagnosis of Breast Cancer, 3rd ed. New York, Gustav Fischer Verlag, 1978
5. Sloane E: Biology of Women. New York, John Wiley and Sons, 1980

25

Surgical Interventions

A person facing surgery, whether of an emergency or elective nature is a person under stress and often in crisis. As stated by Barnes and Tinkham, "to be rendered unconscious and cut with knives is in itself a devastating idea and this anxiety is further exacerbated by the complete surrender of control which surgery implies."[1]

Both males and females must respond by mobilizing their defenses to cope with the overwhelming event of surgery. Techniques of defense vary from one individual to another but often include denial, anger, dependency, and depression. Following surgery, each individual must come to an acceptance of the experience and in so doing reorganize their life.

GENERAL CONCERNS REGARDING SURGERY

Anesthesia

Many people fear general anesthesia because to them it represents a loss of control. The thought of being unconscious is often frightening. There may be fear of what will be done to them as well as concern about what they will do or say or how they will act while unconscious. Some people fear that a mistake will be made in administering the general anesthesia resulting in death or brain damage.

Regional anesthesia, while allowing a person to retain some control, is not without problems. People often fear complications such as postoperative headaches or paralysis and the discomfort they expect with administration of the anesthesia. In addition, there may be concern about being awake during the surgery and how that will be tolerated.

Pain

Pain is usually associated in some way with surgery. When pain is present before surgery the surgical procedure may be seen as a way of easing or ending the discomfort. When a person is relatively well and comfortable before surgery, postoperative pain is usually anticipated. In either case, there is no way to accurately predict the nature, degree, or duration of discomfort a person will experience.

Threat to Life

Impending surgery often brings with it a fear of death or disability. The fear is intensified when cancer is a definite or highly probable diagnosis. For the first time, many people will experience the reality of their own mortality and vulnerability on an emotional rather than a purely intellectual level.

Limitation of Function

Some limitation of a person's normal function can be expected following all but minor surgical procedures. Adaptations will need to be made in many areas of daily living and assistance from others may be necessary.

Dependency

Limitation of function and alteration in usual activities means that some independence must be sacrificed. This may be limited in degree and duration such as following a thyroidectomy, or quite extensive as with a limb amputation or eye surgery.

Body Image

Most surgical procedures are accompanied by actual or feared changes in appearance. The change may be no more than an imperceptible scar but the impact on one's body image may be disproportionate to the size. Surgery is usually perceived as an assault. It often results in loss of organ, limb, or function. Cosmetic or reconstructive surgery would seem to be free of negative impact. Yet, it also results in a change in body image requiring major social, physical, or emotional adjustments.

Financial Concerns

The high cost of surgery and hospitalization cannot be taken lightly. In addition to the direct costs, many people experience a loss of income during part or all of the time of hospitalization and recuperation.

Family Concerns

Whether male or female, a person facing surgery will usually have concerns about the welfare of family members. These concerns may be primarily financial when the person undergoing surgery is the "breadwinner" of the family. A mother contemplating surgery might be particularly concerned with child care during her absence. In many families, partners share in wage earning, household chores, and childcare. Consequently, these individuals will have concerns in overlapping areas of family life.

GYNECOLOGIC AND BREAST SURGERY CONCERNS

In addition to all of the fears and concerns related to any surgical procedure, surgery of the breast or reproductive system involves unique issues. The reproductive and nurturing functions of the uterus and breast give special meaning to these organs. The role they play in female sexuality imparts additional significance to them. Finally, the female's breasts are an important and highly valued aspect of outward physical appearance. Surgery which may alter or remove one or both of these organs is perceived as a threat to a woman's entire being.

Body Image

The loss of a body part results in a real or perceived change in body image whether that part is external or internal. The degree to which that loss is mourned is closely related to the significance placed upon it. The internal genital organs are highly significant to a woman reproductively and sexually. The loss of the uterus or ovaries is strongly felt even though body image is not visually altered. The loss of a breast carries with it the additional problem of an observable change in outward appearance.

Following mastectomy women may feel mutilated, awkward, embarrassed, or defective. An adjustment must be made to the feeling of emptiness where once a breast had been. The scar must eventually be viewed and the impact of that may be profoundly upsetting. If surgery was radical with lymph node dissection, lymphedema of the arm may result in disfigurement and discomfort. The prominence of previously inapparent ribs may be unsettling and repulsive to some women.

Hysterectomy does not bring such outwardly apparent changes. However, myths abound regarding possible physical effects of hysterectomy. Many women fear that postoperatively they will experience weight gain, excessive facial and body hair growth, and physical signs of premature aging such as skin wrinkling and graying hair [2].

Concepts of Femininity

The appearance of female external genitals at birth sets into motion a "cultural blueprint for a feminine gender role."[10] It stimulates the child's parents and others around her to offer experiences of a specific type to reinforce their concept of her future gender role. The young child learns about those characteristics which make her distinctly feminine, and allow her to reproduce and nuture, long before she has any physical evidence of their existence.

By the time the breasts begin to grow and menstruation first occurs, the adolescent has already incorporated the appearance and function of these organs into her concept of femininity. The emphasis placed by our society on the desirability of a voluptuous feminine figure attests to the high value placed on female breasts. The fact that most youngsters are conditioned in early years to regard motherhood as a cherished goal, places equally high value on the uterus and ovaries.

It is easy to understand that surgery involving removal or significant alteration of appearance or function of the breast or reproductive system will be seen as a threat to femininity. A woman whose self-esteem or self-definition centers primarily around her attractiveness may perceive such surgery as particularly devastating. A woman with other sources of self-definition such as intellectual pursuits, career achievements, or other talents and interests usually makes a better adjustment.

Sexuality Concerns

There can be little doubt about the role played by the breasts and reproductive organs in female sexuality. Their role in reproduction is of course closely linked to their sexual role. However, for most women these organs have sexual significance independent of reproductive function. Sexually active women who plan to defer or completely give up childbearing, as well as women who have completed their families, are none the less aware of the sexual meaning these organs have.

Physical sexual response and sensations involve the breast, uterus, vagina, and external genitalia. The ovaries and the hormones produced by them contribute to sexual functioning in a less obvious way. Many women have concerns that their surgery will disturb or disrupt their sexual functioning. In some respects and with some surgeries this will be true. However, many concerns are more myth than reality.

FACTORS AFFECTING PREOPERATIVE ANXIETY

A variety of factors may influence the degree of anxiety felt by a woman facing reproductive or breast surgery. It is wise to assume that some anxiety will be present in all women. Some of the following factors should be taken into consideration when assessing anxiety levels.

Diagnosis

Diagnosis may be an important determinant of anxiety. A feared or confirmed diagnosis of cancer is accompanied by high levels of anxiety. In addition to the jarring reality of one's mortality and vulnerability, there is the ever-present fear of future recurrence.

Time

The duration of time from diagnosis to operative procedure can have an effect on a woman's anxiety. The process of reorganizing one's life patterns, attaining some degree of acceptance, and reintegrating identity seems easier if some time is allowed between diagnosis and surgery. In opposition to this is the tremendous anxiety felt preoperatively by a woman who is undergoing breast surgery and possible mastectomy without prior knowledge of her diagnosis. Allowing some time between diagnosis and major surgery gives her the chance to begin the process leading towards acceptance of the situation. This in turn helps her to deal more effectively with her anxiety.

Self-esteem

Self-esteem is a good indicator of potential anxiety. Women who have a strong sense of self-worth are often able to control and contain their anxiety. Women in whom feelings of self worth are closely linked to their uterus and breasts are likely to have high levels of anxiety.

Coping Mechanisms

The effectiveness of general coping mechanisms and their successful employment in prior stressful situations can often be used to predict the way a woman will cope with surgery. A woman who generally "goes to pieces" under stress is a good candidate for incapacitating preoperative anxiety. A woman who has successfully coped in the past can often apply previously useful techniques to help her through the surgical experience.

Family

Family can either help or hinder a woman in her response to impending surgery. An integrated, adaptable family can often help lessen the anxiety of the mother, wife, daughter, or sister who is ill. This is particularly true if they have previously dealt successfully with a crisis. A family in which individual members are unable to accept and cope with the reality of the illness will be less capable of providing the needed support.

APPROACHES TO PREOPERATIVE CARE

Measures can be undertaken before surgery which can help to decrease the negative impact it will have upon a woman and encourage more rapid and complete postoperative adjustment. These measures include education, emotional support, and identification and utilization of external resources.

Education

Education should include basic anatomy and physiology of the breast and/or reproductive tract. The content and depth of material should be geared to the individual's capacity for understanding and her expressed needs. Some women will want detailed information while others will be more satisfied with basics.

The planned surgery can be discussed within the context of the anatomical and physiological framework. Charts and diagrams are helpful teaching aides. Specific information should be given, i.e., menstruation and conception will no longer occur following hysterectomy, estrogen replacement can be given following oophorectomy, or periods will *not* cease following tubal ligation.

It is helpful to prepare a woman for what she will experience regarding hospital routine and admission procedures. This information might include preoperative skin preparations, medications, dietary restrictions, and bowel preparation. If she will be awake when she is taken into the operating room a description of the room, equipment, and people she will see there will be most helpful. A description of the recovery room area is essential. If it is anticipated that she will wake up with I.V.'s, suction, or drainage tubes, she should be informed of this. A description of any dressing she might have should also be included.

Practice sessions for postoperative exercises are extremely beneficial. These would include coughing, deep breathing, turning, and leg and foot exercises to help prevent thrombophlebitis. The need for elastic stockings, if applicable, should be mentioned. It is helpful to introduce the arm exercises which a woman will use following mastectomy.

Finally, a most important skill can be taught to a woman before her surgery. That skill is the use of a bedpan. This knowledge can reduce the frustration experienced by many women when their first attempt to use a bedpan is while they are still groggy or in pain following surgery.

Emotional Support

There are many forms of emotional support which can be offered by a nurse to a woman who is about to undergo gynecological surgery. Attentive or therapeutic listening is often the most helpful technique. A woman often needs encouragement and permission to vent feelings of anger and fear. Family and friends often do not or cannot tolerate such painful expressions of emotion.

Following expressions of fear and anger the nurse can often help a woman to identify her strengths. A review of past stresses and crises and the ways in which she found to cope with them can often be useful. It sometimes takes an outside, objective observer to point out strengths which can be drawn upon when an individual is feeling overwhelmed.

Finally, the nurse can offer support by sharing illustrations of how others have responded following a similar surgery. She can do this with the authority of one who has observed others with the same diagnosis. When offering emotional support the aim should be to encourage a woman to draw on her own strength and to discourage dependency. By so doing, it is hoped that she will attain mastery of the experience and be able to generalize it to other aspects of her life.

External Resources

The ability of family members to accept the truth, deal with the situation realistically, and offer support are very important to a woman's recovery and eventual resumption of activities. It is helpful to talk with family members and try to identify areas in which they may need help. A discussion with the woman's husband or partner regarding the surgery and its implications to her general health as well as to their sexual relationship is very helpful.

Identification of a support network of friends and community resources can lessen preoperative anxiety and aid in recovery. Needs may include baby sitting, transportation for herself or members of her family, care of pets and plants, or cooking, washing, and housecleaning chores. Seemingly insignificant matters are often the source of greatest concern.

BREAST AND PELVIC SURGERY

Details of immediate physical postoperative care can be found in medical-surgical nursing texts. The skills necessary for helping a woman face the diagnosis of cancer and possible death or the reality of a prolonged recovery period are familiar to nurses. Therefore, neither of these areas will be discussed in detail. Rather a brief description will be given of some of the common major surgical procedures which are unique to women.

Mastectomy

Removal of breast tissue as treatment of primary cancer of the breast may range from removal of only the tumor to extended radical mastectomy. Less extensive surgery may be preceded or followed by radiation or chemotherapy. Endocrine manipulation, either by providing exogenous hormones or by depriving the body of endogenous hormones (through removal of ovaries, adrenals or pituitary) has been found to be helpful in certain types of tumors.

Clinical trials are presently being conducted in many parts of the world to try to determine which treatment method is most effective. The efficacy of a procedure is measured by its survival rate (usually five years) as well as by its rate of local recurrence. A surgeon's primary aims of treatment are to preserve the woman's life, to minimize the chance of recurrence, and to provide optimum functional and cosmetic results. However, the ultimate treatment decision rests with the woman herself.

The *Halsted radical mastectomy* removes the entire breast, skin, major and minor pectoral muscles, axillary lymph nodes, and fat. It results in a flattened or sunken chest wall, extensive scarring, and the possibility of developing lymphedema and shoulder stiffness.

The *extended radical mastectomy* includes the excision of all the structures included in the Halsted. In addition, the internal mammary nodes are excised. In order to reach these nodes, a section of the rib cage usually must be removed.

The *modified radical* removes the breast, some fat, and most of the axillary lymph nodes. The chest muscles are left intact. The cosmetic result is usually better than with the Halsted or extended radicals. Scarring is less and it eliminates the hollowness beneath the clavicle that occurs with the more extensive procedures. It may also reduce the chances of developing lymphedema because fewer lymph vessels are severed. Finally, the arm may be stronger because of the preservation of the chest muscles.

Simple mastectomy sometimes referred to as total mastectomy, takes only the breast tissue leaving pectoral muscles and axillary nodes intact. Prior to this surgery the stage of the disease will be determined. (See chapter 13.) If cancer has spread to the axillary nodes, the simple mastectomy will be followed by radiation or instead a decision may be made to perform a modified or Halsted radical. If cancer develops in the nodes at a later date, they can be surgically removed or irradiated.

Partial mastectomy involves the removal of the tumor and 2-3 centimeters of surrounding tissue. Although this procedure saves some of the breast tissue, it leaves it markedly disfigured. Where appropriate, the breast can later be augmented by plastic surgery. Radiation therapy is usually given following surgery.

Local wide excision, tylectomy, or lumpectomy removes only the tumor mass and a small amount of surrounding breast tissue. It is almost always followed by radiation therapy.

Although cosmetic results of the partial mastectomy and lumpectomy are better than with extensive surgery, many surgeons argue that the multicentricity of breast cancer is not taken into account. They feel it is highly probable that undetectable cancer is present elsewhere in the breast and that there will eventually be local recurrence.

Subcutaneous mastectomy is the removal of the internal breast tissue leaving the skin intact. If the tissue is free of cancer, an implant can be inserted in a subsequent procedure. This is occasionally done in one step. If cancer is found in the removed tissue a more extensive procedure can be done depending upon the state of disease found. Subcutaneous mastectomy is sometimes done as preventive surgery in a woman at high risk or when cancer has been found in one breast and the other has excessive nodularity or cystic disease.

Any surgical procedure may be associated with risks of infection, bleeding, or other medical complications. The various types of mastectomies described are subject to these same risks. The radical types of mastectomies have two additional complications which may occur.

Lymphedema or swelling of the arm from accumulation of excess fluid results from the severing of lymphatic vessels and removal of axillary lymph nodes. This may occur in the immediate postoperative period or many months or years later as a result of injury or infection of the arm on the operative side. It affects 50-70 percent of all radical mastectomy patients to some degree, but is severe in only about 10 percent [13].

Elevation of the arm postoperatively and adequate exercise are helpful preventive measures. Use of a lightweight elastic sleeve during the day is also helpful. Prevention of injury and/or infection of the arm or hand on the operative side is extremely important. A small infection could become serious due to the compromised lymphatic system. These women should be advised of the following:

• Wear gloves when gardening or when using strong detergents.

• Prevent burns by wearing padded gloves when handling hot dishes, avoid sunburn and hold cigarettes with the unaffected hand.

• Shave under the affected arm with an electric razor and avoid harsh deodorants.

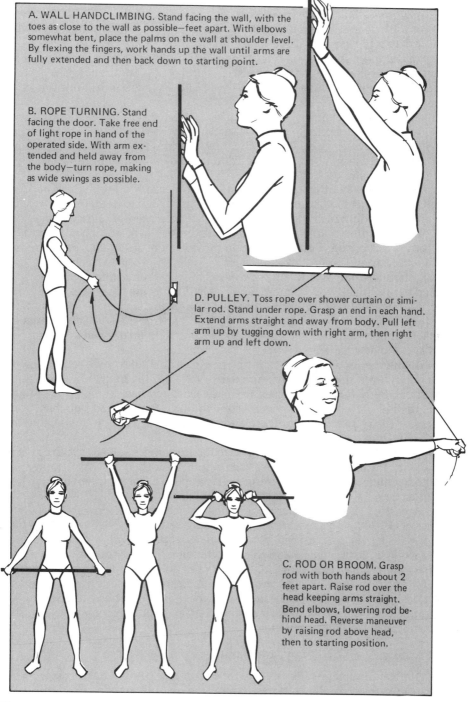

A. WALL HANDCLIMBING. Stand facing the wall, with the toes as close to the wall as possible—feet apart. With elbows somewhat bent, place the palms on the wall at shoulder level. By flexing the fingers, work hands up the wall until arms are fully extended and then back down to starting point.

B. ROPE TURNING. Stand facing the door. Take free end of light rope in hand of the operated side. With arm extended and held away from the body—turn rope, making as wide swings as possible.

D. PULLEY. Toss rope over shower curtain or similar rod. Stand under rope. Grasp an end in each hand. Extend arms straight and away from body. Pull left arm up by tugging down with right arm, then right arm up and left down.

C. ROD OR BROOM. Grasp rod with both hands about 2 feet apart. Raise rod over the head keeping arms straight. Bend elbows, lowering rod behind head. Reverse maneuver by raising rod above head, then to starting position.

Figure 25-1.   Examples of some exercises to help prevent arm and shoulder stiffness following a mastectomy.

- Have injections given and blood pressure taken on the unaffected arm.
- Wear a thimble when sewing.
- Carry purses and heavy items with the unaffected arm.
- Promptly cleanse any injury that does occur and report any unusual swelling or redness to a physician.

Arm and shoulder stiffness may occur as a result of the skin tightness which is caused by the axillary incision. When this is extreme, it is known as *frozen shoulder*. Back and neck pain can also occur as a result of the weight imbalance caused by the loss of the breast.

Arm and shoulder exercises can be started as soon as drainage and healing are adequate as determined by the physician. Mild exercise can be accomplished by normal daily activities such as brushing teeth, face washing, and hair combing using the affected arm. Other exercises that help prevent stiffness as well as lymphedema are illustrated in Figure 25-1.

Radiation and chemotherapy often result in unpleasant side effects. Radiotherapy side effects include fatigue, redness of the irradiated skin, itching or peeling skin, and weakening of the ribs resulting in an increased tendency to fracture. Chemotherapy often results in hair loss but the hair will grow back when the treatment is completed. Both types of therapy often result in nausea, vomiting, diarrhea, and anorexia.

Small, frequent meals and high protein, high carbohydrate snacks may be digested easily. Meals will be more acceptable if foods are chosen carefully with thought for eye and taste appeal. Women experiencing skin changes from radiation should avoid sun exposure and the use of strong soaps, ointments, or creams. Itching is sometimes alleviated by keeping the skin dry and applying corn starch as often as necessary.

A **permanent prosthesis** can usually be worn within four to six weeks following surgery. However, most women begin to use soft padding in the bra while still in the hospital. Permanent prostheses are made from a variety of materials ranging from foam and polyester to heavier silicone or thick, liquid-filled pouches. Some are inserted into a specially made bra and some attach directly to the skin with a special adhesive.

Shopping for a prosthesis can be a traumatic experience since it requires facing the reality of the lost breast as well as sharing this information with another person who is generally a complete stranger. It is important for a woman to have help and guidance with this task.

The American Cancer Society promotes a "Reach to Recovery" program. Volunteers who have themselves experienced mastectomy are available to help women with all aspects of their recovery. The volunteer often makes her first contact while the woman is still in the hospital. She can provide information and encouragement on a wide range of subjects including exercises, side effects of radiation or chemotherapy, and prostheses. A Reach to Recovery volunteer can be found by contacting the local American Cancer Society. They can also provide information and other resources that the woman and her family may need during the time of postoperative adjustment.

Hysterectomy, Oophorectomy, and Salpingectomy

The surgical removal of the uterus, tubes, or ovaries may be necessary for a variety of reasons. These include malignancy, excessive, uncontrolled bleeding, severe pelvic inflammatory disease, or benign tumors such as leiomyomas which are causing severe problems.

Total hysterectomy refers to removal of just the uterus. This can be done when malignancy is not a possibility and when preservation of the ovaries is desirable such as in a premenopausal woman. Surgery can be done by means of an abdominal or vaginal incision.

The abdominal approach is always used when malignancy has been confirmed or strongly suspected. This allows exploration for possible extension of the tumor. In some cases a low transverse incision can be made but when extensive exploration will be necessary a vertical incision will be required. Vaginal hysterectomy has the advantage of leaving no visible scar.

Oophorectomy is the removal of an ovary and can be either unilateral or bilateral depending on the diagnosis. In a young woman every effort will be made to save some ovarian tissue. If surgery does not require hysterectomy, childbearing function is preserved and the need for hormone replacement avoided. When bilateral oophorectomy is performed in a premenopausal woman, an abrupt surgical menopause will occur. Estrogen replacement therapy will be required.

Salpingectomy is the removal of the Fallopian tube and can be partial or total, unilateral or bilateral. This procedure is usually done in conjunction with oophorectomy or hysterectomy. When all involved organs are removed, the operation is called hysterectomy with bilateral salpingo-oophorectomy.

Recovery from surgery when an abdominal approach has been used is somewhat slower than when a vaginal approach has been used. More pain will be involved and ambulation will be more difficult. However, within six weeks, most women will have resumed their normal functions and activities. Intercourse can also be resumed after six weeks. Tub baths and douches must be avoided for the same length of time to avoid contamination of the vaginal incision.

Some women do not realize that removal of the uterus and/or both ovaries means that menstrual periods will cease and they will become sterile. Once this is understood, a woman may need help adjusting to this reality. The capacity for sexual function and sexual sensations is not altered by these surgeries. However, the fear that sexual pleasure may be diminished often leads to impaired sexual functioning postoperatively.

Depression following hysterectomy has often been reported. This may be related to perceived alteration in sexual function [2]. It may also be that it is related to the loss of fertility, need for years of hormonal therapy, and/or the seriousness of the problem requiring surgery.

Following hysterectomy a woman should be encouraged to continue having regular gynecological examinations. The need for Pap smears does not stop following surgery. Smears done from the vaginal vault may detect early vaginal malignancies. Considerations of radiation and chemotherapy were discussed with mastectomy and would be similar following hysterectomy.

Repair of Cystocele, Rectocele, and Uterine Prolapse

A-P repair is an inclusive term meaning anterior-posterior repair of weakened vaginal walls. This type of operation is technically more difficult to perform than a hysterectomy. It also results in more postoperative pain than does a vaginal hysterectomy. This is due to the more extensive incisions and sutures required. Postoperative recovery and instructions are similar to those for vaginal hysterectomy but intercourse may need to be delayed longer.

Dilatation and Curettage

D and C may be done for a variety of reasons including abortion, control of heavy bleeding, or diagnostic purposes. After dilating the cervical os a curette is used to remove the endometrium. Recovery from this procedure is rapid and a woman can usually be discharged from the hospital the following day. A slight amount of bleeding is normal. Tampons, douches, tub baths, and intercourse must be avoided for two or three weeks.

Laparoscopy

Laparoscopy may be used as a diagnostic method to view the pelvic organs or to perform sterilization by tubal ligation or fulgaration. A general anesthesia is usually preferred but some clinics do perform laparoscopic sterilization under local anesthesia.

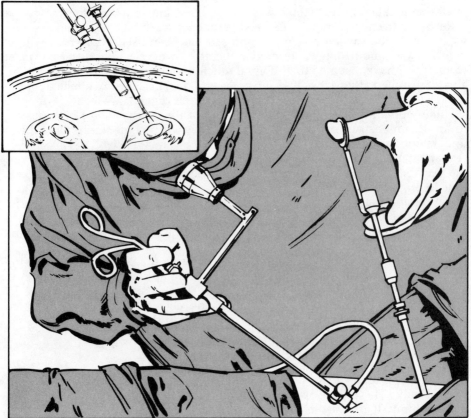

Figure 25-2.   The surgeon views the abdominal organs through the laparoscope (right hand) while performing the procedure through the trocar sleeve (left hand).

Approximately 3 liters of carbon dioxide or nitrous oxide are infused into the peritoneal cavity through a needle inserted under the umbilicus. After withdrawing the needle, a trocar is placed through the same incision and a laparoscope placed through the sleeve of the trocar. This provides the surgeon an excellent view of the pelvic organs. If biopsies or sterilization are to be performed, the instruments can be introduced through a second incision or through a channel in the laparoscope. Incisions are small and usually require only a few stitches, thus the name "bandaid surgery." See Figure 25-2.

Postoperative incisional pain is minimal. However, a woman should be advised that she may have shoulder and chest pain caused by the gas in the abdomen for twenty-four to forty-eight hours after the surgery. Resting for one to two days is advised but normal activities can usually be resumed in two to three days. Bathing and showering can be done at any time after surgery. Intercourse may be resumed as soon as it is comfortable to do so.

REFERENCES

1. Barnes A, Tinkham C: Surgical gynecology. *In* Notman M, Nadelson C (eds): The Woman Patient: Medical and Psychological Interfaces, Volume I, Sexual and Reproductive Aspects of Women's Health Care. New York, Plenum Press, 1978
2. Dennerstein L et al: Sexual response following hysterectomy and oophorectomy. Obstetrics and Gynecology, Vol. 49 No. 1, January 1977
3. Euster S: Rehabilitation after mastectomy: The group process. Social Work in Health Care, Vol. 4 No. 3, Spring 1979
4. Hamilton A, Kelley P: An education program for hysterectomy patients. Supervisor Nurse, Vol. 10 No. 4, April 1979
5. Levinger G: Working through recovery after mastectomy. American Journal of Nursing, Vol. 80 No. 6, June 1980
6. Merkatz R, Smith D, Seitz P: Preoperative teaching for gynecologic patients. American Journal of Nursing, Vol. 74 No. 6, June 1974
7. Moidel H, Giblin E, Wagner B: Nursing Care of the Patient with Medical-Surgical Disorders, 2nd ed. New York, McGraw-Hill, 1976
8. Notman M: A Psychological consideration of mastectomy. *In* Notman M, Nadelson C (eds): The Woman Patient: Medical and Psychological Interfaces. New York, Plenum Press, 1978
9. Pierson E, D'Antonio W: Female and Male: Dimensions of Human Sexuality. Philadelphia, J. B. Lippincott, 1974
10. Roeske N: Hysterectomy and other gynecological surgeries: A psychological view. *In* Notman M, Nadelson C (eds): The Woman Patient: Medical and Psychological Interfaces. New York, Plenum Press, 1978
11. Sredl D: Is there sex after . . . ? The Journal of Practical Nursing, No. 9, September 1976
12. Stillman MJ: Helping your patient through elective hysterectomy. R.N., Vol. 42 No. 2, February 1979
13. U.S. Department of Health, Education and Welfare: The Breast Cancer Digest. DHEW Publication No. NIH 79-1691, Bethesda, MD, Office of Cancer Communications, 1979
14. Welch D: Assessing psychosocial needs involved in cancer care during treatment. Oncology Nursing Forum, Vol. 6 No. 1, January 1979
15. Williams MA: Cultural patterning of the feminine role. Nursing Forum, Vol. 12, 1973

26

Referrals, References, and Resources

Peggy H. Roeder, Carmine M. Valente, and Nancy M. O'Hara

The material in the preceding chapters gives a basic background of information for many topics related to women's health. Those who wish to expand on this knowledge as well as to keep abreast of new knowledge may find this chapter helpful. In addition to the resources listed here, local libraries, telephone directories, medical, and other health related associations, local health departments, and social action groups provide updated, often free, information and help.

Major topics are listed in alphabetical order. A select listing of books, pamphlets, audiovisual material, and agencies is included for each topic. We recognize that our listing is not inclusive. It is meant to give direction for both professional and client education. *A master list of addresses for ordering the pamphlets and films which are included can be found at the end of the chapter.*

ABORTION

Books

See local medical and community libraries.

Pamphlets

Abortion: A Woman's Right to Choose. Women's Health and Abortion Information.
Abortion: Health Resource Guide. National Women's Health Network.

Audiovisual

Early Abortion. Film distributed by Perennial Education.

Agencies

National Abortion Federation
110 East 59th Street
New York, New York 10022
(212) 688-8516
Consumer Hotline 1-800-223-0618

National Abortion Rights Action League (NARAL)
825 15th Street, NW
Washington, D.C. 20005
(202) 347-7774

ADOPTION

Books

_____*Adoption of Children 3rd ed.* Evanston, Ill: American Academy of Pediatrics, 1973.
  Wishard L: *Adoption: The Grafted Tree.* San Francisco: Cragmont, 1980
  Lashik R: *A Parent's Guide to Adoption.* New York: Sterling, 1979

Pamphlets

Adopting a Child. Public Affairs Pamphlets.

Agencies

National Adoption Information Exchange System (NAIES)
67 Irving Place
New York, New York 10003
(212) 254-7410

BREAST

Books

  Brennan M: *Breast Cancer: New Concepts in Etiology and Control.* New York, Academic Press, 1980
  Golfarb J: *Breastfeeding Handbook: Practical Reference for Physicians, Nurses, and Other Health Professionals.* Hillside, New Jersey, Enslow, 1980
  Kushner Rose: *Why Me?* New York, New American Library, 1977
  Morra M: *Choices: Realistic Alternatives in Cancer Treatment.* New York, Avon, 1980

Pamphlets

Breast Cancer: Health Resources Guide. National Women's Health Network

Breast Cancer Digest. DHEW, 80-1691
Facts on Breast Cancer. American Cancer Society
How to Examine Your Breasts. American Cancer Society
Progress Against Breast Cancer. DHEW, 78-1621
What You Need to Know About Cancer of the Breast. DHEW, 79-15556

Audiovisual

Betsi Breast. OMNI Education
   A model for teaching breast examination.
Breast Cancer and Mastectomy. Filmstrip, Trainex
Breast Self Examination. A teaching model and audio cassette, Spenco

Agencies

American Cancer Society
777 3rd Avenue
New York, New York 10017
(212) 371-2900
See phone directory for local chapters.

Cancer Information Service (CIS)
National Cancer Institute
Bethesda, Maryland
National Toll Free Number 1-800-638-6694
Alaska and Hawaii 1-800-638-6070
Maryland 1-800-492-6600

Cancer Information Clearing House
Bethesda, Maryland
(301) 496-9536

LaLeche League International
9616 Minneapolis Avenue
Franklin Park, Illinois 60131
See phone directory for local chapters.

CHILD ABUSE

Books

   Armstrong Louise: *Kiss Daddy Goodnight: A Speakout on Incest.* New York, Pocket Books, 1979
   Geiser R: *Hidden Victims: The Sexual Abuse of Children.* Boston, Beacon Press, 1980
   Rush F: *Best Kept Secret.* Englewood Cliffs, New Jersey, Prentice Hall, 1980

Pamphlets

The Abused Child. Hoffman-LaRoche
To Combat Child Abuse and Neglect, Public Affairs Pamphlet
What Everyone Should Know About Child Abuse. Channing L. Bete

Agencies

Clearinghouse on Child Abuse and Neglect Information
Hotline (202) 628-3228

National Committee for Prevention of Child Abuse (NCPCA)
332 So. Michigan Avenue
Chicago, Illinois 60604
(312) 565-1100

Parents Anonymous
22330 Hawthorne Avenue
Torrance, California 90505
(213) 371-3501

CONTRACEPTION

Books

Billings J: *Natural Family Planning: Ovulation Method, 3rd ed.* Collegeville, Minnesota, Liturgical Press, 1975
Boston Women's Health Collective, *Our Bodies Ourselves, 2nd ed.,* New York, Simon and Schuster, 1976
Dickey Richard: *Managing Contraceptive Pill Patients.* Aspen, Colorado, Creative Infomatics, Inc., 1977
Hatcher R, et al: *Contraceptive Technology, 1980-81,* 10th ed. New York, Irvington Publishers, 1980

Pamphlets

A Book About Birth Control. Montreal Health Press, Inc.
Catalogue of Family Planning Materials (and supplement). DHEW, 79-5606.
Family Planning and Health. DHEW, 79-5657.
Family Planning Methods of Contraception. DHEW, 80-5646.
Sterilization by Laparoscopy. ACOG.
The Man Who Cares. DHEW, 79-5651.

Audiovisuals

The Choice is Yours. 16 mm or videocassette, color 32 min., National Audiovisual Center.

Family Planning. Filmstrip with cassette or record, color, Spanish version available, Trainex.

Hope is Not a Method II. 8mm, 16mm, or videocassette, color, 17 min. Perennial Education.

Agencies

Couple to Couple League
P.O. Box 11084
Cincinnati, Ohio 42511
(Provides help with Natural Family Planning.)

The Human Life Foundation of America and the Natural Family Planning Federation of America
1511 K Street, NW
Washington, D.C. 20005

The National Clearinghouse for Family Planning Information
DHEW
(301) 443-2430

Planned Parenthood Federation of America
810 7th Avenue
New York, New York 10019
(212) 541-7800
Check phone directory for local chapter.

DEVELOPMENTAL ISSUES

Books

Allman L and Jaffee D (eds): *Readings in Adult Psychology: Contemporary Perspectives.* New York, Harper and Row, New edition available yearly.

Lesnoff-Caravaglia G: *Health Care of the Elderly.* New York, Human Sciences Press, 1980

Lopata H: *Women as Widows: Support Systems.* New York, Elsevier, 1979

Rivers C, Barnett R and Baruch G: *Beyond Sugar and Spice: How Women Grow, Learn, and Thrive.* New York, G. P. Putnam's Sons, 1979

Sheehy G: *Passages: Predictable Crises of Adult Life.* New York, E. P. Dutton and Co., 1976

Troll L: *Early and Middle Adulthood.* Monterey, California, Brooks/Cole Publishing Co., 1975

Pamphlets

After 65: Resources for Self Reliance. Public Affairs Pamphlets.
Getting Ready to Retire. Public Affairs Pamphlets.

Where Older People Live: Living Arrangements for the Elderly. Public Affairs Pamphlets.

Audiovisuals

Good Girl. 16mm, color, 45 min., Filmmakers Library, Inc.
Peege. 16mm, 40 min., color, Phoenix Films.
Sometimes I Wonder Who I Am. 16mm, black and white, New Day Films.
Smiles. 16mm., color, 20 min., University of Maryland, Health Education Dept.

Agencies

Gray Panthers
3635 Chestnut Street
Philadelphia, Penn. 19104
(215) 382-3300

National Association of Older Americans (NAOA)
12 Electric Street
West Alexandria, Ohio 45381
(513) 839-4619

National Clearinghouse on Aging
330 Independence Avenue, SW
Washington, D.C. 20201
(202) 245-0669

National Organization for Women (NOW)
Check phone book for local chapters.

GENERAL HEALTH

Books

Chenevert M: *Special Techniques in Assertiveness Training for Women in the Health Professions.* St. Louis: Mosby Co., 1978
Fogel C: *Health Care of Women: A Nursing Perspective.* St. Louis: Mosby, 1981
Kjervik D and Martinson I: *Women In Stress: A Nursing Perspective.* New York, Appleton-Century-Crofts, 1979

Agencies

National Health Information Clearinghouse
P.O. Box 1133
Washington, D.C.
1-800-336-4797

National Women's Health Network
224 7th Street, SE
Washington, D.C. 20003

Tel Med, Inc.
Medical Health Information by phone
Check local phone directory or call
(714) 825-6034

Women and Health Roundtable
2000 P Street, NW
Washington, D.C.

Women U.S.A.
76 Beaver Street
New York, New York 10005
1-800-221-4945

GENETIC COUNSELING

Pamphlets

Clinical Genetic Service Centers: A National Listing. DHHS
Genetic Counseling. National Foundation March of Dimes
Questions and Answers on Birth Defects. National Foundation March of Dimes.
Unprescribed Drugs and Birth Defects Prevention. National Foundation March of Dimes.

Audiovisual

Wednesday's Child. 16mm., 25 min., Human Betterment League of North Carolina, Inc.

Agencies

Center for Sickle Cell Disease
Howard University
Washington, D.C.

National Clearinghouse for Human Genetic Diseases
1776 East Jefferson Street
Rockville, Maryland 20852
(301) 279-4642

National Foundation March of Dimes
1275 Mamaroneck Avenue
White Plains, New York 10605
(914) 428-7100

National Genetics Foundation
555 W. 57th Street
New York, New York 10019
(212) 586-5800

National Tay Sachs and Allied Diseases Association, Inc.
122 E. 42nd Street
New York, New York 10017

HOLISTIC HEALTH AND NATURAL REMEDIES

Books

Allen R and Hyde D: *Investigations in Stress Control.* Minneapolis, Burgess Pub. Co., 1980
Ardell D: *High Level Wellness.* Emmaus, Pa., Rodale Press, 1977
——*Baltimore-Washington Healing Resources,* Silver Spring, Md., Healing Resources, Inc., 1977
Bloomfield H: *Inner Joy.* New York, Harper and Row, 1980
Brown D: *American Yoga.* New York, World Press, 1980
Buchman D: *Complete Herbal Guide to Natural Health and Beauty.* New York, Doubleday, 1973
Parvati J: *Hygeia: A Woman's Herbal.* Berkeley, Cal., Freestone Collective, 1978
Rose J: *The Herbal Body Book.* New York, Grosset and Dunlap, 1976
Schock N: *Holistic Assessment of the Healthy Aged.* New York, Wiley, 1980
Sorochan W: *Personal Health Appraisal.* New York, Wiley, 1976
Whitehouse GT: *Everywoman's Guide to Natural Health, 3rd ed.* Wellingborough, Northamptonshire, Thorsen's Publishers Limited, 1979

LESBIANS

Books

Baetz R: *Lesbian Crossroads.* West Caldwell, New Jersey, Morrow, 1980
Califia P: *Sapphistry: The Book of Lesbian Sexuality.* Weatherby Lake, Missouri, 1980
Ettore E: *Lesbians, Women, and Society.* Boston, Rutledge and Kegan, 1980
O'Donnell M et al: *Lesbian Health Matters!* Santa Cruz, Cal., Santa Cruz Women's Health Collective, 1979
Vida G: *Our Right to Love: A Lesbian Resource Book.* Englewood Cliffs, New Jersey, Prentice-Hall, 1978

Pamphlets

Changing View of Homosexuality. Public Affairs Pamphlets.
Homosexuality in Our Society. Public Affairs Pamphlets.

Audiovisuals

Holding. 16mm, Focus Film Productions.
Homosexuals. 16mm, Association Films.
Lavender. 16mm, Perennial Education.

Agencies

Gay Hotline
Washington, D.C.
(202) 547-7601

National Gay Health Coalition
P.O. Box 677
Old Chelsea Station
New York, New York 10011

MENOPAUSE

Books

Fuchs E: *Second Season: Life, Love, and Sex in the Middle Years*. New York, Double-day, 1977
Rose L (ed): *The Menopause Book*. New York, Hawthorn, 1977
Reitz R: *Menopause: A Positive Approach*. Radmore, Pa., Chelton, 1977

Pamphlets

Menopause. National Women's Health Network.
Menopause: The Experts Speak. DHEW 75-756.

Audiovisual

Menopause: Myths and Realities. 16mm, Perennial Education.

MENSTRUATION

Books

Dan A: *Menstrual Cycle*. New York, Springer, 1980
Gardner L: *Period*. San Francisco, New Glide, 1980
Maddox H: *Menstruation*. Villanova, Pa., Tobey, 1975

Pamphlets

Accent on You: Your Personal Questions Answered About Menstruation. Tampax, Inc.

From Fiction to Fact: A Teaching Guide on Menstruation and Menstrual Health. Tampax, Inc.

Practical Guide for Teaching Menstrual Hygiene. Kimberly-Clark.

Questions and Answers About Dysmenorrhea. Reprint from *The Female Patient,* August, 1977.

Toxic Shock Syndrome and Tampons. DHHS 81-4025.

Audiovisual

Linda's Film-Menstruation. 16mm, color, 18 min., Phoenix Films.

PELVIS

Books

Gifford-Jones W: *What Every Woman Should Know About Hysterectomy.* New York, Funk and Wagnalls, 1977

Pamphlets

Hysterectomy: Health Resources Guide. National Women's Health Network.

Questions and Answers About DES Exposure During Pregnancy and Before Birth. DHHS, 80-1118.

Stay Healthy! Learn About Uterine Cancer. American Cancer Society, 2062-LE.

The PAP Test. Searle and Co.

What Will Happen to Me During a Pelvic Exam? The Alameda County Health Care Services Agency.

Audiovisual

Gynny. OMNI Education. Life scale model for learning to perform pelvic examination.

Lindi. OMNI Education. Plastic pelvic model for client education.

Agencies

American Cancer Society
777 3rd Ave.
New York, New York 10017
See phone book for local chapters.

Cancer Information Clearinghouse
Bethesda, Maryland
(301) 496-9536

Cancer Information Service
National Cancer Institute
Bethesda, Maryland
1-800-638-6694
Alaska and Hawaii 1-800-638-6070
Maryland 1-800-492-6600

DES Action/New York
Long Island Jewish-Hillside Medical Center
New Hyde Park, New York 11042

See phone directory for local Self Help Groups.

PREGNANCY

Books

Berezin N: *The Gentle Birth Book.* New York, Simon and Schuster, 1980
Bradley R: *Husband-Coached Childbirth.* New York, Harper and Row, 1974
Dick-Read G: *Childbirth Without Fear.* New York, Harper and Row, 1970
Kitzinger S: *Complete Book of Pregnancy and Childbirth.* New York, Knopf, 1980
Nilsson L: *A Child Is Born.* New York, Delacorte Press, 1977
Schwartz L: *Environment of the Pregnant Year: Guide to Prenatal Bonding for Expectant Parents.* New York, Merek, 1980

Pamphlets

Be Good to Your Baby Before it is Born. National Foundation March of Dimes.
Prenatal Care. American Medical Association.
Prenatal Care. DHEW.
Preparation for Childbearing. Maternity Center Association.
So You're Going to Have a Baby. Channing L. Bete, Co.
What To Do About Minor Discomforts of Pregnancy. Ross Laboratories.

Audiovisual

Birth. 16mm, black and white, 40 min., Filmmakers Library, Inc.
A Family is Born. 16mm, Association Films.
When Life Begins. 16mm, color, 12 min., McGraw-Hill Films.

Agencies

International Childbirth Education Association, Inc.
P.O. Box 70258
Seattle, Washington 98107
Check phone directory for local chapter.

LaLeche League, International
9616 Minneapolis Ave.
Franklin Park, Illinois 60131
Check phone directory for local chapter.

Maternity Center Association
48 E. 92nd Street
New York, New York 10028

SEXUALLY TRANSMITTED DISEASES

Books

Boston Women's Health Collective, *Our Bodies, Ourselves, 2nd ed.* New York, Simon and Schuster, 1976
  Corsaro M: *STD: A Commonsense Guide.* New York, St. Martin's Press, 1980
  Hamilton R: *The Herpes Book.* Los Angeles, J. P. Tarcher Co., 1980
  Keith L: *Sexually Transmitted Diseases.* Aspen, Colorado, Creative Infomatics, 1978

Pamphlets

Facts You Should Know About VD But Probably Don't. Metropolitan Life Insurance Co.
  Sexually Transmitted Diseases. DHEW 79-909
  The Helper. American Social Health Association.
  Vaginal Problems: A Quick Guide. San Francisco Family Planning Council.
  Vaginitis. Alameda County Health Care Services Agency.
  VD Handbook. Montreal Health Press, Inc.

Audiovisual

Look What's Going Around. 8mm, color, 16 min., Churchill Films, Spanish version available.

Agencies

American Social Health Association (ASHA)
P.O. Box 100
Palo Alto, California 03432

Center for Disease Control (CDC)
Atlanta, Georgia
(404) 329-3534
Local CDC may be found in large metropolitan area phone books.

National VD Hotline
1-800-227-8922

SEXUALITY

Books

Kennedy E: *Sexual Counseling: Practical Guide for Nonprofessional Counselors.* New York, Continuum, 1980
Mayle P: *What's Happening To Me?* Secaucus, New Jersey, Lyle Stuart, 1975
Mayle P: *Where Did I Come From?* Secaucus, New Jersey, Lyle Stuart, 1973
Salk L: *What Every Child Would Like His Parents To Know.* New York, David McKay, 1973
Starr B and Weiner M: *Report on Sex and Sexuality in the Mature Years.* New York, Paddington, 1980

Pamphlets

Changes and Choices: Your Children and Sex. DHEW
Choices: You and Sex. DHEW
Sex Education: The Parent's Role. Public Affairs Pamphlets.

Agencies

American Association of Sex Educators, Counselors, and Therapists (AASECT)
5010 Wisconsin Ave., NW
Washington, D.C. 20016

Planned Parenthood World Population
810 7th Avenue
New York, New York 10019
See phone book for local listings.

Sex Information and Education Council of the U.S. (SIECUS)
84 5th Ave.
New York, New York 10011
(212) 929-2300

SPOUSE ABUSE

Books

Basset S: *Battered Rich.* Port Washington, New York, Ashley Books, 1980
Fleming J: *Stopping Wife Abuse.* New York, Anchor Press, 1979
Langley R: *Wifebeating.* New York, E. P. Dutton, 1977
Martin D: *Battered Wives.* San Francisco, New Glide Publications, 1976
Walker L: *Battered Women.* New York, Harper and Row, 1980

Pamphlets

Battered: A Survival Manual for Battered Women. Maryland Commission for Women.
Intimate Victims: Study of Violence Among Friends and Relatives. U.S. Department of Justice.
Resource Kit on Battered Women. Women's Bureau, Department of Labor.

Agencies

House of Ruth
459 Massachusetts Ave., NW
Washington, D.C. 20001
(202) 842-0192
See phone book for local listings.

National Clearinghouse on Domestic Violence
Rockville, Maryland

RAPE

Books

Burgess A and Holmstrom L: *Rape: Crisis and Recovery.* Bowie, Maryland, Robert J. Brady, Co., 1979
Mills P: *Rape Intervention Resource Manual.* Ann Arbor, Michigan, C. C. Thomas, 1977
Storaska F: *How To Say No To a Rapist and Survive.* New York, Warner Books, 1976

Pamphlets

Assault on Women: Rape and Wife Beating. Public Affairs Pamphlets.

Basic Guidelines for Victims of Rape and Sexual Offenses. Maryland Commission for Women.

How to Protect Yourself Against Sexual Assault. Department of Justice.

Rape and Older Women: Guide to Prevention and Protection. National Institute of Mental Health.

Audiovisual

How to Say No to a Rapist and Survive. 16mm, color, 52 min., Learning Corporation of America.

Agencies

National Rape Information Clearinghouse
Rockville, Maryland
Check phone book for local Rape Crisis Centers.

DISTRIBUTORS

Pamphlets

Alameda County Health Care Services Agency
499 5th Street
Oakland, California 94607

American Cancer Society (ACS)
219 E. 42nd Street
New York, New York 10017

American College of Obstetricians & Gynecologists (ACOG)
One East Wacker Drive
Chicago, Illinois 60601

American Medical Association
535 N. Dearborn Street
Chicago, Illinois 60610

American Social Health Association (ASHA)
260 Sheridan Avenue
Palo Alto, California 94306

Channing L. Bete Co., Inc.
45 Federal Street
Greenfield, Massachusetts 01301

Department of Health, Education, and Welfare (DHEW)
Public Health Services
Health Services Administration
Rockville, Maryland 20857

Government Printing Office (GPO)
710 North Capital Street
Washington, D.C.
(202) 783-3238

Hoffman-LaRoche, Inc.
Nutley, New Jersey 07118

Kimberly-Clark
Neenah, Wisconsin

Maryland Commission for Women
Baltimore, Maryland

Maternity Center Association
48 E. 92nd Street
New York, New York 10028
(212) 369-7300

Metropolitan Life Insurance Co.
1 Madison Avenue
New York, New York 10010

Montreal Health Press, Inc.
P.O. Box 1200 Station G
Montreal, Quebec H2W2N1 Canada
(514) 272-5441

National Foundation March of Dimes
1275 Mamaroneck Ave.
White Plains, New York 10605
(914) 428-7100

National Institutes of Health (NIH) and National Institute of Mental Health
(NIMH)
9000 Rockville Pike
Bethesda, Maryland

National Women's Health Network
224 7th Street, SE
Washington, D.C. 20003

Public Affairs Pamphlets
22 E. 38th Street
New York, New York 10016

Ross Laboratories
Box 1317
Columbus, Ohio 43216

San Francisco Family Planning Council
1490 Mason Street
San Francisco, California 94133

Searle and Co.
San Juan, Puerto Rico 00936

Tampax, Inc.
Educational Department
5 Dakota Drive
Lake Success, New York

United States Department of Justice
10th and Constitution Ave., NW
Washington, D.C.

Women's Bureau—Labor Department
200 Constitution Ave., NW
Washington, D.C.

Films and Models

Association Films
333 Adelaide Street, West
Toronto, Ontario, Canada

Churchill Films
662 North Robertson Blvd.
Los Angeles, California 90069

Filmakers Library, Inc.
133 E. 58th Street
New York, New York 10022

Focus Film Production
1385 Westwood Boulevard
Los Angeles, California 90024

Human Betterment League of North Carolina, Inc.
P.O. Box 3036
Winston-Salem, North Carolina 27102

Learning Corporation of America
1350 Avenue of the Americas
New York, New York 10019

McGraw-Hill Films
1221 Avenue of the Americas
New York, New York 10020

National Audiovisual Center
General Services Administration
Capitol Heights, Maryland
(301) 763-1896

New Day Films
P.O. Box 315
Franklin Lakes, New Jersey 07417

OMNI Education
190 West Main Street
Somerville, New York 08876

Perennial Education, Inc.
477 Roger Williams
P.O. Box 855, Ravinia
Highland Park, Illinois 60035

Spenco Medical Corporation
P.O. Box 8113
Waco, Texas 76710

Trainex Corporation
P.O. Box 116
Garden Grove, California 92642

University of Maryland
Department of Health Education
College Park, Maryland 20742

inclusion, 33, 255
Nabothian, 240–241
needle aspiration of fluid, 319
ovarian, 219
sebaceous, 177, 255
vaginal-inclusion, 240
Cystic disease, *see* Fibrocystic breast disease
Cystic ovarian tumor(s), 222–223
functional, 222–223
neoplastic, 223
Cystitis, 273, 373
diagnosis of, 275
etiology of, 274
honeymoon, 274, 276
prevention of, 276
symptoms and signs of, 274–275
treatment of, 275–276
Cystocele, 132, 157, 309
problems associated with, 157–158
repair of, 330–240
Cytology, cervical-vaginal, 301

D5W, 326
D&C, 222, 225, 262, 265, 285, 320, 327, 340
purpose of, 340
suction, 325
Danazol, for treatment of endometriosis, 271
Data base, 4
Data gathering, methods for, 4
see also Assessment
Dating mores, changes in, 165
Death, fear of, surgery and, 330
Death rate, associated with birth and birth control, 214f
Deep fascia, 22, 23
Deep vein(s), of breast, 24
Deficiency disease theory, related to emotional symptoms of menopause, 161–162
Deoxyribonucleic acid (DNA), transcription, 56
Dependency, fear of, surgery and, 330
Depression, 163, 271, 293
following abortion, 327
Dermoid cyst, 223
Desire phase, of sexual response, 290
disorders of, 290
Detrusor muscle, 40
Development
physical, *see* Physical development
prenatal, *see* Prenatal development
psychosocial, *see* Psychosocial growth
stages of, 138
Diabetes, 230, 274
Diagnosis, related to surgery, concerns in, 332
Diaphragm (anatomic)
pelvic, *see* Pelvic diaphragm
urogenital, *see* Urogenital diaphragm
Diaphragm (contraceptive), 197, 198, 227, 241
insertion and removal of, technique for, 196f, 197
instructions for use, 198, 199–200
questions regarding, 200
rim styles and sizes, 197, 198f
use of, during premenopause, 156
Dienestrol, use of, 102, 103
Diethylstilbesterol (DES), 206, 241, 287, 302
defined, 313

exposure to
effects of, 314
examination and follow up for, 314
purpose of, 313
symptoms and signs of, 314
types of, 313
Digestive problem(s), 158
Dilatation and curettage, *see* D & C
Dilator(s), 296
Diplococcus, intracellular, 234, 235f
Disability, fear of, surgery and, 330
Discharge, vaginal, *see* Vaginal discharge
Discussion group(s), for menopausal women, 166
Diverticulitis, 219
Divorce, midlife, 165
Dorsal nerve, of clitoris, 53
Douche, douching, 227, 229, 243
as form of contraceptive, 186
procedure for, 243–244, 244f
substances used, 243
Dowager's hump, 158
Down's syndrome, 155
Draping of patient, for gynecological examination, 310, 311f
Drug(s), 292
Duct(s), of breast, 19, 20, 21f, 21
Ductal carcinoma, 179
Dysfunctional uterine bleeding (DUB), 264
in absence of ovulation, 265
associated with ovulatory cycle, 264–265
causes of, 264
Dysmenorrhea, 267
primary, 267, 267t, 268–270
secondary, 267, 267f, 270–271
Dyspareunia, 31, 219, 270
in older women, 157
Dysuria, 249, 277

E₂, 70
E. coli, 218, 220, 274
Economic situation, changes in, during menopause, 165
Ectasia, mammary duct, 178
Ectocervix, polyps of, 240
Ectoderm, 19
Ectopic pregnancy, 219
IUD use and, 209
Education, 302
of elderly, 168
on health issues, in childhood, 93
see also Sex education
for menopausal women, 166
preoperative adjustment and, 333–334
Effectiveness
theoretical, 185–186
use, 186
Egg(s), 64
expulsion of, 71
fertilization of, 64, 69
transport of, 72
viability of, 189
Ego integrity, sense of, 166
Ejaculation, disorders in, 290
Ejaculatory duct, 11
Electrolyte(s), 49, 326
Embarrassment, 8
related to pelvic examination, 302
Embryo, sex differentiation of, 20f
Embryology, *see* Prenatal development
Emotion(s), 129, 261

Emotional need(s), meeting of, 143
Emotional response(s), following abortion, 326, 327
Emotional support, preoperative, 334
Emotional symptom(s), related to menopause, 161–164
Empty nest syndrome, menopause symptoms and, 163
Endocervical cell(s), obtaining of, 306–307, 308f
Endocervical epithelium, changes in, during pregnancy, 133
Endocervical gland(s), 33
Endocervix, 38
curettage of, 225
Endocrine gland, 55
Endocrine system, function of, 77
during childhood, 77
Endometrial-biopsy curette, 320
Endometrial carcinoma, 224–225, 261
diagnosis of, 225
staging of, 225
symptoms of, 225
treatment of, 225
Endometrial hyperplasia, 222, 261–262
Endometrial polyp(s), 222
diagnosis and treatment of, 222
symptoms of, 222
Endometrial tissue, biopsy of, 317f, 320
procedure for, 320
Endometrioma(s), 223, 270, 271
Endometriosis, 223, 270
diagnosis of, 270–271
origin of, 270
sites for, 270
symptoms of, 270
treatment of, 271
Endometriotic cyst(s), 240
Endometritis, 218
Endometrium, 39, 49, 69, 72
abnormal bleeding in, 264
build-up of, 112
changes in, from aging, 156
curettage of, 225
inadequate, creation of, 201
infection of, 218
prostaglandin levels in, 269
removal of, 340
sloughing of, 264
structure of, 37
Endopelvic fascia, 44, 45, 46
anatomic relationships of, 43f
Endoscope, 98
Environment, nursing process and, 5–6, 6f
Enzyme(s), production of, 56
Episiotomy, 31
Epithelial cell(s), 81
of breast, 19, 20
vaginal, 31
changes in, 31, 33
function of, 31
Epithelium, 42
abnormal, 316
endocervical, changes in, during pregnancy, 133
vaginal
changes in, from aging, 156
during puberty, 114
of newborn, 79
see also Mucous membrane
see also Squamous epithelium
Erectile tissue, 62
Erythromycin, 233
Estradiol, 61, 69, 70
levels of
infancy to mid school age, 80, 81
in puberty, 112

production of, 40
decline in, 151
Estriol, 70, 78
excretion of, 78
formation of, 69
Estrogen(s), 19, 31, 36, 37, 56, 61, 64, 69, 70, 132, 149, 178, 192, 202, 261, 269
deficiency of, 158
effects of, 69, 71t, 77
prenatal, 80
hypothalamus sensitivity to, 150
levels of
during pregnancy, 77, 78
fetal health and, 78
during puberty, 112, 113, 114, 115
in fetus, 78
menopause and, 151
in newborn, 79
rise in, 69
production of, 56, 69
pathways for, 70
release of, from placenta, 78
role in endometrial carcinoma, 244–225
source of, 151
stimulation of
interruption of, 261, 264
prolonged, 265
use in contraception, 206
Estrogen cream(s), 157
Estrogen/progesterone balance, 70
Estrogen-progestin oral contraceptive, 264, 271
Estrogen replacement therapy (ERT), 149–150, 222, 225
for menopausal symptoms, 152–153
regime for, 153–154
risks in, 154
side effects of, 154
osteoporosis and, 158
Estrone, 70
levels of
during pregnancy, 112
infancy to mid school age, 80
Evaluation, as part of nursing process, 3, 5
Examination, 8
pelvic, *see* Pelvic examination
for physical assault of children, 107
Excitement phase, of sexual response, 157, 291
Excretory duct(s), of breast, 19, 20, 21, 21f
Exercise, 8, 129
postoperative, 334
Exhaustion, 279
Exocervix, 38
Extended radical mastectomy, 335
External genital problem(s), 247
benign tumors, Bartholin's cyst, 254f, 255
folliculitis, 254
inclusion and sebaceous cysts, 255
infection
condyloma accuminata, 250–251
herpes genitalis, 247–250
molluscum contagiosum, 252
vulvitis, 250
infestations
pediculosis pubis (crabs), 252, 252f, 253
scabies, 253–254
trauma, 256
vulvar malignancies, 255–256
External genitalia, 9, 14, 62, 332
characteristics of
during infancy to mid school

implementation, 5
planning, 5
Nursing skills, used in nursing
process, 4t
Nutrition, 8, 26, 129, 131, 132 *see
also* Malnutrition

Obesity, 261
see also Overweight
Oligomenorrhea, 261
treatment of, 261–262
Oncologic agent(s), 181
Oophorectomy, 338, 339
see also Salpingo-oophorectomy
Oophoritis, 218
Oral contraceptive(s), 155, 224,
262, 265, 287
action of, 200–201
complications and side effects
of, 201, 202
contraindications for use, 201–
202
effectiveness of, 202–203
instructions for use and follow-
up, 203–204
mini-pill, 205
questions about, 204–205
for treatment of endometriosis,
271
use for dysmenorrhea, 269
Oral-genital stimulation, as form
of contraception, 188
Organism(s)
causing cystitis, 274
in vaginal wall, 132
Orgasm, 61, 132
holding back of, contraception
and, 186
lack of, 290
muscular contractions in, 290
vaginal vs. clitoral, 292
Orgasmic dysfunction, 290
levels of therapy for, 295–296
primary, 295
secondary, 295
Orgasmic phase, of sexual
response, 157, 291–292
Orgasmic platform, 291
Os, 133
cervical, 325, 340
external, 38, 133
internal, 46
Osteoporosis, 158
causes of, 158
incidence of, 158
symptoms of, 158
treatment of, 158–159
Otoscope, 99, 101
Ovarian artery(ies), 47, 49
Ovarian cancer, 225–226
diagnosis, of, 226
symptoms of, 226
treatment of, 226
Ovarian cortex, of newborn, 80
Ovarian cyst, 219
Ovarian follicle(s), 64, 81
Ovarian tumor(s)
cystic, 222–223
solid
diagnosis of, 224
symptoms of, 223–224
treatment of, 224
types of, 223
Ovary(ies), 9, 11, 15, 31, 39, 47,
53, 55, 56, 332
anatomy of, 39–40
blood supply to, 49, 50f
changes in
during pregnancy, 133
menopause and, 151
characteristics of
during infancy to mid school
age, 81

during puberty, 115
disorders of, 262
endometriomas of, 271
examination, of, 310
infection of, 218
ligaments of, 45
of newborn, 80
prenatal development of, 9
removal of, *see* Oophorectomy
tissue layers of, 40
Overweight, in puberty,
hormone levels and, 112
see also Obesity
Ovulation, 64, 69, 70, 112, 113,
176
absence of, *see* Anovulation
action of prostaglandins on, 71
body temperature and, 190
documentation of, 261
during premenopause, 155
estrogen levels and, 151
inhibition of, 200
period of
awareness of, 192
predicting of, 189
regulation of, 115
suppression of, 262
Ovum, *see* Egg
Oxidation product(s), 69
Oxytocin, 56
action of, 56
milk secretion and, 62

Pacemaker(s), myometrium
contraction and, 37
Pain, fear of, related to surgery,
329
Pap smear, 133, 225, 226, 241,
242, 305, 306
purpose of, 306
repeat of, 307
results of, reporting of, 307
scheduling for, 301
technique for, 306–307, 308f
Papilloma, intraductal, 179
Parabasal cell(s), 81
Parametrium, *see* Peritoneum
Parasympathetic fiber(s), 40
Parasympathetic nervous
system, innervation of, 53
Partial mastectomy, 336
Patient's Bill of Rights, 2, 3
nurse's role in, 3
Pectoralis major, 123
Pectoralis minor, 23
Pediculosis pedis, 252, 252f, 254
causes of, 253
diagnosis of, 253
influencing factors in, 253
prognosis of, 253
signs and symptoms of, 253
treatment of, 253
Pelvic basin, formation of, 43
Pelvic bone(s), 25, 43–44
landmarks formed by, 43
Pelvic diaphragm, 45, 47
anatomy of, 45, 46–47
Pelvic examination, 8, 226, 325
attitudes toward, 301, 302
bimanual, 308–309, 309f, 310
gonorrhea culture, 307
humanizing of, 310, 311f, 312
draping of patient in, 310, 312
inspection
of external genitalia, 303
of vagina and cervix, 303, 305,
305f, 306f
Pap smear, 305, 306–307, 308f
patient preparation for, 302
routine, 301
special considerations in
DES exposed women, 313–314
vaginismus, 313

virginal or tight hymen, 312–
313
Pelvic floor, 44
divisions of, 45, 46f
pelvic diaphragm, 45, 46–47
urogenital diaphragm, 46f, 47
Pelvic girdle, 132
Pelvic inflammatory disease
(PID), 131
acute phase of, 218
chronic phase of, 218
diagnosis of, 219
pyogenic, 220
risk factors and sequellae, 219–
220
signs and symptoms of, 219
spread of, routes of, 217f, 218
treatment of, 219
tuberculous, 218
Pelvic organs
in reproductive function, 63–64
reproductive physiology of, 55,
59f
sexual function and, 59f, 62–63
Pelvic plexus, 53
Pelvic space(s), 42, 43f
anatomic relationships of, 43f
Pelvic surgery, *see* Gynecologic
and breast surgery
Pelvic ultrasonography, 324
Pelvic wall, 43, 45
Pelvis
abscess in, 219
coordinating structures of
blood supply to, 47–49, 50f
lymphatic system of, 45, 49,
51f, 52
disorders of, *see* Upper
reproductive tract disorders,
Pelvic inflammatory disease
external genitalia, 26–231
false, 80
infection in, 270
IUD use and, 208
internal genitalia, 31–40
lymph nodes of, 51, 52
major ligaments of, 44–45
nerve supply to, 52–53, 54f, 55
pain in, 219
pelvic floor, 45–47
perineal muscles, 47
peritoneum of, 45
relaxation of, *see* Dyspareunia
spaces of, 42–43
structure of
in older women, 157
support, 43, 44f, 44
urinary and intestinal, 40–42
Penicillinase, 235
Penis, 14
glans of, 11
surgical creation of, 16
Peptostreptococcus, 220
Perineal body, 30, 31
Perineal muscle(s), 44
Perineal structure(s), blood
supply to, 49
Perineum, 26, 42, 45, 47, 81, 113
bacteria in, 274
depression of, 308
muscles of, 47
nerve supply to, 53, 54f
structure of, 30, 31
Peripheral nervous system
(PNS), 53, 56
Peritoneum, 38, 42, 44, 270
abdominal, 39
anatomy of, 36, 44f
function of, 45
anatomic relationships of, 43f
Periurethral duct(s), *see* Skene's
glands and ducts
Permission, related to sex
therapy, 294, 295, 296
Personal identity, during
adolescence, 118, 119, 121

Personality
behavior and, 138
development of, 83, 84, 88
lack of competency and, 123f
mature, 137
Ph, 38
in newborn, 79
vaginal, 81
changes in, 157
from aging, 156
during puberty, 114
during reproductive years, 132
Pharyngeal infection(s), 235
Phenazopyridine HC1, 276
Physical development, 7, 77, 82,
90
during infancy to mid school
age, 80–82
in neonate, 77–80
Physical process, effect of, on
female behavior, 139
Physiologic change(s), associated
with aging, 158
see also Menopause
Physiology, *see* Reproductive
physiology
Pigmentation
of breasts, 19
during pregnancy, 133, 134
Pituitary adenoma, 262
Pituitary gland, 55
anterior, 69, 150
function of, 69
hormones secreted by, 40, 55–
56
Pituitary tumor, 264
Placenta, 55, 56, 77
estrogen release from, 78
hormones of, 40, 79
Planning, as part of nursing
process, 3, 5, 7
Plateau phase, of sexual
response, 157, 291
Podophyllin treatment(s), for
treatment of condyloma
accuminata, 251
Polycystic ovary disease, 261
Polymenorrhea, 264–265
Polyp(s), 270
cervical, 240
endometrial, 222
Posterior cul-de-sac, 31
Posterior fornix, 31
Postmenopause, 149, 226
Potential, accomplishment of, 91
Precocious puberty, 104–105
organic cause of, 105
pseudo, 105
true, 105
Pregnancy, 7, 55, 69, 124, 132,
222, 233, 274
during premenopause, risks in,
155
dysmenorrhea and, 268
ectopic, *see* Ectopic pregnancy
estrogen levels during, 77, 78
herpes genitalis and, 250
IUD use and, 208–209
lactation and, 61
physical changes in, 133–134
splash, 187
toxemia in, 72
unplanned, *see* Unplanned
pregnancy
Premarin, use of, 102, 103
Premature andrenarche, 105
Premature pubarche, 105
Premature telarche, 105
Premenopause
contraception during, 155–156
menstrual periods during, 151
risk of pregnancy during, 155
Premenstrual spotting, 264
Prenatal development, 2, 16
abnormalities
adrenogenital syndrome